Advances in Neurosurgery 2

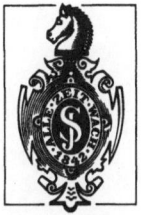

Meningiomas

Diagnostic and Therapeutic Problems

Multiple Sclerosis

Misdiagnosis

Forensic Problems in Neurosurgery

Edited by
W. Klug · M. Brock · M. Klinger · O. Spoerri

With 200 Figures and 86 Tables

Springer-Verlag Berlin Heidelberg GmbH 1975

Proceedings of the 25th Annual Meeting
of the "Deutsche Gesellschaft für Neurochirurgie"
Bochum, September 22–25, 1974

ISBN 978-3-540-07237-9   ISBN 978-3-642-66118-1 (eBook)
DOI 10.1007/978-3-642-66118-1

Library of Congress Cataloging in Publication Data. Deutsche Gesellschaft für Neurochirurgie. Meningiomas: diagnostic and therapeutic problems. (Advances in neurosurgery; 2) "Proceedings of the 25th annual meeting of the Deutsche Gesellschaft für
Neurochirurgie, Bochum, September 22–25, 1974." Bibliography: p. Includes index.
1. Meningioma –Congresses. 2. Multiple sclerosis –Congresses. 3. Forensic neurology.
I. Klug, Wilhelm, 1910–. II. Title. III. Series. (DNLM: 1. Diagnostic errors – Congresses.
2. Malpractice – Congresses. 3. Meningioma – Congresses. 4. Multiple sclerosis –
Diagnosis – Congresses. 5. Neurosurgery – Congresses. W1 AD684N v. 2/WL368
D436m) RC663.D48   1975.   616.9'92'8   75-8941

Preface

On this occasion we look back on 25 years of the Deutsche Gesellschaft für Neuro-chirurgie. They hold a great deal: founding and development of the society, comple-tion and extension, communication between the individual members and contacts to other societies beyond our borders.

They also stand for close co-operation with those who transfer their patients to us – the neurologists and specialists in internal medicine, the ophthalmologists and ear-nose-and throat specialists as well as the general surgeons.

This 25th annual meeting will deal with two examples of diseases that present common problems to the neurologist and to the neurosurgeon, namely meningiomas and multiple sclerosis.

In view of their long histories often going back over many years, both of these lesions lead to diagnostic errors and indequate treatment. And yet it should be possible to recognize meningiomas at an early date and to initiate the only possible treatment, the operation,if all diagnostic measures are repeatedly carried out.

The diagnosis MS, on the other hand, with the multiplicity of symptoms which are peculiar to this disease, should continue to be re-examined until every other lesion has been excluded with certainty.

The increasing number of legal proceedings because of diagnostic and therapeutic measures as well as the doctor-patient talk preceding the written consent for these measures are further problems in need of discussion. For this reason, the topic „medical liability in special reference to the neurosurgeon" was chosen for this meeting.

Many questions necessitate many answers.

May each participant in this congress find a satisfactory solution to his own problem in the multitude of answers.

W. KLUG

Welcoming Address
to Mark the Opening of the 25th Congress of the German Society for Neurosurgery

W. KLUG

Our today's opening of the 25th Congress of the German Society for Neurosurgery here in Bochum would be incomplete without our first conducting a review of the past.

In 1824, that is exactly 150 years ago, KARL-ARNOLD KORTUM, the well-known physician, satirist, technical writer and local politician, died in Bochum. 40 years previously, 1784, he had published the 1st part of his "Jobsiade" with which we are all familiar, either from the original text or from the work of WILHELM BUSCH.

Exactly 100 years later, on November 25, 1884, GODLEE performed the first operation on a cerebral tumour in a 25 year-old man with paralysis of the left hand and the fingers as well as paresis of the left leg. He removed a smooth, solid, well-demarcated tumour the size of a walnut. 4 days following the operation a suppuration supervened, then a prolapse. Three weeks after the operation the patient died. Despite this outcome, the operation was a trail-blazing event, perhaps the first indication of there being new territory ahead, to which more attention should be paid.

In actual fact surgeons and neurologists increasingly concerned themselves in the ensuing period systematically with this branch of medicine, the progress of which up to the stage of its becoming an independent entity was still to require many years.

Names such as FEDOR KRAUSE, HARVEY CUSHING, OTFRIED FOERSTER etc. represent milestones along the path leading towards the independence of our special medical sector. Not to be forgotten is the pioneering work of ERNST VON BERGMANN, whose work *"Lehre von den Kopfverletzungen"*, published in 1880 by the firm of F. Enke, Stuttgart, must be rated as a summary of his experience in the battles of Weissenburg and Wörth in the Franco-Prussian War as well as at Plevna in the Russo-Turkish War. But that was not all. His book on the *Chirurgische Behandlung von Hirnkrankheiten*, printed in the *Archiv für Klinische Chirurgie 36*, was published in 1888 as an independent work in 2nd edition by the August Hirschwald publishing-house, Berlin, and issued in a considerably expanded form 11 years later in 3rd edition by the same publishers.

Those who have read these books are aware that the generation of doctors who lived a good century ago knew very well how to observe and to draw conclusions from what they observed. We who are living today can only learn from this use of our five senses! Notwithstanding the pleasure we feel about the steadily advancing development of our technology and improvements to our instrumentarium, we should never forget the eminent accomplishments of our great masters. Their activities of that time constitute the foundation of our present-day knowledge and skills, and just as our hypothesis of today already harbour the errors of tomorrow, we should judge the events of the past that have proved to be erroneous in the light of present-day perceptions with that degree of tolerance that is befitting for a western civilisation that has its roots in antiquity and christianity.

Since then German neurosurgery, thanks to the dynamism and abilities of a WILHELM TÖNNIS and the cordial and generous assistance of his teacher, FRITZ KÖNIG, has succeeded in finding its own path so that we may all look back with pride and satisfaction on the emergence of neurosurgery in Germany as an independent branch of medicine.

Here in Germany neurosurgery has advanced to the stage where it has become an established, acknowledged constituent of medical science as a whole. More than that, it has succeeded in re-establishing the contact with its international counterparts lost during the Second World War, and can present itself today as ranking equal to them.

It combines the good of the past with the better of present-day advances, and is paving a path for itself into the future that is full of hope. Could a tradition that has grown up on the basis of long and fruitful experience present a better image of itself than by retaining that which has proved to be good and jettisoning that which has not been found to be meaningful, or even wrong?

The public at large, but especially the sick, those requiring help, should be grateful to the majority of doctors for not having complied with the frequently expressed wish for change also in this direction. A *good* conservative attitude is of greater value than any form of doubtful experimenting with its uncertain outcome, in particular when this relates to the sick person.

As is to be expected, these ideas, which in part have their origin in pure ideologies, come almost entirely from healthy people. They know neither the world of the sick, nor are they able to put themselves into their position. How rapidly these frequently totally practiceremote notions collapse is usually shown whenever the loaded question is asked: "Who would you like to operate on you, if necessary"? The intern, the surgeon who has already carried out several similar operations, the head surgeon, or perhaps the senior medical officer, who has in the meantime become the whipping-boy of a whole horde of papers, but who has nevertheless the most experience at his disposal, or perhaps, if one asks "Who is to decide about your illness, your treatment, a team of doctors or one responsible doctor"? After all responsibility is not divisible. But it is out of this that a mission arises, which generations of medical practitioners have taken very seriously. For them, apart from the illness to be treated there was also the patient that wanted to be cared for. And since the one and same illness of 100 years ago does not differ one iota from the one of today, the anxiety of the sufferers has always remained and will always remain the same, the treatment can only be directed towards two things: 1. the diagnosis and therapy of the illness as such, and 2. to the treatment, concurrently, of the individual as a human-being.

These are facts that no one can pass over without seing them. The demand for full mechanisation of hospitals is justifiable for organisational reasons. It promotes the flow of the work processes.

The steady reduction in the working hours, on the other hand, encourages personnel to watch the clock; the 5-day week, from the viewpoint of the hospital, by comparison with other professions that can afford it, induces staff to press for an ever-longer week-end off. Nobody will be able to stop this general tendency, but it should be made quite clear that illnesses and injuries do not cease to exist just because the week-end has come around.

In the hospital it is just one of those things that special tasks are in the foreground, these having very much to do with ethics, humanity and personal help, but very little to do with politics, ideologies or even empty verbosity, which can neither help the sick nor give them hope.

The patient, with his understandable hypersensitivity, most certainly notices the shift or sliding duty arrangements or whatever other term might be used. It is only with difficulty that he gets used to the changing number of staff nursing and attending to him.

Those who are in a position to critically judge the case of the sick in former times and today will come to the conclusion that the work in the wards has become a necessary service branch and is no longer a genuine nursing of the sick that comes from the heart.

Perhaps I may express this in slightly different words. No two-way communications system, no control desk with individual parameter monitoring, no optic or acoustic information on the condition of the patient can replace the friendly chat with him, the touching of his hand to re-assure him. The personal ties of the patient with the doctor treating him and vice versa are the best foundation for his recovery. A patient who has trust in his doctor is well off, one who believes in him is even better off. These are facts that every experienced doctor is familiar with.

What do those healthy people, who are able to avail themselves of medical help at any time, know of the inner self of a doctor? Of his decisions that very often have to be taken alone, and which many a time involve life or death, and which no one can lift from his shoulders? What do they know of his worries and cares about a patient, his frequently nocturnal deliberations when it is a question of the pros and cons regarding a high-risk operation? What do they know of his involvement in the experience and suffering of a patient whom he has come to have a feeling for, also in human terms, but whom he is no longer able to help? What do they know of his feelings when he has to break the news to parents that their only child can no longer be saved, that the life of the young mother can no longer be preserved?

And then there are also those intellectual critics who, against their better knowledge and belief, perhaps only because they have had some negative personal experience with a rather unsympathetic doctor, whom we too know, by making generalisations about a whole profession, would like to imprint upon all the stamp of amoral conduct. In doing so, they contribute not only to the discrimination of a whole professional group, but above all to undermining the patient-doctor relationship. The fact that at the same time, however, also the confidence relationship between the two partners suffers in consequence, and accordingly the decisive and most important pre-requisite for every successful treatment is destroyed, appears to have escaped their attention.

How many members of that professional group, which again and again demand from us a full clarification, ask neither for the exact diagnosis nor for the prognosis when they themselves are the persons involved. A large number of patients would with certainty refuse an operation, which despite all risks could prove successful, if they were given information in advance about every detail of diagnostic or therapeutic methods.

Thus all the more to be welcomed are those tactful publications free from every sensation-mongering tendency of our mass media, which report on new perfected processes or techniques that have been discussed with their originators, and accordingly help to bring these innovations more quickly to the attention of the sick than we are able to do.

All too frequently in the past hopes have been raised in the population by distorting reports that simply could not be realised, if only for the reason that they were factually incorrect.

How often are collections made even these days for sick people and big sacrifices made for them on the assumption that their salvation lies only on the other side of the ocean, whereas any well-read layman knows that this help could be had just as well in a nearby German town.

In all these questions meaningful cooperation between the mass media and doctors would be better than working against one another and thus be a true help for the sick, whom in the final instance is involved.

Let us hope that the discussion of the problems to be dealt with will proceed in the same spirit: as a valuable answer to critical questions for the benefit of the patients entrusted to our care!

Contents

Meningiomas

Diagnostic and Therapeutic Problems

XII

Forensic Problems in Neurosurgery

Free Communications

List of Contributors

ABTAHI, H., Neurochirurgische Universitätsklinik, Gießen (BRD)

ABU BAKR, K., Neurochirurgische Klinik, Krankenhaus St. Jürgenstr., Bremen (BRD)

ALTHOFF, P. H., Abteilung für Endokrinologie, Johann Wolfgang Goethe-Universität, Frankfurt/Main (BRD)

ARNOLD, H., Neurochirurgische Universitätsklinik, Krankenhaus Hamburg-Eppendorf, Hamburg (BRD)

ARTMANN, H., Neurochirurgische Klinik, Krankenhaus St. Jürgenstr., Bremen (BRD)

ASSMUS, H., Neurochirurgische Abteilung, Chirurgische Universitätsklinik, Heidelberg (BRD)

BARZ, D., Neurochirurgische Klinik, Städt. Krankenhaus Neukölln, Berlin (BRD)

BAUER, H. J., Neurologische Universitätsklinik, Göttingen (BRD)

BOCK, W. J., Neurochirurgische Universitätsklinik, Essen (BRD)

BÖCKEM, F. K., Neurochirurgische Abteilung, Nervenkrankenhaus, Günzburg/Ulm (BRD)

BOCKHORN, J., Neurochirurgische Universitätsklinik, Göttingen (BRD)

BRAUN, W., Neurochirurgische Klinik, Krankenhaus Bethesda, Wuppertal-Elberfeld (BRD)

BRENDEL, A., Neurochirurgische Universitätsklinik, Freiburg/Breisgau (BRD)

BRKIC, J., Neurochirurgische Universitätsklinik, Essen (BRD)

BROCK, M., Neurochirurgische Klinik, Medizinische Hochschule, Hannover (BRD)

CASTRO, A., Neurochirurgische Klinik, Knappschaftskrankenhaus, Bochum-Langendreer (BRD)

CERVÓS-NAVARRO, J., Abteilung für Neuropathologie, Klinikum Steglitz der Freien Universität, Berlin (BRD)

COLLMANN, H., Neurochirurgische Universitätsklinik, Westend, Berlin (BRD)

DEISENHAMMER, E., Abteilung für Nuklearmedizin, Wagner-Jauregg-Krankenhaus, Linz (Österreich)

DELANK, H. W., Neurologische Klinik, Berufsgenossenschaftliche Krankenanstalt, Bergmannsheil, Bochum (BRD)

DEMIREL, T., Neurochirurgische Klinik, Krankenhaus Bethesda, Wuppertal-Elberfeld (BRD)

DRAGOUN, P., Neurochirurgische Universitätsklinik, Essen (BRD)

EFFINOWICZ, H., Neurochirurgische Universitätsklinik, Frankfurt/Main (BRD)

ELIES, W., Neurochirurgische Universitätsklinik, Tübingen (BRD)

ENGELMANN, U., Neurochirurgische Universitätsklinik, Erlangen (BRD)

ENTZIAN, W., Neurochirurgische Universitätsklinik, Bonn (BRD)

ERBS, G., Institut für Nuklearmedizin, DKFZ, Heidelberg (BRD)

FARHOUMAND, E., Neurochirurgische Klinik, Knappschaftskrankenhaus, Bochum-Langendreer (BRD)

FEIGL, W., Pathologisches Institut, Universität, Wien (Österreich)

FRIEDRICH, H., Neurochirurgische Universitätsklinik, Freiburg/Breisgau (BRD)

FROMM, H., Neurochirurgische Universitätsklinik, Frankfurt/Main (BRD)

FROWEIN, R. A., Neurochirurgische Universitätsklinik, Köln (BRD)

FUCHS, E. C., Neurochirurgische Klinik, Klinikum Westend, Freie Universität, Berlin (BRD)

FUKUSHIMA, T., Neurochirurgische Klinik, Klinikum Steglitz, Freie Universität, Berlin (BRD)

GAAB, M., Neurochirurgische Universitätsklinik, Würzburg (BRD)

GALOW, W., Neurochirurgische Universitätsklinik, Frankfurt (BRD)

GEORGI, P., Institut für Nuklearmedizin, Deutsches Krebsforschungscenter, Heidelberg (BRD)

GRAEF, G., Neurochirurgische Klinik, Klinikum Westend, Freie Universität, Berlin (BRD)

GRUMME, TH., Neurochirurgische Klinik, Klinikum Westend, Freie Universität, Berlin (BRD)

GULLOTTA, F., Institut für Neuropathologie, Universität Bonn, Bonn (BRD)

GUND, A., Neurochirurgische Klinik, Wagner-Jauregg-Krankenhaus, Linz (Österreich)

HALVES, E., Neurochirurgische Universitätsklinik, Göttingen (BRD)

HAMEL, E., Neurochirurgische Universitätsklinik, Köln (BRD)

HAMMER, B., Röntgeninstitut, Wagner-Jauregg-Krankenhaus, Linz (Österreich)

HAPP, J., Abteilung für Endokrinologie, Johann Wolfgang Goethe-Universität, Frankfurt/Main (BRD)

HARTMANN, K., Neurochirurgische Klinik, Knappschaftskrankenhaus, Bochum-Langendreer (BRD)

HARTROTT, H. H., v., Abteilung für Klinische Neurophysiologie, Klinikum Westend, Freie Universität, Berlin (BRD)

HASCHEMI, M., Neurochirurgische Klinik, Knappschaftskrankenhaus, Bochum-Langendreer (BRD)

HEUCK, F., Röntgeninstitut, Katharinenhospital, Stuttgart (BRD)

HOFFMANN, F. D., Abteilung für Neurochirurgie, Johann Wolfgang Goethe-Universität, Frankfurt/Main (BRD)

HOHELÜCHTER, K. L., Neurochirurgische Universitätsklinik, Bonn (BRD)

HOLBACH, K. H., Neurochirurgische Universitätsklinik, Bonn (BRD)

HOPMAN, H., Neurochirurgische Universitätsklinik, München (BRD)

HÜNEFELD, G., Neurochirurgische Klinik, MHH, Hannover (BRD)

IIZUKA, I., Neurochirurgische Universitätsklinik, Bonn (BRD)

ISCHEBECK, W., Neurochirurgische Universitätsklinik, Düsseldorf (BRD)

JANSEN, J., Neurochirurgische Universitätsklinik, Göttingen (BRD)

KAHL, R. I., Neurochirurgische Universitätsklinik, Mainz (BRD)

KALM, H., Neurologische Klinik, Städtische Krankenanstalten, Dortmund (BRD)

KANZOW, E., Physiologisches Institut, Universität Göttingen, Göttingen (BRD)

KARIMI-NEJAD, A., Neurochirurgische Universitätsklinik, Köln (BRD)

KAZNER, E., Neurochirurgische Universitätsklinik, München (BRD)

KERSTING, G., Institut für Neuropathologie, Universität Bonn, Bonn (BRD)

KERSTING, H. W., Neurochirurgische Klinik, MHH, Hannover (BRD)

KIENECKER, E. W., Neurochirurgische Klinik, Krankenhaus St. Jürgenstr., Bremen (BRD)

KIRCHHOFF, D., Neurochirurgische Universitätsklinik, Gießen (BRD)

KISCH, G., Neurologische Klinik Dr. Schmieder, Gailingen (BRD)

KLEIN, J., Neurochirurgische Klinik, Krankenhaus St. Jürgenstr., Bremen (BRD)

KLETTER, G., Neurochirurgische Universitätsklinik, Wien (BRD)

KLINGER, M., Neurochirurgische Universitätsklinik, Erlangen (BRD)

KLUG, N., Neurochirurgische Universitätsklinik, Mainz (BRD)

KLUG, W., Neurochirurgische Klinik, Knappschaftskrankenhaus, Bochum-Langendreer (BRD)

KNÜPLING, R., Neurochirurgische Klinik, Klinikum Westend, Freie Universität, Berlin (BRD)

KOOS, W. TH., Neurochirurgische Universitätsklinik, Wien (Österreich)

KRENKEL, W., Neurochirurgische Klinik, Rheinisch-Westfälische Technische Hochschule, Aachen (BRD)

KROPPEN, H., Oberlandesgericht, Düsseldorf (BRD)

KUHLENDAHL, H., Neurochirurgische Universitätsklinik, Düsseldorf (BRD)

KÜHNER, A., Neurochirurgische Abteilung, Chirurgische Universitätsklinik, Heidelberg (BRD)

KUSKE, I., Neurochirurgische Universitätsklinik, Düsseldorf (BRD)

LAUSBERG, G., Neurochirurgische Universitätsklinik, Gießen (BRD)

LAZARO, M. C., Abteilung für Neuropathologie, Klinikum Steglitz der Freien Universität, Berlin (BRD)

LEDINSKI, G., Zentralinstitut für Tumoren, Zagreb (Jugoslawien)

LEITHOLF, O., Neurologische Klinik Dr. Schmieder, Gailingen (BRD)

LINKE, D., Neurochirurgische Universitätsklinik, Bonn (BRD)

LOPEZ-BRUGOS, C., Neurochirurgische Klinik, Knappschaftskrankenhaus, Bochum-Langendreer (BRD)

LORENZ, R., Neurochirurgische Universitätsklinik, Gießen (BRD)

MALLIN, J. P., Neurologische Klinik, Klinikum Steglitz, Freie Universität, Berlin (BRD)

MARKAKIS, E., Neurochirurgische Klinik, MHH, Hannover (BRD)

MARTINS, L. F., Abteilung für Neuropathologie, Klinikum Steglitz der Freien Universität, Berlin (BRD)

MAYAMAGI, Y., Neurochirurgische Klinik, Klinikum Steglitz, Freie Universität, Berlin (BRD)

MEESE, W., Neurochirurgische Klinik, Klinikum Westend, Freie Universität, Berlin (BRD)

MENZEL, J., Neurochirurgische Abteilung, Chirurgische Universitätsklinik, Heidelberg (BRD)

MEYERMANN, R., Neuropathologisches Institut, Univ. Göttingen, Göttingen (BRD)

MOISSL, G., Abteilung für Neuroradiologie, Universität Würzburg, Würzburg (BRD)

NADJMI, M., Abteilung für Neuroradiologie, Universität Würzburg, Würzburg (BRD)

NEUBAUER, M., Abteilung für Endokrinologie, Johann Wolfgang Goethe-Universität, Frankfurt/Main (BRD)

NICOLA, N., Neurochirurgische Universitätsklinik, Düsseldorf (BRD)

NIEDERMEIER, B., Neurochirurgische Universitätsklinik, Essen (BRD)

NITTNER, K., Neurochirurgische Universitätsklinik, Köln (BRD)

OLDENKOTT, P., Neurochirurgische Universitätsklinik, Tübingen (BRD)

ORTHNER, H., Abteilung für Neuropathologie, Universität Göttingen, Göttingen (BRD)

PALLESKE, H., Neurochirurgische Universitätsklinik, Homburg-Saar (BRD)

PALM, K. V., Neurochirurgische Klinik, Krankenhaus St. Jürgenstr., Bremen (BRD)

PENDL, G., Neurochirurgische Universitätsklinik, Kiel (BRD)

PERNECZKY, A., Neurochirurgische Universitätsklinik, Wien (Österreich)

PFEIFFER, J., Institut für Hirnforschung, Universität Tübingen, Tübingen (BRD)

PISCOL, K., Neurochirurgische Klinik, Krankenhaus St. Jürgenstr., Bremen (BRD)

POSER, S., Neurologische Universitätsklinik, Göttingen (BRD)

POTTHOFF, P. C., Neurochirurgische Abteilung, Nervenkrankenhaus, Günzburg/Ulm (BRD)

RATZKA, M., Abteilung für Neuroradiologie, Universität Würzburg, Würzburg (BRD)

REICHENBACH, M., Allianzversicherung München, München (BRD)

RICHARD, K. E., Neurochirurgische Universitätsklinik, Köln (BRD)

SATTLEGGER, R., Neurochirurgische Klinik, Knappschaftskrankenhaus, Bochum-Langendreer (BRD)

SCHAAKE, TH., Neurochirurgische Universitätsklinik, Göttingen (BRD)

SCHÄFER, M., Neurochirurgische Universitätsklinik, Frankfurt/Main (BRD)

SCHEPELMANN, F., Neurochirurgische Universitätsklinik, Gießen (BRD)

SCHIRMER, M., Neurochirurgische Klinik, Städtisches Krankenhaus Neukölln, Berlin (BRD)

SCHMIDT, H., Pathologisches Institut, Universität Erlangen, Erlangen (BRD)

SCHMIDT, K., Neurochirurgische Abteilung, Nervenkrankenhaus, Günzburg/Ulm (BRD)

SCHUSTER, H., Neurochirurgische Universitätsklinik, Wien (Österreich)

SEBOLDT, H., Abteilung für Herz-, Thorax- und Gefäßchirurgie, Universität Tübingen, Tübingen (BRD)

SHAABAN, M., Neurochirurgische Klinik, Krankenhaus St. Jürgenstr., Bremen (BRD)

SIMON, G., Neurochirurgische Klinik, Krankenhaus Hamburg-Heidelberg, Hamburg (BRD)

SINN, H., Institut für Nuklearmedizin, DKFZ, Heidelberg (BRD)

SINZINGER, H., Anatomisches Institut der Universität, Wien (Österreich)

SOLLMANN, H., Neurochirurgische Abteilung, Nervenkrankenhaus Günzburg/Ulm, Günzburg/Ulm (BRD)

STOCHDORPH, O., Abteilung für Neuropathologie, Pathologisches Institut, Universität München, München (BRD)

STÖLZEL, R., Abteilung für klinische Neurophysiologie, Klinikum Westend, Freie Universität, Berlin (BRD)

STÖWSAND, D., Neurochirurgische Universitätsklinik, Kiel (BRD)

THOMALSKE, G., Neurochirurgische Universitätsklinik, Frankfurt (BRD)

TZONOS, T., Neurochirurgische Klinik, Katharinenhospital, Stuttgart (BRD)

VAHAR-MATIAR, H., Neurologische Universitätsklinik, Bonn (BRD)

VITZTHUM, H., Abteilung für Neuropathologie, Max-Planck-Institut für Hirnforschung, Frankfurt/Main (BRD)

VOGEL, B., Neurochirurgische Universitätsklinik, München (BRD)

VOGT, H., Neurochirurgische Universitätsklinik, Göttingen (BRD)

WALDBAUR, H., Neurochirurgische Universitätsklinik, Erlangen (BRD)

WALKENHORST, A., Neurochirurgische Klinik, Knappschaftskrankenhaus, Bochum-Langendreer (BRD)

WASSMANN, H., Neurochirurgische Universitätsklinik, Bonn (BRD)

WEISNER, B., Neurologische Universitätsklinik, Krankenhaus Hamburg-Eppendorf, Hamburg (BRD)

WENKER, H., Neurochirurgische Klinik, Städtisches Krankenhaus Neukölln, Berlin (BRD)

WICHBOLD, J., Neurochirurgische Universitätsklinik, Göttingen (BRD)

WILCKE, O., Neurochirurgische Universitätsklinik, Köln (BRD)

WILD, K., v., Abteilung für Neurochirurgie, Johann Wolfgang-Goethe-Universität, Frankfurt/Main (BRD)

WIMMER, B., Institut für Nuklearmedizin, DKFZ, Heidelberg (BRD)

WINKELMÜLLER, W., Neurochirurgische Klinik, MHH, Hannover (BRD)

WISPLINGHOFF, K. P., Neurochirurgische Universitätsklinik, Köln (BRD)

ZAMANI, SCH., Neurochirurgische Klinik, Knappschaftskrankenhaus, Bochum-Langendreer (BRD)

ZIEMANN, B., Neurochirurgische Universitätsklinik, Bonn (BRD)

ZIERSKI, J., Neurochirurgische Universitätsklinik, Gießen (BRD)

ZÜLCH, K. J., Abteilung für Allgemeine Neurologie, Städtische Krankenanstalten, Köln-Merheim (BRD)

ZUMER, M., Neurochirurgische Klinik, Ljubljana (Jugoslawien)

Meningiomas

Diagnostic and Therapeutic Problems

Meningiomas and their Problems: A Neuropathologist's Remarks

O. STOCHDORPH

1. Meningiomas are commonly thought to be derived from a meningo-
thelial (5) matrix, i. e. from the cellular layer covering the
arachnoidal membranes and their trabecula. The term of dural endothelioma has become obsolete, all the more so because most textbooks mention a subdural capillary space between the inner surface
of the dura and the outer aspect of the pia-arachnoid, and deny
the existence of a cellular layer on the inner surface of the dura.
Electron-microscopic observations, however, indicate a 'neurothelial' cell layer between dura proper and pia-arachnoid (1). These
cells appear to be very easily damaged by mechanical tear and
autolytic changes. This cell layer can be identified on preparations from human leptomeningeal tissue removed during operation
(7). Therefore, the question of histogenetic derivation of meningioma tissue should be re-evaluated.

2. In some instances, meningioma cells of apparently fusiform shape
can be identified as sections through flattened cell bodies arranged in stacks.

3. Vacuolated cell bodies, sometimes with hyaline inclusions, might
correspond to neurothelial cells.

4. Highly vascular meningiomas should not be lumped together with
hemangioblastomas of the CNS (4) and hemangiopericytomas of the
meninges (3, 6).

5. Concerning pathogenesis of meningiomas, the discovery of abnormal
chromosomal pattern with loss of one G 22 chromosome (8, 10) might
be connected with the presence of a virus belonging to the papova
group (11).

6. The unique observation of a sarcoma in the mouse induced by human
spinal meningioma implant (2) might be another hint at a possibly
viral origin of some meningiomas.

7. Grading appears to be a useful tool for differentiating between
meningiomas of different prognostic value. Thus, meningioma grade 1
does not exceed usual degrees of insinuation between other tissue
structures. Meningioma grade 2 is characterized by cellular and
nuclear polymorphism and/or mitotic activity. Meningioma grade 3
reveals definite infiltrative and destructive growth. The aspect
of meningioma grade 4 conforms to sarcoma with a recognizable derivation from meningioma. Meningioma grade 4 has also been called
meningosarcoma (9).

8. Grading should be applied within a single tumor species only, not
to a hodgepodge of different tumor species.

REFERENCES

1. ANDRES, K. H.: Über die Feinstruktur der Arachnoidea und Dura mater von Mammalia. Z. Zellforsch. 79, 272 - 295 (1967).

2. ANIGSTEIN, L., ANIGSTEIN, D. M., UNTERHARNSCHEIDT, F. J.: Mouse transplantable tumor induced by human spinal meningioma implant in mice inoculated with human antithymus antiserum. Tex. Rep. Biol. Med. 27, 341 - 266 (1969).

3. BEGG, Ch. F., GARRETT, R.: Hemangiopericytoma occurring in the meninges. Cancer 7, 602 - 606 (1954).

4. CERVOS-NAVARRO, J.: Elektronenmikroskopie der Hämangioblastome des ZNS und der angioblastischen Meningeome. Acta neuropath. (Berlin) 19, 184 - 207 (1971).

5. CUSHING, H.: The meningiomas. Their source and favoured seats of origin. Brain 14, 282 - 316 (1922).

6. KRUSE, F.: Hemangiopericytoma of the meninges (angioblastic meningioma of CUSHING and EISENHARDT). Neurology (Minn.) 11, 771 - 777 (1961).

7. LOPES, C. A. S., MAIR, W. G. P.: Untrastructure of the arachnoid membrane in man. Acta neuropath. (Berl.) 28, 167 - 173 (1974).

8. MARK, H., LEVAN, G., MITELMAN, F.: Identification by fluorescence of the G chromosome lost in human meningiomas. Hereditas (Lund) 71, 163 - 168 (1972).

9. MATAKAS, F., CERVOS-NAVARRO, J.: Die Feinstruktur sog. maligner Meningeome. Verh. Dtsch. Ges. Path. 57, 418 (1973).

10. ZANG, K.: Chromosomal constitution of meningiomas. Nature 216, 84 - 85 (1967).

11. ZANG, K.: Personal communication.

Malignant Meningiomas

K. J. ZÜLCH and H. D. MENNEL

A critical evaluation of malignancy in meningiomas presupposes the definition of malignancy. Malignancy has some significance in our current daily work; its meaning, however, is not always clear, especially if we deal with tumors of the nervous system.

I. Historical Evolution

In the field of neurological sciences LEBERT (11) was the first to state, in 1851, that fibroblastic and sarcomatous tumors of the intracranial cavity have different survival times. Fibroblastic tumors appeared to be more benign. This was the first correlation of histological classification and prognosis. BAILEY and CUSHING (1) tried to establish the correlation of survival time and morphology for the tumors of the glioma group. Their observations form the basis of our present day knowledge (21, 23). The evaluation of malignancy for the different groups of meningiomas by CUSHING and EISENHARDT (4) was not so clearly elaborated. However, these authors pointed to the particular problems of malignancy in meningiomas when they reported the famous case of Dorothy May Russell, who had been operated on 17 times for a recurrent meningioma and finally died from a metastasis in the lung. This case illustrated that a very long history does not contradict the eventual malignant transformation of a tumor of this group. We were able to report a very similar case from our own collection, in which a metastasis in the lungs weighting more than 1 kg was found 22 years after the first operation. This case was considered as not benign from the beginning because of the angiographic findings and because of the in vitro growth of tumor cells in tissue culture (25). However, metastases from meningiomas to remote sites have always been considered rarities (5, 6, 7, 19, 20).

II. Malignancy in Neurooncology

In neurooncology there is no particular histological feature decisive for the diagnosis of malignancy for all tumors in question. On the contrary, malignancy has to be defined for each tumor entity by a correlated clinico-pathological investigation. By this procedure histological criteria may be found for each tumor group, which allow a definition of its biological behaviour. Yet this procedure is complicated by the fact that the pure clinical malignancy, derived from the peculiarities of the central nervous system, has to be ruled out, and that growth properties have to be judged somewhat theoretically (24).

In the attempts of the World Health Organization to establish a new classification, this point of view was taken to define the biological behaviour of the different groups. A group of experts is working out a new classification of tumors of the brain and spinal cord which will be acceptable as a worldwide compromise. This work is in progress and all major problems seem to be solved to date.

In the preliminary draft a malignant variant for all groups of tumors is foreseen (Table 1). In the work of the WHO "anaplasia" (or "malignancy") is defined as including all morphological pecularities which, according to our clinical experience, presumably lead to malignant growth. These features are: pleomorphism, increased cellularity, growth by invasion, numerous mitotic figures, particularly atypical forms, poor differentiation, giant cells, abnormal stroma reactions, especially vascular proliferations, pseudopalisades, necroses and, in some cases, metastases through the cerebralspinal pathways and even outside the central nervous system.

Table 1. Anaplasia or malignancy according to the preliminary draft of the WHO classification of tumors of the central nervous system

---

Pleomorphism
increased cellularity
numerous mitotic figures, particularly atypical forms
poor differentiation

Abnormous stroma reaction, especially vascular proliferation
giant cells
pseudopalisades
necroses

Growth by invasion
metastasis   through the spinal pathway
                    outside the central nervous system

This is a rather pragmatic definition of anaplasia and/or malignancy by enumerating features which may be present together or in various combinations. They are, then, considered to be the histological equivalent of malignant growth. One difficulty consists in the synonymous use of the terms anaplasia and malignancy, which, however, may be considered preliminary.

III. Concept of Malignancy Applied to Meningiomas

According to our clinical experience, these general peculiarities are the signs of rapid, anaplastic and malignant growth. These signs may be more or less prominent in the different entities, but it is nor required for all of them to be present. Therefore, a combination of several of these features may be decisive for malignant growth in each tumor group. In the case of the meningiomas (Table 2) the most important indicator of anaplasia apparently is an increasing number of mitoses, i. e. "polymitotic" growth. Another rather important point consists in the infiltrative growth into the surrounding brain tissue. However, infiltrative growth has to be demonstrated histologically; fingerlike extensions into the surroundings, as often seen in tumors of the Sylvian area or the temporal base, are not considered to be an invasion, neither is the not unusual growth within mesenchymal tissue, e. g. the dura, cranium or temporal muscle.

On the other hand, cellular pleomorphism in meningiomas alone does not indicate higher malignancy. This had been stated by CUSHING and EISEN-

4

HARDT (4); in our group, MARCOS (12) has shown that in the V 2 variant, a subgroup of angiomatous meningioma, cellular pleomorphism, may be very prominent without any tendency towards malignancy.

Table 2. Anaplasia or malignancy in meningiomas; only few of the generally adopted criteria are valuable

High number of mitoses, especially atypical
low differentiation
cellular pleomorphism *combined* with
numerous mitoses
infiltrative growth
metastases

Cellular pleomorphism is a malignant sign in the meningioma group only if combined with other indications of rapid growth. The pattern of histological features associated with malignancy in meningiomas is therefore the following:
1. high number of mitoses, especially atypical ones,
2. low differentiation i. e. breakdown of organoid structures,
3. infiltrative growth and metastases, and
4. cellular pleomorphism *combined* with high mitotic rate.

IV. Grading of Malignancy in Meningiomas

Grading schemes have proved to be helpful in diagnostic work during the last 25 years. We adopted a IV-grade scale of malignancy, which is similar to the grading scheme of KERNOHAN and coworkers (8), but does not introduce a continuous grading for each tumor group. For instance, we may have only two grades for most gliomas, e. g. semibenign and semimalignant (or "polymorphic"), three or even four grades for other groups and only one grade for the glioblastoma or medulloblastoma (IV: "malignant").

In this scheme meningiomas are generally considered to be benign. Malignant or anaplastic meningiomas belong to the groups II (semibenign) or even III (semimalignant) of our scale. Group IV (malignant) is reserved for the true primary fibrosarcomas of the meninges. Some, probably secondary very malignant meningiomas, mostly recurrent tumors of former benign meningiomas, have to be classified as sarcomatous meningiomas and belong to this group; they grew infiltrating and eventually metastasized.

Using this grading scheme, we adopt a rough subgrouping of benign and anaplastic meningiomas. Since our material is not yet fully analyzed statistically, and follow up studies have not yet been performed, this subgrouping cannot be but preliminary. We used this grading as the basis of a statistical analysis dealt with later on.

This subgrouping contains (Fig. 1):

1. The benign meningiomas including the (benign!) polymorphic types and the so-called angiomatous or angioblastic types.
2. Polymitotic meningiomas with transitional forms from benign to semibenign and semimalignant.
3. The metastasizing and infiltrative meningiomas which in general have to be considered as at least semimalignant.
4. The primary fibrosarcoma of the meninges.

It has long been noted that in angioblastic meningiomas the frequency of recurrences is apparently higher (4). This, however, has been contested by several authors (3, 16). The splitting-up of the group of socalled angioblastic meningiomas into angiomatous meningiomas, hemangioblastic meningiomas and hemangiopericytic meningiomas may prove useful in solving this question (18). The preliminary draft of the WHO-nomenclature has introduced these three types as meningioma subgroups (Table 3). It has been reported by some authorities that only the hemangiopericytic type of meningioma is more prone to recur (9). This statement has to be reviewed after additional work on the basis of the WHO-classification. No general conclusions may be drawn from the participation of the stroma in this tumor group.

Table 3. Subclassification of meningiomas according to the preliminary classification scheme of the WHO

Meningiomas

1. meningotheliomatous (endotheliomatous, syncytial)
2. fibrous (fibroblastic)
3. transitional (mixed)
4. psammomatous
5. angiomatous
6. hemangioblastic
7. hemangiopericytic

8. anaplastic (malignant)

Primary fibrosarcomas of the meninges may be considered to be the truly malignant counterparts of the benign meningiomas. They have been introduced as the primary meningeal sarcomatosis into the WHO classification. Their growth is invasive and infiltrating, their vasculature is not very prominent, necroses are generally not associated with stroma reaction. This is quite different from the features seen in glioblastoma, where all sorts of vascular hyperplasia up to the formation of glomerula are found. However, the isomorphic monotony of cellular growth in fibrosarcomas may be interrupted by the occurrence of chromatin-dense multinucleated giant cells. The number of mitoses, on the other hand, is the same in other tumors of this group in the body.

Inbetween the benign tumors on one side, and the malignant sarcomas on the other, we find the different forms of polymitotic, rapidly growing, partly invasive meningiomas which exhibit the malignant character in different expressions. Both these groups, in our grading scheme II (semibenign) and III (semimalignant), are the main subject of the following statistical evaluation.

V. Statistical Data

In our collection of 9000 tumors of the nervous system, 1492 are meningiomas, i. e. 16.6 %; 532 were found in males and 960 in females.

Statistical analysis was only possible in the cases collected from 1958 on. In the time between 1958 and 1974 we classified 624 cases as meningiomas, 57 of which, i. e. 9.1 %, were malignant according to our definition mentioned above.

In our grading scheme (Table 4) 32 of these 57 anaplastic or malignant
tumors were considered to be of grade II with some cellular pleomorphism and mitoses; 20 were considered to be of grade III with very numerous, partly atypical, mitoses and pronounced pleomorphism. Sometimes these tumors showed a prominent intercellular fiber production,
as usually seen in reticulum cell sarcomas. Only 5 tumors were thought
to be of grade IV. These are some of the recurrences of former benign
meningiomas which became sarcomas as mentioned above.

Table 4. Grading of 624 meningiomas

I benign	II semibenign	III semimalignant	IV malignant
	32	20	5
567 = 90,9 %		57 = 9.1 %	

The sex distribution of meningiomas in our collection shows the well
known female preponderance. For this group of 624 tumors we have found
a rate of approximately 2 : 1. Interestingly enough, in the malignant
form there is a preference for the male sex; the relation is about
3 : 2. This is apparently consistent with a general trend in neurooncology (Fig. 2). Malignant forms occur predominantly in males, the
benign in females (23).

In contrast, the age incidence of the 567 benign and 57 malignant tumors is almost identical. This shows quite clearly that malignant
meningiomas are by no means sarcomas, which have no age peak when occurring in the central nervous system.

The length of preoperative history could be evaluated only in a part
of our material. There were no major differences in benign and less
benign forms. However, in the malignant form short preoperative histories prevail. This may be explained partly by the fact that only
6 % of the benign forms were already recurring meningiomas, while in
the anaplastic tumors 21 % were first, second or more recurrences.

As to the localization of the benign and malignant forms, the tumors
of the spinal region are much more frequent (14 %) in the benign than
in the malignant (4 %) form. One explanation of this fact may be seen
in the high frequency of benign psammomatous meningiomas in the spinal
region, which almost exclusively occur in women in the age between 50
and 65 (10, 22). Malignant meningiomas are, in contrast, more frequent
in the intracranial cavity, especially with a frontal site.

VI. Malignancy of Meningiomas in General Neurooncology

General neurooncology has been broadly influenced by the experimental
result of tumor induction with resorptive carcinogens. Peculiar facts
of these experiments are, for instance, the occurrence of multiple tumors in these animals and the higher malignancy of induced tumors.
These results, therefore, have stressed once more the discussion of
malignancy in neurooncology as well as the discussion of multiplicity
of tumor growth.

One example of this higher malignancy is the fact that in the experiments with resorptive carcinogenes almost no true benign meningiomas

have been found. If tumors occurred in the meninges, they were almost exclusively malignant meningeal sarcomas, which, however, were not very numerous in these experiments. In contrast, they were regularly induced by topic application of carcinogenic carbohydrates as well as in viral carcinogenesis in the central nervous system.

Meningeal sarcomas, found sporadically in rats treated with resorptive carcinogens, were constituted by spindle cells and had a strong participation of collagen and reticulin fibers. Cells explanted in vitro behaved like fibroblasts without, however, showing contact inhibition. In vitro production of reticulin fibers was observed at the beginning of in vitro growth. Tumors could be transplanted successfully. They grew subcutaneously as well as in the cranial cavity. In this latter site they grew only within the meninges and infiltrated the brain through the perivascular space.

Neurooncogenic viruses, on the other hand, almost regularly produce very malignant tumors of the meninges. One of the last results is that of OGAWA (15), who employed adenovirus 12, which induces tumors starting from the meninges and growing into the brain not unlike the human fibrosarcomas. These tumors exhibit the highest cellular pleomorphism.

One other remark on the field of theoretical oncology: meningiomas are, together with the chronic myeloic leucemia, one of the few examples known which have almost constant cheomosome aberrations (17). One chromosome of the G-group is lacking. MARK (13, 14) has identified this chromosome as being number 22. BENEDICT and coworkers (2), and MARK (13, 14), showed tumors which had more chromosome aberrations than this mentioned pattern; both authors tried to correlate this karyotype to recurrence and malignancy.

VII. General Conclusions

We think we can state the following points as a general conclusion for the malignancy of meningiomas:

1. The risk of recurrence apparently correlates better with the totality of removal than with the histological subgroups or histologically observed anaplasias.
2. Our criteria of malignancy in meningiomas are pragmatic. We took over the preliminary definition of anaplasia of the WHO. In meningiomas, however, this definition is only of value if the tumor is totally removed.
3. Up to now, the significance of different subgroups of meningiomas as to the prognosis does not seem to be established with sufficient certainty.
4. Comparable follow-up studies are only reasonable on the base of a commonly accepted classification. Yet these studies are urgently needed to clarify the different points not solved up to now.

REFERENCES

1. BAILEY, P., CUSHING, H.: Tumors of the glioma group. Philadelphia: I. B. Lippincott Co. 1926.
2. BENEDICT, B. F., PORTER, I. H., BROWN, C. H. D., FLORENTIN, R. A.: Cytogenetic diagnosis of malignancy in recurrent meningioma. Lancet 1, 971 - 973 (1970).

3. CROMPTON, M. R., GAUTIER-SMITH, P. C.: The predilection of recurrence in meningiomas. J. Neurol. Neurosurg. Psychiat. 33, 80 - 87 (1970).

4. CUSHING, H., EISENHARDT, L.: Meningiomas: Their classification, regional behaviour, life history, and surgical end results. Springfield, Ill.: C. Thomas 1938.

5. GESSAGA, E.: Über einen Fall eines malignen Meningeomes mit extrakranialen Metastasen. Sistema Nervoso 20, 258 - 270 (1969).

6. HOFFMANN, G. T., EARLE, K. M.: Meningioma with malignant transformation and implantation in the subarachnoid space. J. Neurosurg. 17, 486 - 492 (1960).

7. KALM, H.: Ein malignes Tentoriummeningeom mit Metastasierung in die Medulla oblongata und in die subarachnoidalen Liquorräume. Dtsch. Zschr. Nervenhk. 163, 131 - 140 (1950).

8. KERNOHAN, J. W., MABON, R. F., SVIEN, H. J., ADSON, A. W.: A simplified classification of the gliomas. Proc. Staff Meet. Mayo Clin. 24, 71 - 75 (1949).

9. KRUSE, F.: Hemangiopericytoma of the meninges. Neurology 11, 771 - 777 (1961).

10. LAPRESLE, J., NETSKY, M. G., ZIMMERMAN, H.: The pathology of meningeomas, a study of 121 cases. Amer. J. Path. 28, 757 - 791 (1952).

11. LEBERT, H.: Über Krebs und die mit Krebs verwechselten Geschwülste im Gehirn und seinen Hüllen. Virch. Arch. 3, 463 - 569 (1851).

12. MARCOS, F.: Über ein hochgradig polymorphes Meningeom mit langsamem Wachstum. Zbl. Neurochir. 14, 304 - 307 (1954).

13. MARK, H.: Karyotype patterns in human meningiomas. A comparison between studies with G- and Q-banding techniques. Hereditas 75, 213 - 220 (1973).

14. MARK, J.: Origin of the ring chromosome in a human recurrent meningioma studied with G-band technique. Acta path. microbiol. scand. 81, 591 - 592 (1973).

15. OGAWA, K.: Personal Communication.

16. SIMPSON, D.: The recurrence of intracranial meningiomas after surgical treatment. J. Neurol. Neurosurg. Psychiat. 20, 20 - 39 (1957).

17. SINGER, H., ZANG, K. D.: Cytologische Untersuchungen an Hirntumoren. Humangenetik 9, 172 - 184 (1970).

18. SKULLERUD, K., LÖKEN, A. C.: The prognosis in meningiomas. Acta Neuropath. ...

19. STRANG, R. R., TOVI, D., NORDENSTAM, H.: Meningioma with intracerebral, cerebellar and visceral metastases. J. Neurosurg. 21, 1098 - 1102 (1964).

20. WINKELMAN, N. W., CASSEL, C., SCHLESINGER, B.: Intracranial tumors with extracranial metastases. J. Neuropath. 11, 149 - 168 (1952).

21. ZÜLCH, K. J.: Biologie und Pathologie der Hirngeschwülste. In: Handbuch der Neurochirurgie, Bd. III. Berlin-Göttingen-Heidelberg: Springer 1956.

22. ZÜLCH, K. J., HOSSMANN, K.-A.: Die spinalen psammomatösen Meningeome der Frau. Neurochirurgie 9, 106 - 113 (1966).

23. ZÜLCH, K. J., MENNEL, H. D.: The biology of brain tumors. In: Handbook of Clinical Neurology, Vol. 16 (eds. P. J. VINKEN, G. W. BRUYN) pp. 1 - 55. Amsterdam: North-Holland Publ. Comp. 1974.

24. ZÜLCH, K. J., MENNEL, H. D., ZIMMERMANN, V.: Intracranial hypertension. In: Handbook of Clinical Neurology, Vol. 16 (eds. P. J. VINKEN, G. W. BRUYN) pp. 89 - 149. Amsterdam. North-Holland Publ. Comp. 1974.

25. ZÜLCH, K. J., POMPEU, F., PINTO, F.: Über die Metastasierung der Meningeome. Zbl. Neurochir. 14, 253 - 260 (1954).

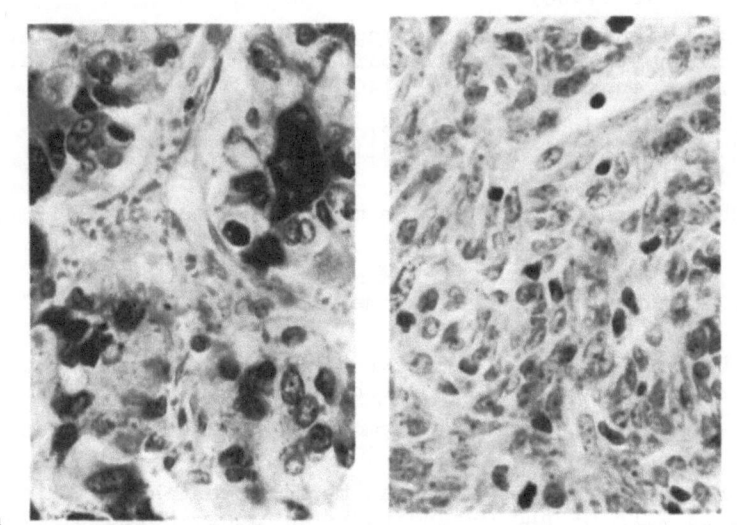

a

b

Fig. 1 a. Marked variation in cell size and shape is not considered as sign of malignancy unless other indications of rapid growth are present. Case 5631, H & E 500 x

Fig. 1 b. Numerous mitoses are the most important indicator of increasing malignancy in meningiomas. Case % 4635, cresyl violet, 500 x

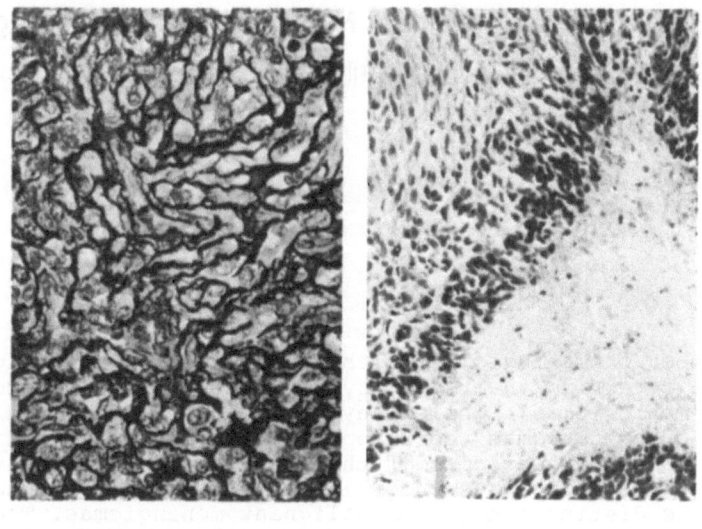

c   d

Fig. 1 c. In anaplastic meningiomas a dense reticulin network may be present. Case E 6821, Tibor Pap, 500 x

Fig. 1 d. In the sarcomas of the meninges, necroses are - in contrast to glioblastomas - not followed by major stromal reactions. Case 148, cresyl violet, 250 x

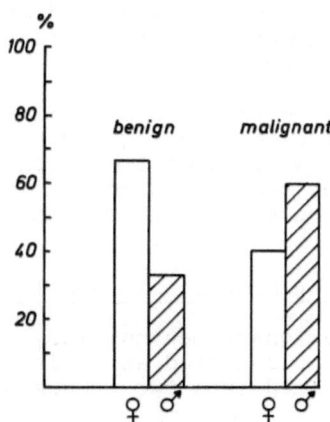

Fig. 2. Sex distribution in benign and malignant meningiomas

Ultrastructure of Malignant Meningioma and Meningosarcoma*

J. Cervós-Navarro, L. F. Martins, and M. C. Lazaro

A number of meningiomas which showed histological signs of malignancy, while retaining their primary structures, were diagnosed as "malignant meningiomas". While many of the cases described in the literature as "meningosarcomas" correspond to the malignant meningiomas, there is a number of sarcomas of the meninges which display no primary meningioma-like structures under light microscopic examination, and can thus be distinguished from malignant meningiomas. They are also called fibrosarcomas (24, 27, 6) or fibrosarcomas of the dura (14, 32, 10, 2).

The purpose of the electron microscopic examination of malignant meningiomas was to determine ultrastructural criteria of malignancy in these tumors and to establish their relationship to the sarcomas of the meninges.

Material and Methods

Four tumors diagnosed under the light microscope as malignant meningiomas, and one diagnosed as a meningosarcoma, were examined. 26 endotheliomatous or fibroblastic meningiomas were available as comparison material (5).

Table 1 gives a summary of the duration of illness, localization, and histological findings. During the operation, several pieces (about 1 mm^3) were taken from each tumor, fixed for 4 hours in 5 % glutaraldehyde, then in isotonic 1 % OsO_4. The embedding was done in Vestopal W in cases 1 and 6, and in Mikropal in the other cases.

Electron Microscopic Results

The malignant meningiomas, which, in spite of a certain variability, can be classified as a single group under the light microscope, can be divided into two groups with the electron microscope.

Group 1 (cases 1 and 2)

The cells are elongated, nearly parallel, and closely packed (Fig. 1). The nuclei have both elliptic-roundish and irregular pointed profiles. In 40 % of the nuclear sections, there are one or two nucleoli. Most of them lie directly on the nuclear membrane (Fig. 1).

The cytoplasm is arranged as a fringe around the nucleus, extending processes in all directions, but above all toward the pole. They ex-

---

*The study is dedicated to Prof. H. SELBACH on his 65th birthday.

Table 1

No. Age Sex	Time first symptom - operation	Location	Histological diagnosis	Mitoses	Necrosis Necrobiosis	Invasion of neighbouring tissues	Time of survival
1 17 y m.	4 months	Clivus	Malignant endothelio-matous meningioma	+	+	dura	15 months recurrence
2 46 y f.	10 months	Parasagittal	"	+	–	dura and skull	16 months recurrence no autopsy
3 36 y m.	5 years	sphenoidal ridge	"	+	+	dura	3 months circumscrib. purulent meningitis
4 62 y f.	1 year first op. 9 years second op.	sinus sag. sup. occipital falx	"	+	+	dura skull	alive, 3, 5 years after operation
5 50 y m.	5 weeks	precentral	meningeal sarcoma	+	+	dura brain	6 weeks after operation

tend parallel to each other, and may also intermesh, with the processes of neighbouring cells. The mitochondria display a distinct polymorphy.

Monstrous mitochondria appear which attain, in the second case, a size
of 5 µ (Fig. 2).

Golgi zones are seldomly encountered. The endoplasmatic reticulum is
sparsely developed and almost exclusively of the granular type. Glycogen granules are ubiquitous, frequently in dense accumulations
(Fig. 2). Solitary lysosomes are found. The cytofilaments are loosely
aligned or run in narrow trains. In a few areas of case 2, they are
more developed and clustered in some regions of the cytoplasm. Here
the cells display a more developed Golgi apparatus and an increase in
the number and size of nuclear bodies. The plasma membranes frequently show pinocytotic bubbles. Desmosomes between neighbouring plasma
membranes are numerous, but mostly only 50 - 100 nm long (Fig. 2).

Group II (cases 3 and 4)

Both tumors display an extensive similarity in their cytological characteristics and, to some extent, in their structural principles. In
case 3 one observes areas with closely fitting, elongated cells, mostly lying parallel, with a tendency to spiral (Fig. 3). In case 4 there
are also areas in which the cells lie close to each other in groups.
They are, however, not elongated, but polygonal, and the short extensions have no tendency to form whorls (Fig. 4). The principle of
the enclosure of a tumor cell by processes from neighbouring cells is
distinctly noticeable. In both cases the connective tissue has so
greatly increased that the tumor cells have been pushed apart and lie
isolated between the connective tissue processes.

The nuclei display an irregular, usually poligonal (in case 3 also
elongated) profile with occasional indentations.

The most obvious finding in the cytoplasm of the tumor cells is the
abundance of cytofilaments, which run through the cytoplasm frequently in whorls, and pushed the other organelles to the periphery (Fig. 5 a).
The latter consist mostly of granulated endoplasmatic reticulum. Its
cisterns contain a homogenous, slightly adielectric substance. Free
ribosomes, arranged in rosettes, are numerous in some areas.

The mitochondria have, as a rule, a regular structure. Extensive Golgi
zones are frequent, partly in the immediate neighbourhood of the nucleus, but also between the structures surrounding the cytofilaments.

In the areas rich in connective tissue, the cells are solitary or lie
in small groups.

In many of the cell sections, there were regressive changes. These
consisting of a change of the endoplasmic reticulum, whose ribosomes
are lost and whose narrowed cisterns, without adielectric content,
display circular or elliptical patterns. The cytoplasm has few organelles, and few or no filaments (Fig. 5 b). Glycogen clumps may
appear. Lysosomes and occasional fat vacuoles are also present. Sometimes there are pyknotic nuclei, which are surrounded by a very dark,
narrow cytoplasmic border.

Group III (Case 5)

The tumor cells lie in dense clusters without any definite order
(Fig. 6 a). Between the group of tumor cells is a broad intercellular

space, whose content is a very loose ground substance. In a few places
a spiral pattern of the tumor cells occurs. This always involves a
central cell, which is more or less completely surrounded by a few
other cells (Fig. 6 b). The nuclei have irregular, mostly polygonal
sometimes lobulated profiles. The chromatin is homogenously distrib-
uted. Nucleoli are mostly small and appear in only a few nuclear sections (Fig. 6 b).

The cytoplasm represents only a thin layer around the cell nucleus,
but can also display broad spreading. The mitochondria appear regularly, but not in clumps. They are mostly small and have regularly formed
cristae. But there are some monstrous mitochondria with scarcely any
peripheral cristae. Golgi zones appear broadly spread. The granular
endoplasmic reticulum is sparsely present. Free ribosomes are also
present only in small numbers. In a few places, one sees greatly degenerated cells, in which there are many lysosomes. The plasma membranes lie close together, and very small desmosomes may sometimes
be recognized. They form short finger-like extensions into the broad
intercellular space. The endothelial cells of the vessels are large
and plump and contain ample endoplasmic reticulum and mitochondria.
The basal membrane around the vessels is frequently multilayered.

Discussion

The ultrastructural architectonic principles in the cases of *group I*
correspond to those which we described for endotheliomatous and fibroblastic meningiomas (5).

The cytological differences are simply a matter of the number and
size of the nucleoli, as well as of the number and polymorphy of the
mitochondria.

An increase in the size of the nucleoli was found in the second removal of a meningioma, compared with the material from the first (1). For
a number of tumors, the size of the nucleolus was seen as a criterion
for malignancy (19) or simply as an expression of active protein synthesis (28). Differential evaluation of the ultrastructures of nucleoli (26, 29) show that the results from one type of cells and its tumors cannot be extrapolated to other cells. Within one type of cells,
the increase in the nucleolus is an expression of rapid growth.

The large number of mitochondria and their polymorphy have been described in rapidly growing tissues (3). The significance of the giant
mitochondria, which have been examined in many tissues under various
conditions (8), has not yet been fully explained. The cytological
differences between the tumors examined here and the control material
indicate a rapid growth of the tumors in the present group. This is
also indicated by the short case histories of 4 to 10 months, and the
postoperative reappearence after little more than a year. The tumors
of this group represent the genuine malignant meningiomas. Their morphological appearence permits to correlate the presence of their recurrence in spite of adequate surgical treatment (15, 7).

The cases in *group II* differ from the ordinary meningiomas both in
their structural principles and in their cytological characteristics.
The structural principle of endotheliomatous meningioma can only be
recognized in some areas of case 3.

The increase in the space occupied by connective tissue does not occur
in the manner of the fibroblastic type of tumor, in which one finds
layers of only a few cells or sometimes even a single cell process.

In case 4 the lack of long cytoplasmic processes precludes such a structural principle. In case 3 the connective tissue appears in lacunar spaces, which are bordered by broad cellular areas. In addition, one seldom finds microfibrils in the connective tissue areas. For the most part, only collagen fibers are found, which is the reverse of the situation in fibroblastic meningiomas. It cannot be decided whether the considerable collagen development should be considered only a regressive sign, or if it represents the participation of the invaded dura in the construction of the tumor. However, the fact that areas with greater connective tissue development also contain degenerative cells and many lysosomes suggests that a regression is occuring. The high degree of development of the Golgi zones and the endoplasmic reticulum is related to the abundance of cytofilaments. While the endoplasmic reticulum plays the major role in protein synthesis (11), the Golgi zone is responsible for the synthesis of mucopolysacharides (12). An excessive abundance of cytofilaments of 11 mm diameter was described in ageing cultures of carcinoma of the breast. This was interpreted as a symptom of a degenerative process. It can be hypothesized that mutations occur in degenerative tumors, and that clones of these tumors grow with an increased rate of division.

The long history of the cases of this group may support the conclusion that they were benign tumors originally. In the third case the short postoperative survival certainly cannot be regarded as indication for a tumor recurrence. The long survival of the fourth case proves that the histological signs of apparent malignancy were only the manifestation of degenerative changes. Meningiomas with histological signs of malignancy but a benign clinical course were repeatedly observed with the light microscope by early authors (8, 4, 16, 25). The existence of apparently malignant meningiomas of this type is responsible for the fact that this correlation is not an absolute one.

The cytological characteristics of our meningosarcoma correspond to those of immature tissue or undifferentiated sarcoma (21, 31, 12). They are also similar to those of the circumscribed sarcoma of the cerebellum (22) and of the medulloblastomas (20). However, in some places of our case, there is definite organization of the tumor cells in whorls, that sarcomas do not display. On the contrary this architectural organization is very characteristic of meningiomas. It is even observed among meningioma cells in tissue culture (18), and indicates the close relationship between the histogenesis of the meningosarcoma and the meningioma.

The only fibrosarcoma of the dura known to us, which has been examined under the electron microscope (17) displayed the same degenerative phenomena as several cells from our group II. Otherwise, nothing can be established from a comparison between it and the various tumors we examined. Particularly the disposition to form whorls seems to be wholly lacking. These tumors must be considered sarcomas as was postulated by (23), although they originate from the same cell types as meningiomas.

Summary

The malignant meningiomas can be divided into two groups on the basis of their ultrastructural characteristics. The first group differs from the benign meningiomas by the number and size of the nucleoli as well as by the amount and polymorphism of mitochondria. Their morphological appearance correlated with their rapid growth, especially with the richness in cytofilaments and increase of connective tissue. These features may be attributed to degeneration.

The cells of meningeal sarcomas are characterized by high dedifferentiation. The ultrastructural features of these cells correspond to those of immature tissue or undifferentiated sarcomas. However, in some places the architectonic organization of meningeomatous whorls can be seen.

REFERENCES

1. ARNOULD, J., LEPOIRE, J., PIERSON, B., BARRUCAND, D.: Memoires originaux, les meningiomes malins (A propos d'une observation). Revue Neurol. 105, 469 - 477 (1961).

2. BAILEY, O. T., INGRAHAM, F. D.: Intracranial fibrosarcomas of the dura mater in childhood: Pathologic characteristics and surgical management. J. Neurosurg. 2, 1 - 15 (1945).

3. BASS, R., NEUBERT, D., MORRIS, H. P.: Thymidin-Einbau in die Mitochondrien-DNS von Rattenleber und hepatocellulären Tumoren. Arch. Pharm. exp. Path. 255, 2 - 3 (1966).

4. BERTRAND, I., GUILLAUME, J., OLTEANU, I.: Etude histologique de 130 meningiomes. Rev. Neurol. 80, 81 - 99 (1948).

5. CERVOS-NAVARRO, J., VAZQUEZ, J. J.: An electron microscopic study of meningiomas. Acta neuropath. (Berl.) 13, 301 - 323 (1969).

6. CHRISTENSEN, E., KLAER, W., WINBLAD, S.: Meningeal tumors with extracerebral metastasis. Brit. J. Cancer 3, 485 - 493 (1949).

7. CROMPTON, M. R., GAUTTIER-SMITH, P. C.: The prediction of recurrence in meningiomas. J. Neurol. Neurosurg. Psychiat. 33, 80 - 87 (1970).

8. CUSHING, H., EISENHARDT, L.: Meningeomas (Reprint). New York: Hafner Public. Co. 1962.

9. DAVID, H.: Zellschädigung und Dysfunktion. Protoplasmatologia, Bd. X/1. Wien - New York: Springer 1970.

10. DUBLIN, W. B.: Metastasizing intracranial tumors. Northwestern Med. 43, 83 - 84 (1944).

11. FAWCETT, D. W.: The cell. Its organelles and inclusions, p. 135. Philadelphia - London: W. B. Saunders Co. 1967.

12. FRIEDMAN, B., GOLD, H.: Ultrastructure of Ewing's sarcoma of bone. Cancer 22, 307 - 322 (1968).

13. GHADIALLY, F. N., PRAN, N. M.: Ultrastructure of osteogenic sarcoma. Cancer 25, 1457 - 1467 (1970).

14. GOLDMAN, M., ADAMS, R. D.: Fibrosarcoma of the sphenoid bone, producing the syndrome of the lateral wall of the cavernous sinus - a case report. J. Neuropath. Exp. Neurol. 5, 155 - 159 (1946).

15. GULLOTTA, F., WÜLLENWEBER, R.: Zur Frage der malignen Entartung bei Meningeom und Meningeom-Rezidiv. Acta neurochir. 18, 15, 27 (1968).

16. HENSCHEN, F.: Tumoren des Zentralnervensystems und seiner Hüllen. In: Hdb. d. spez. path. Anat. u. Hist. (Hrsg. HENKE-LUBARSCH-RÖSSLE), Bd. 13/III. Berlin-Göttingen-Heidelberg: Springer 1955.

17. HIZAWA, K., WECHSLER, W.: Zur Feinstruktur des Fibrosarcoms der Dura. Beitr. pathol. Anat. u. Allg. Pathol. 134, 449 - 463 (1966).

18. KERSTING, G., LENNARTZ, H., FINKEMEYER, H.: Über die Züchtung von Hirngeschwülsten als Gewebskultur. Ein Beitrag zur experimentellen Neuropathologie. Dtsch. Med. Wschr. 82, 968 - 970 (1957).

19. MACCARTY, W. C.: The value of the macronucleolus in the cancer problem. Amer. J. of Cancer 26, 337 - 344 (1968).

20. MATAKAS, F.: Färbemethoden und histochemische Reaktionen an Kunststoffdünnschnitten für lichtmikroskopische Untersuchungen. Mikroskopie 23, 337 - 344 (1968).

21. MATSUI, K.: Ultrastructure of reticulosarcoma. Fourth Intern. Symp. on Reticulo-endothelial System, pp. 36 - 37. Otsuo-Kyoto 1964.

22. RAMSEY, H. J., KERNOHAN, J. W.: Circumscribed sarcoma of the cerebellum. An electron microscopic study. J. Neuropathol. Exp. Neurol. 23, 706 - 718 (1964).

23. RUSSEL, D. S., RUBINSTEIN, L. J.: Pathology of tumors of the nervous system. 22nd edition. London: Arnold Publ. Ltd. 1963.

24. RUSSEL, W. D., SACHS, E.: Fibrosarcoma of arachnoidal origin with metastases. Report of 4 cases with necropsy. Arch. Path. 34, 240 - 261 (1942).

25. SIMPSON, D.: The recurrence of intracranial meningiomas after surgical treatment. J. Neurol. Neurosurg. Psychiat. 20, 22 - 39 (1957).

26. SMETANA, K., GYORKEY, F., GYORKEY, Ph., BUSCH, H.: Studies on nucleoli and cytoplamic fibrillar bodies of human hepatocellular carcinomas. Cancer Res. 32, 925 - 932 (1972).

27. SWINGLE, A. J.: Meningosarcoma with pulmonary metastasis. Arch. Neurol. Psychiat. 61, 65 - 72 (1949).

28. STOWELL, R. E.: The relationship of nucleolar mass to protein synthesis. Exp. Cell Res. 9, 164 - 169 (1963).

29. STUDZINSKI, G. P., GIERTHY, J. F.: Cytologic appearance of the nucleolus of normal and neoplastic cells in relation to the synthesis of RNA. Acta Cytologica 16, 245 - 248 (1972).

30. TUMILOWICZ, J. J., SARKAR, N. H.: Accumulation of filaments and other ultrastructural aspects of declining cell structure derived from human breast tumors. Exp. Mole. Path. 16, 210 - 221 (1972).

31. WEINBERGER, M. A., BANFIERLD, W. G.: Fine structure of a transplantable reticulum cell sarcoma. I. Light and electron microscopy of viable and necrotic tumor cells. J. nat. Cancer Inst. 34, 459 - 479 (1965).

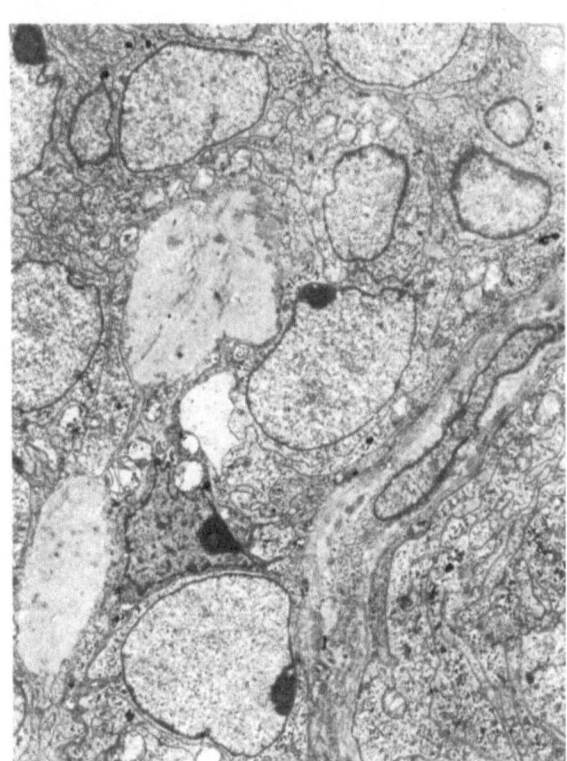

Fig. 1. Case 1. Meningioma
cells are closely packed and
the cell boundaries are
interlocking. The nucleoli
lie directly on the nuclear
membrane. 6.000 x

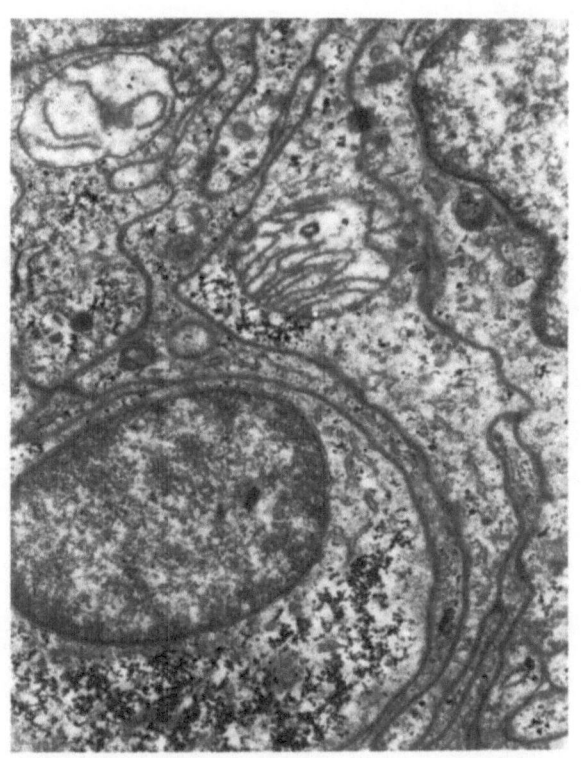

Fig. 2. Case 2. Meningioma
cells with accumulation of
glycogen granules. The cytoplasmic processes are interlocking with those of
neighbouring cells. 24.000 x

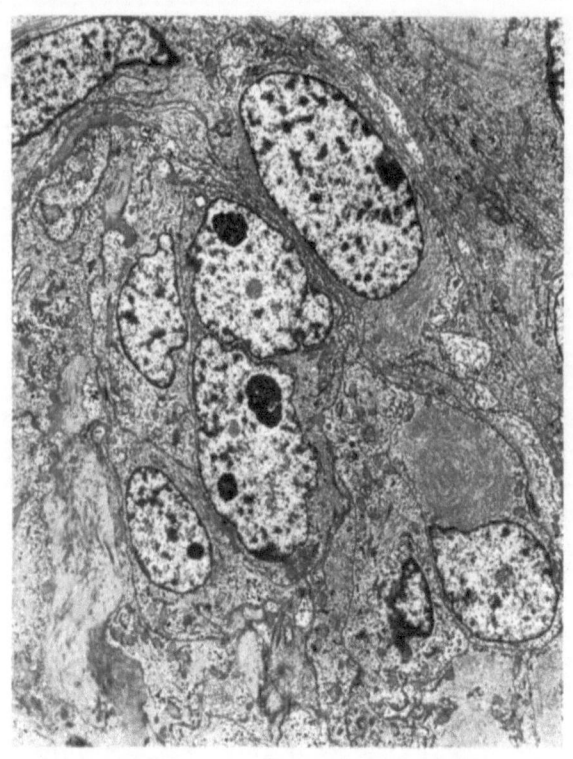

Fig. 3. Case 3.
The meningioma cells are elongated. The main nuclei contain nucleoli and spheroid bodies . Large areas of the cytoplasm are occupied by cyto-filaments. 4.500 x

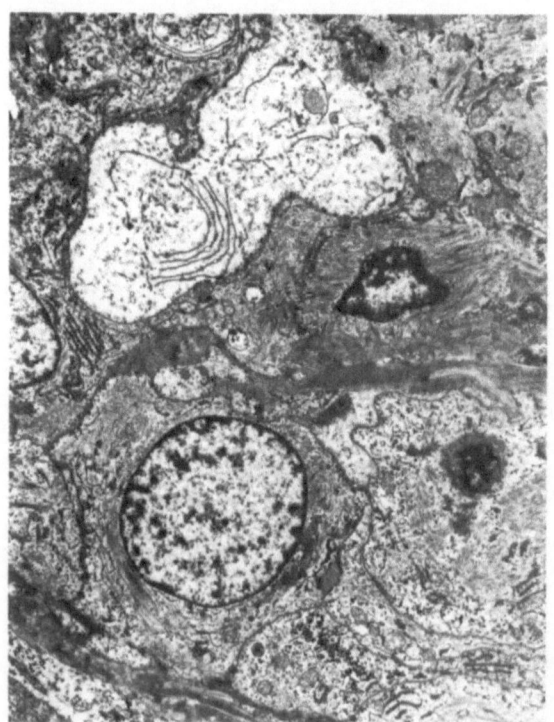

Fig. 4. Case 4.
The meningioma cells are polygonal with short pro-cesses. Above: cell section with regressive changes. 5.000 x

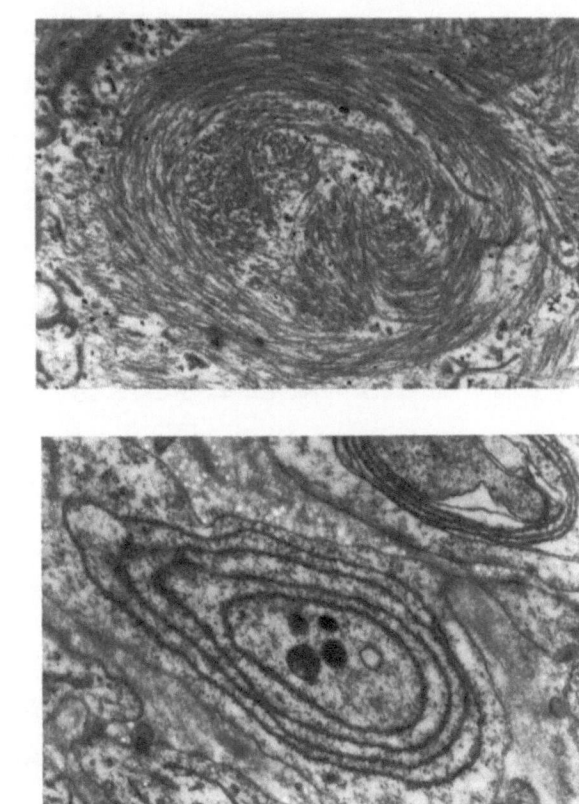

a

b

Fig. 5 a). Case 4. Whorl of cytofilaments. 25.000 x
Fig. 5 b). Endoplasmic reticulum with narrowed cisterns that display
elliptical patterns. 25.000 x

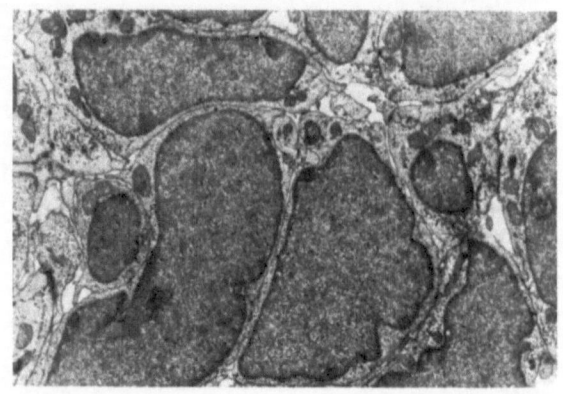

a

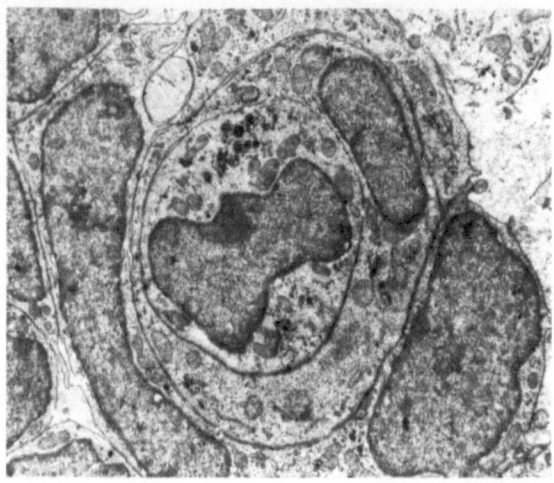

b

Fig. 6 a). Case 5. Clusters of tumor cells. The cytoplasm is only a thin layer surrounding the nucleus. 10.000 x
Fig. 6 b). Case 5. The tumor cells display a whorl pattern. 10.000 x

Unusual Course of Surgically Treated Intracranial Meningiomas, with Special Reference to their Malignant Degeneration

H. Fromm, M. Schäfer, and H. Gräfin Vitzthum

It is difficult for the pathologist to judge the rate of growth or the possible malignancy of a meningioma solely by its histological appearance. On the other hand the surgeon appreciates confirmation of his prognosis by the pathologist, if this is at all possible.

We have investigated the incidence of recurrence in 300 cases of intracranial meningioma, which were operated upon in the neurosurgical clinic of Frankfurt (1954 - 1973).

20 of these 300 patients returned once or several times for the operation of a relapse. In 14 of the 20 cases a macroscopically total removal of the tumor had not been possible at the initial operation or had to be abandoned for functional reasons. These cases in which the tumor continued to grow will not be considered here.

In all of the remaining 6 cases the meningiomatous tissue had been totally removed at operation. The tumors recurred between one and three times. In patients who had to have several operations the time intervals between subsequent relapses shortened progessively (Table 1).

Histopathologically these totally removed recurrent meningiomas presented different aspects, which will be demonstrated briefly in the following three examples:

Case 5 (G. N.):

This was a partly endotheliomatous, partly fibromatous meningioma with mitoses and small foci of necrosis but without infiltrating growth. The recurrent tumors appeared polymorphous and showed many typical and several atypical mitoses as well as focal infiltrations into the nervous parenchyma.

In view of the fact that the relapses occurred each time after an interval of about one year and that the total survival time of the patient amounted to three years we would classify this tumor as a rapidly growing meningioma with malignant transformation.

Case 6 (K. H.):

The tumor, an angioblastic meningioma, with three relapses, was initially surrounded by a partly infiltrated capsule; at a later stage, however, the tumor growth became undoubtedly infiltrating. The recurrent tumors are, in places, more cellular than the initial growth and of a moderately polymorphic cell type. Mitoses occurred from the start.

Table 1. Recurrences of completely removed meningiomas

Nr.	Sex	Localisation	Histology	Nr of operated Recurrences	Interval in Months		
1	M	(diagram)	endothel.	1	29		
2	M	(diagram)	endothel.	1	34		
3	F	(diagram)	fibroblast.	1	33		
4	F	(diagram)	endothel. + fibroblast.	2	22	6	
5	M	(diagram)	endothel. + fibroblast.	2	13	11	
6	F	(diagram)	angioblast.	3	54	22	10

In accordance with the increasingly shorter intervals of 54, 22, and 10 months between relapses, it seems justified to talk of a slowly progressive transformation of this tumor.

Case 1 (W. H.):

Within the otherwise homogenous picture of a typical endotheliomatous meningioma there was, seen in retrospect, a small circumscribed sector of a polymorphous character. The tumor infiltrated the brain substance from the start and showed numerous mitoses. Later on there was infiltration of the galea and the temporal muscles although mitotic figures did not increase in number.

The question arises, whether or not in a survival time of seven years this tumor should be called a sarcoma or an agressively growing malignant meningioma.

Microscopically, in 4 out of these 6 cases there was, at least in parts, an infiltrating growth from the beginning. In 5 of these cases mitoses were found in each biopsy, whilst in the 6th case there was an obvious increase in the number of mitoses at a later stage.

Metastatic dissemination to other parts of the body, which is regarded as extremely rare, has not been observed in our patients.

Discussion

There is, in the literature, no uniform opinion regarding the question of malignant meningiomas. ZÜLCH (6, 7) defines the malignant meningioma as a rapidly growing, encapsulated growth, which, though not invading the brain substance, will rapidly infiltrate mesodermal tissues, which recurs rapidly and, in exceptional cases, may lead to metastases in other parts of the body. The primary fibrosarcoma of the dura, on the other hand, grows, according to ZÜLCH (6), by invading the brain substance from the very beginning. In the Anglo-Saxon literature, represented by RUSSELL and RUBINSTEIN (3), CROMPTON and GAUTIER-SMITH (1), SIMPSON (4), TYTUS et al. (5) and MORLEY (2) the concept is advanced that increased mitoses, nuclear polymorphism, focal necroses, and infiltrating growth into the brain substance without the formation of a capsule, are to be regarded as the most common signs of malignancy.

Our three examples are meant to demonstrate that, in a small percentage of cases, the meningiomas, as primary benign tumors, may change their prognostic valuation towards a malignant degeneration. Although the time intervals between successive recurrences become progessively shorter, these tumors may not always fulfil all the criteria of a sarcomatous transformation. Conversely, tumors may occure which, from the beginning, show the characteristics of sarcomatous, aggressively growing forms, but still have a relatively long survival time.

References

1. CROMPTON, M. R., GAUTIER-SMITH, P. C.: The prediction of recurrence in meningiomas. J. Neurol. Neurosurg. Psychiat. 33, 80 - 87 (1970).

2. MORLEY, T. P.: Tumors of the cranial meninges. In: Neurological Surgery, Vol. III (ed. J. R. YOUMANS), pp. 1394 - 1396. Philadelphia - London - Toronto 1973.

3. RUSSELL, D. S., RUBINSTEIN, L. J.: Pathology of the Tumors of the Nervous System. London 1959.

4. SIMPSON, D.: The recurrence of intracranial meningiomas after surgical treatment. J. Neurol. Neurosurg. Psychiat. 20, 22 - 39 (1957).

5. TYTUS, J. S., LASERSOHN, J. T., REIFEL, E.: The problem of malignancy in meningiomas. J. Neurosurg. 22, 551 - 557 (1967).

6. ZÜLCH, K. J.: Biologie und Pathologie der Hirngeschwülste. In: Handbuch der Neurochirurgie, Bd. III (Hrsg. H. OLIVECRONA, W. TÖNNIS), S. 399 - 468. Berlin - Göttingen - Heidelberg: Springer 1956.

7. ZÜLCH, K. J.: Atlas of the Histology of Brain Tumors. Berlin - Heidelberg - New York: Springer 1971.

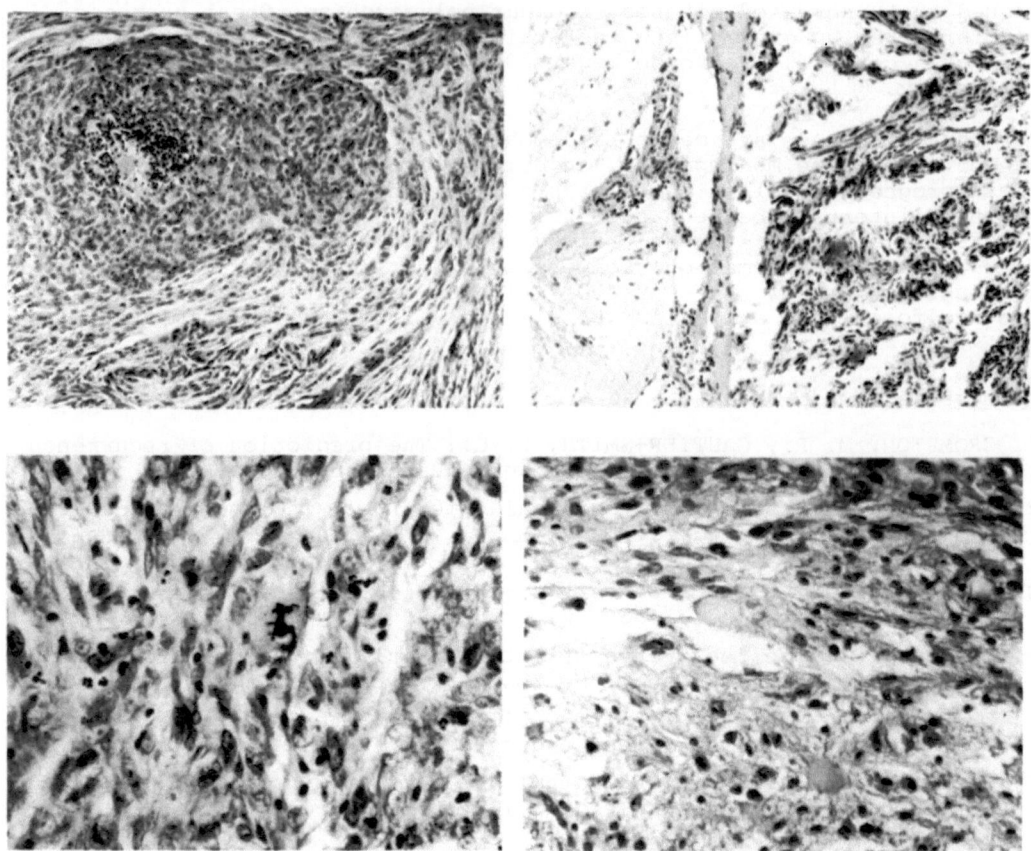

Fig. 1. Case 5, G. N. ♂, born 1906. E 3694/70. Upper left: Endotheliomatous and fibromatous meningioma with focal necrosis. Haematoxylin
and Eosin, x 140. Upper right: Capsule separating tumor (on right)
from brain substance. H + E, x 140. - E 4005/71, 1st relapse. Lower
left: Malignant transformation with polymorphism and atypical mitoses.
Cresylviolet, x 400. Lower right: Infiltrating tumor without capsule,
reactive gliosis in the brain substance (bottom half). H + E, x 360

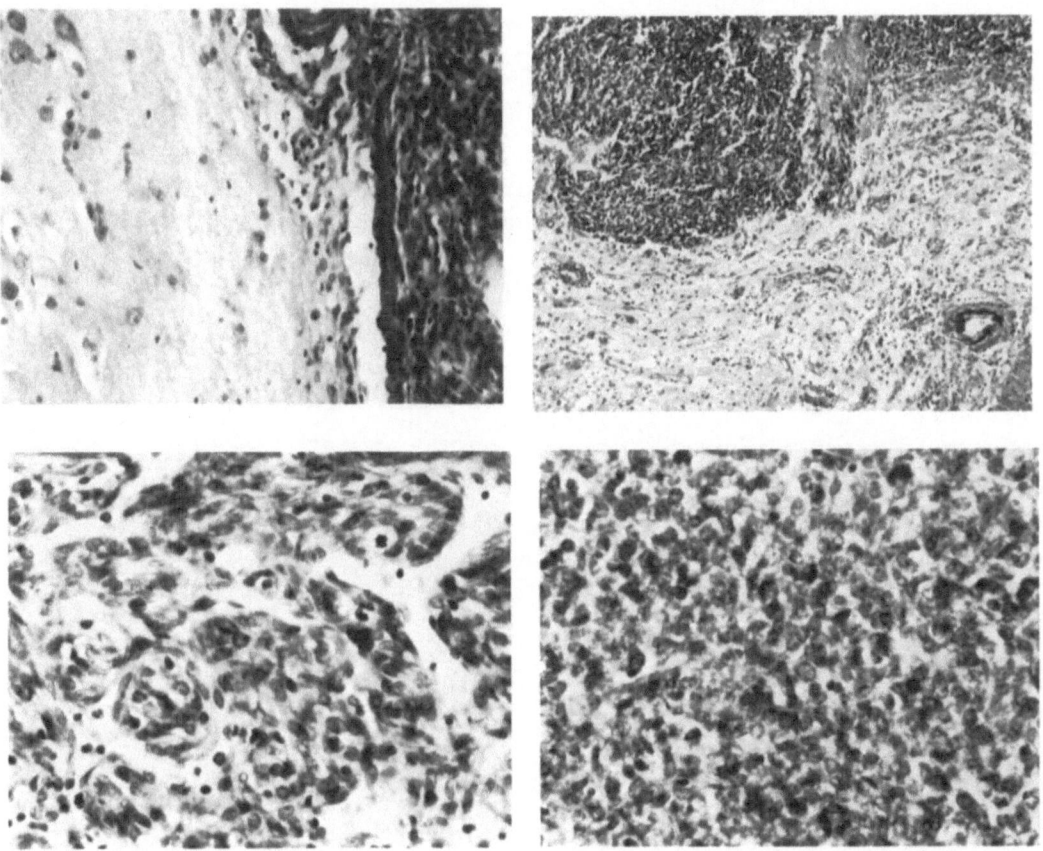

Fig. 2. Case 6, K. H. ♀, born 1900. Upper left: NK 5010/59. Capsule separating tumor from brain substance. Elastica-van Gieson, x 200. Upper right: E 2131/64. 1st relapse. Invasive growth into the brain substance. EvG, x 125. Lower left: NK 5010/59. Primary tumor, an angio-blastic meningioma with mitoses. EvG, x 500. Lower right: E 2131/64, 1st relapse. Increased cellularity in the recurrent tumor. EvG, x 500

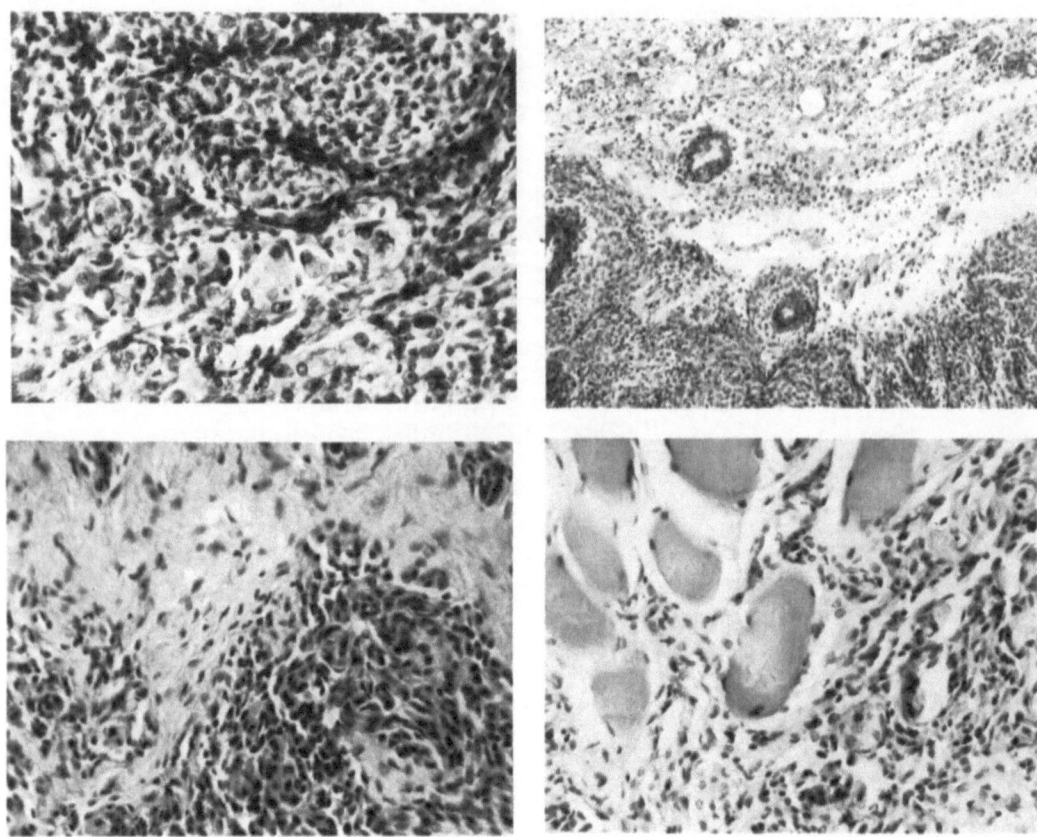

Fig. 3. Case 1, W. H. ♂, born 1916. E 2619/66. Upper left: Predominantly endotheliomatous meningioma with a polymorphous area (bottom half) in the 1st biopsy. H + E, x 310. Upper right: Invasive growth into the CNS with reactive gliosis. EvG, x 140. - E 3287/68, 1st relapse. Lower left: Invasive growth into the galea. H + E, x 310. Lower right: Infiltration of the temporal muscles. H + E, x 310

Mass Movements in Brain Tumors – Tissue Culture Investigation with Time Lapse Cinematography

G. KERSTING

During the past years experimental cancerology was enriched by such a number of new and interesting findings that the knowledge of tumor pathology and, especially, of brain tumor pathology has been greatly enlarged. The utilization of this knowledge, however, presents some difficulties due to the abundance of new informations. Although the fundamental reflections of ancient investigators seem to be extrapolated to more recent findings easily, the differences between the experimentally produced and the original human brain tumors are so evident that further conclusions are hardly possible. This emphasizes the need of further immediate information about human brain tumors. Tumor culture is well able to provide this information through comparative pathomorphological investigations.

Technique: The carefully removed tumor material is divided into four fragments. The first fragment is submitted to deep freezing in liquid nitrogen for enzymatic histochemical investigations. The second fragment is fixed for electron microscopy, the third is submitted to routine paraffin histology and the fourth is explanted in tissue culture. The new cell colonies are cultivated for some weeks - the time of cultivation depending on the aim of the experiment. During this period of cultivation, time lapse cinematographic recordings of living cultures, in phase contrast can be obtained, and cytological tests, immunological or virological studies, etc. can be performed. At the end of the cultivation period the in vitro formations of tumor cells can be compared with the initial tissue by staining one part of the cultures by means of the usual histological methods, while another undergoes enzymatic histochemical studies, and a third part is submitted to electron microscopy.

Our aim is to segregate tumor from the individuality of the bearer, and to give the proliferating tissues the opportunity to show, in vitro, their autochthonous capabilities in the absence of any organ bound influence. The disadvantage of the artificial milieu is more than compensated by the possibility of exact comparison of the various tumor tissues under the same standard conditions. The cell colonies newly formed in vitro show the characteristics of the tumor elements more clearly than they do in histological preparations. Thus they can be used in differential diagnosis. This unobjectionable way of diagnosis of the various brain tumors in vitro is the main premise of this investigation.

Questions can be posed to these cultures, which will be answered the more exactly the better they have been adapted to the in vitro circumstances. We have been able to demonstrate several typical examples: medulloblastoma, mixed gliomas of childhood, grading of astrocytomas, the problem of malignancy etc. At present we are concerned with another problem of the term of cultivation itself: the visibility of movements within the tumor cell colonies, and primarily the motion within cultures the proliferation of which has already come to an end. Only under these conditions can one be sure that the rate of cell motion is not influenced by cell growth, and that the direction of the cell movement is not influenced by the proliferation of the explant. It can be shown that under such "stationary" conditions the sum of many single motions results in a mass movement of whole cell formations.

Concerning the technique, it may be added that coverslip cultures grown in tubes are transferred to culture chambers which can be observed under a phase contrast microscope allowing time lapse cinematographic recordings. The optical conditions of the set-up are demonstrated.

The presented film shows the typical movements of astrocytoma, glioblastoma multiforme, meningioma, primary sarcoma of the brain, pituitary adenoma, carcinoma, as well as microglia and white blood cells. The 15 minutes of the film correspond to a real time of about three weeks.

The recorded movements of the mentioned tumor groups in vitro are distinctly different. In astrocytomas there are nearly motionless cell bodies with strong undulating membranes along and on top of the processes, true locomotion being observed only in macrophages and fibroblasts. In glioblastoma multiforme there is an extremely strong locomotion of the irregularly shaped cells with few undulating membranes and only slight movements of the nuclei within the cytoplasm. The cells wander to and fro through the culture chamber without signs of contact inhibition. In meningiomas, with strong movement of macrophages, only slight movements of tumor cells occur after days, resulting in a completely different organization of the monolayer without any cellular growth. Interesting are the rotating movements of the explanted whorls with the release of macrophages. In proliferating meningiomas there is slight rotation of nuclei previous to mitosis. Reticulosarcomas seem to be characterized by remarkable counter movements due to the proliferation of spindle shaped cells. The pituitary adenoma forms an epithelial monolayer with marked gliding movements in the zone of proliferation. Many rotations of resting nuclei as well as vertical rolling movements of nuclei are observed previous to mitosis. There is a marked contact inhibition. A permanently carcinomatous cell line differs from the mentioned brain tumors by lack of organization, no locomotion of the cells themselves, strong undulating membranes and pinocytosis. The movements of microglia differ from those of wandering leucocytes by only slight locomotion fixed to one point, by strong undulation of membranes and by many pseudopodes.

On the Course of the Disease of Intracranial Meningioma

H. KALM

In order to deal with my task of characterizing the course of intra-cranial meningiomas from the neurological point of view, I make refer-ence to the appropriate literature, to 55 observations of my own made from 1.10.1958 to 30.6.1974 in a total of about 20.000 in-patients and to 9 case histories of recurrent meningiomas, made available to me by Dr. Klug.

Every review of a large group of patients confirms (3, 4, 9, 17) that, as a rule, the usual age of a meningioma patient lies between 40 and 60 years (Fig. 1). If the age of the patient at the first symptom of a meningioma is correlated to the site of the tumor, no significant differences are found for the individual localizations. At most, it can be said that the meningiomas in the medial region of the wings of the sphenoid bone, and those at the tuberculum sellae, are more frequently discovered in younger patients, that is, between the ages of 30 and 40 years. All the reports in the literature emphasize the predominance of women at a ratio of 2 : 1 or 3 : 1. Basal meningiomas occur even considerably more frequently in women. In Dortmund and the surrounding areas (served by its hospitals), the meningioma seems to "favour" particularly women - of 55 patients 46 were women.

Site of the meningioma	women	men
Wing of the sphenoid bone	19	-
Orbits	3	-
Olfactory nerve	1	1
Cerebellopontine angle	1	-
Falx cerebri	4	2
Parasagittal region	11	5
Convexity	13	4
	52	12

The clinical syndrome and the course of the disease, on the other hand, are largely determined by the site of the meningioma. In con-sequence of their close physical proximity to the optic chiasm, the optic nerve and the orbits, the sphenoid bone meningioma, the menin-gioma of the roof of the orbit and the orbit, and also olfactory meningiomas, give rise to very similar clinical manifestations. The rare meningiomas at the exit openings of the basal cerebral nerves and the meningioma of the cerebellopontine angle are usually only solitary observations, such rarities as a meningioma in the internal auditory meatus also being known. The remaining meningiomas of the posterior cranial fossa, such as the meningioma of the tentorium, the meningioma of the convexity of the cerebellum, of the clivus and of the occipital foramen are also not frequently seen. The observations

in neurosurgical departments, made over a considerable period of time,
usually do not go beyond 10 cases. Initially, the meningiomas of the
posterior cranial fossa often present considerable difficulties in
the diagnosis. The initial, intermittent headaches, changes in personality and hydrocephalic crises without local symptoms usually lead
to a different diagnosis until a cerebellar ataxia, quadrigeminal
symptoms, functional "drop-outs" of cerebral nerves and signs of increased intracranial pressure reveal the situation of the process in
the posterior cranial fossa. It is my intention to report on the more
common processes and I shall, therefore, not concern myself with the
plexus meningioma or the multiple meningiomas including diffuse meningiomatosis.

Of 19 cases of *meningioma of the sphenoid bone*, all were women. The
duration of the disease, from the time of the first subjective disturbances to the surgical operation can be expressed in two frequent
periods - 1 to 4 months and 1 to 4 years. The longest duration of
disease in our observations was 26 years. Among the subjective symptoms, disturbances of vision, usually taking the form of a loss of
visual power and a reduction in the field of vision that can progress
to blindness, largely predominate. Only at a relatively late stage do
single-sided disturbances occur, only rarely are temporal lobe attacks
to be seen, and only occasionally does the patient complain of headaches or manifest a change of personality. At the time of admission
to the hospital, the patient almost always presents with disturbances
of vision, sometimes accompanied by single-sided disturbances and
cerebro-organic personality changes. An examination of the electrical
activity of the brain now usually reveals a focal lesion. In all meningiomas, the figures for protein in the cerebrospinal fluid are all
within the normal range, or are only slightly elevated, so that from
these findings an indication as to an intracranial process is only
rarely found. The highest value I have seen in this connection was a
figure of 107 mg % in the case of a large convexity meningioma; among
the sphenoid bone meningiomas, the figures all fall within the normal
range with the exception of two somewhat elevated figures of 63 and
69 mg %. In about 20 to 30 % of the cases, the sphenoid bone meningiomas revealed bony changes in the radiography (Fig. 2)[1] and thus, in
conjunction with the clinical symptoms, allow a diagnosis to be made
without any further measures being necessary. The reports of other
authors quote a higher rate of involvement of the bones of the skull.
On the site of the meningioma in the sphenoid bone, however, depends
the question as to whether the visual disturbances are associated
with an exophthalmus, or whether, with the primary site at the greater
wing of the sphenoid, a hyperostosis is already manifested by a bulging
in the temporal region (5, 10, 11, 13).

A particular diagnostic problem is presented by the meningiomas of the
anterior clinoid processes, which would better be termed medial sphenoid bone meningiomas. The disturbances of vision which, as a rule,
begin on one side and which manifest an uncharacteristic limitation
of the field of vision, initially caused the patient to consult an
ophthalmologist (14). The neurological examination brings no further
information, unless good X-ray pictures reveal a sclerosis. At the
beginning of the follow-up period, we have such diagnoses as neuritis
nervi optici or papillits, despite the fact that the age of the patient at the time of contracting the disease (about 50 years) should
give rise to grave doubts.

[1] I am indebted to Professor Fassbender, Director of the Radiological
Department of the Municipal Hospitals, Dortmund, who kindly lent me
the radiographs.

The occurrence of a neuritis nervi optici as the first sign of a disseminated encephalomyelitis at this age must be considered a great
rarity. Since, however, as already mentioned, the patients with meningiomas of the medial part of the wing of the sphenoid bone not infrequently contract the disease at an earlier age, the difficulties in
differential diagnosis can be resolved only by the follow-up observations of the patient. A further tip is that even a single-sided
neuritis nervi optici does not usually give rise to changes in the
cerebrospinal fluid. In our observations, the duration of the disease
is 18 months to 2 years. The diagnosis of a suprasellar spaceconsuming
process is unequivocally given by the angiographic and air-encephalo-
graphic findings. As far as early diagnosis is concerned, we cannot
expect any aid from cerebral scintigraphy since a tumor having the
size of only 2 to 3 grams and located at the base of the skull, is
hardly likely to be differentiated from the bones of the skull. In
our survey, the smallest sphenoid bone meningioma that was demonstrated scintigraphically and removed by surgical operation weighed 14
grams; of interest in this connection is the fact that we have employed this technique systematically since 1969.

The predominant symptoms in the case of meningioma of the orbit, which
often originates in the roof of the orbit, is exophthalmus. The patients consult the doctor only after a considerable delay, and then
often only because such symptoms as a feeling of pressure and pain
behind the eye is experienced. If, at the first examination, X-ray
studies do not reveal a thickening of the roof of the orbit, or of
the lesser wing of the sphenoid bone (Fig. 3), the diagnosis of endocrine exophthalmus or a unilateral ocular myositis suggests itself
and gives rise to appropriate therapeutic measures. The duration of
the process is usually three to six years, but can be as long as 20
years. In the case of an exophthalmus, the physician should not neglect
to carry out an examination of the family photo album. Relatives and
the patient himself often cannot indicate with accuracy the beginning
of exophthalmus and often relate its appearance to the first symptoms. A confirmed exophthalmus existing over a period of years does
not comply with the picture of endocrine exophthalmus. In the follow-
up period of observation, radiographic screening should not be neglected. An incipient thickening of the walls of the orbit must be
taken as a reason to consider the presence of a meningioma. This all
the more so since the future of the patient depends upon an operation
being carried out in good time. The size and the origin of the meningioma in the wall of the orbit can often be recognized in carotid
angiography and in the filling of the orbital veins.

It probably depends upon the "site of attachment" of the socalled
meningioma of the olfactory nerve as to whether the sense of smell
disappears first or whether disturbances of vision are initially re-
marked. The fact that a disturbance in the sense of smell occasions
relatively little subjective significance makes it possible for a
meningioma of the olfactory nerve to develop to a considerable size
before "falling into the hands" of the neurosurgeon. Unfortunately,
with increasing size of the meningioma, the risk of surgery also increases, together with the extent of the persisting frontal lobe syndrome. Here, too, one can often obtain an indication in the X-ray
picture of the skull, with atrophy of the sella, decalcification of
the crista galli, hyperostosis or atrophy of the roof of the orbit (7).

In the case of *convexity meningiomas*, the cerebro-organic focal
and generalized epileptic attacks, often with post-convulsive, re-
mitting hemiparesis, are the first clinical signs until, finally, in
the course of 1 to 4 years, a progressive hemiparesis develops. It

is frequently the motor or sensory focal disturbances that cause the
patient to consult a doctor for a thorough clinical examination, before the occurrence of a hemiparesis. In one to two-thirds of all
cases, the radiographic picture of the skull reveals atrophy of the
bones, dilated vessel canals, hyperostosis or bulging of the skull
as a result of tumor infiltrations (15) (Fig. 4). Almost always, the
record of the electrical waves produced by the brain (EEG) indicate a
local lesion or slow waves, or intermediate waves, predominately on
one side. On the size of the tumor depend such general signs of increased intracranial pressure as papilloedema and cerebro-organic
personality changes accompanied by loss of concentration, difficulty
in remembering things, and a fall-off in the critical faculty. We
have never seen a meningioma that did not manifest itself in the scintigram of the brain. The smallest convexity meningioma did, admittedly, weigh only 25 grams. In cases of doubt, the technique of subtraction can clarify the question as to the presence of a blood supply
via external vessels and reveal the site of the tumor (Fig. 5).

In three patients, hemiparesis had developed during the course of 4
to 12 months. After the removal of the meningioma, the paralysis improved, as did the psychic changes. A recurrence revealed itself by
the augmentation of the hemiparesis after an interval of several
years (2 to 8 years). In every case, the personality changes increased
with every sign of a renewed elevation of the intracranial pressure.

The meningioma involving the falx cerebri, with its clinical course
of 6 months to 6 years, initially gives rise to headaches and loss of
concentration. There follow focal disturbances and progressive hemiparesis. On admission to hospital, the patient often presents a papilloedema, and unilateral disturbances associated, in almost all cases,
with signs of a focal lesion in the electroencephalogram.

In cases of *parasagittal meningioma*, the majority of patients are
usually clinically diagnosed after a duration of the disease of 1 to
2 years. They complain of headaches and are subject to focal disturbances, frequently limited to the leg, followed by permanent pareses,
predominantly leg-orientated; or a flaccid cortical extensor paralysis
of the foot develops which is not infrequently misdiagnosed as a peroneal paralysis, with the result that even a laminectomy might be
performed to "improve" the condition. It goes without saying that the
decisive point is the establishment of the correct findings and for
this purpose, electric stimulating equipment is indispensable. If
the parasagittal meningioma has already reached the space-consuming
stage, papillary changes, usually in the form of papilloedema, are
found when the patient is admitted to hospital. The main clinical
symptom is hemiparesis, with the leg being predominantly affected.
The focal findings in the electroencephalogram pattern and in the
scintigram of the brain pinpoint the site of the space-consuming process. Again, in 20 % of the cases the parasagittal meningiomas reveal
themselves by calcifications, even in the plain X-ray (Fig. 6), while
we all know how difficult it is to recognize the parasagittal space-
consuming process from the course of the A. cerebri anterior in a. p.
projection. If it were not for the support provided by the airence-
phalographic findings, and the brain scan, we would more frequently be in danger of misinterpreting the space-consuming process as a
disturbance in cerebral blood flow, especially in view of the fact
that, not infrequently, marked improvements of a hemiparesis can be
observed under the clinical therapy. The parasagittal meningioma, however, due to its relationship to the sagittal sinus, has a strong
tendency to recur. Dr. Klug has kindly allowed me to study the case
histories of 6 of his patients. In each of 2 patients, 2 operations

for the removal of recurrent tumors had to be carried out at intervals of 7 and 3 months and 2 1/2 and 1 1/2 years, while in single repeat operation for recurrences, intervals of 10, 7 and even 16 years were observed. The symptoms for recurrent meningiomas were the renewed occurrence of focal, rarely generalized, disturbances, or a gradually worsening hemiparesis (unilateral paralysis).

If we compare the meningiomas on the basis of the early symptoms, and if we classify the tumors into the three groups

meningiomas of the anterior cranial fossa and the sphenoid
meningiomas of the posterior cranial fossa and
meningiomas of the falx cerebri, the parasagittal region and the convexity as supratentorial tumors

we find that the initial pathological signs for the first group comprise unilateral disturbances and exophthalmus, for the second group hydrocephalic, and for the third group headaches, focal or generalized epileptic attacks with temporary hemiparesis. The generally slow growth of the tumors may result in the absence of severe headaches, with the exception of the tumors in the posterior cranial fossa. For all meningiomas, it can be said that the patient presents with localized symptoms and also complains of a loss of efficiency, a reduction in drive, a reduction in his contact to his environment, and that the amount of work that he could previously get through in a day is now impossible to manage. Of course, such complaints associated with headaches are frequently heard from 50 to 60-year-olds and it is only in a relatively small number of patients that the cause is to be found to be an intracranial meningioma. How is it possible to secure an early diagnosis? The thorough establishment of the case history and dealing earnestly with the symptoms most quickly reveals a decrease in vitality. At this stage, however, the physician has the duty to make a radiographic examination of the skull, and, if necessary, to repeat it, to investigate the bony changes mentioned, further, not to neglect an electroencephalographic examination and to effect scintigraphy, under certain circumstances, repeatedly. It is not known how much time a meningioma requires at the various locations to grow to a point where it gives rise to clinical symptoms. Perhaps we are justified in assuming, on average, a period of 1 to 3 years, since, in general, this period of time usually passes from the first evaluable clinical symptom until the surgical intervention. All in all, this is a period of time in which the question as to the organic cause, even of uncharacteristic disturbances in the patient's well-being - which might also stem from an intracranial meningioma - must repeatedly be asked.

Summary

In a review, the clinical symptomatology and the course of the disease of supratentorial meningiomas, the meningiomas of the posterior cranial fossa and of the base of the skull, are characterized with reference to 64 observations made by the author. With an average duration of the disease of 1 - 3 years, predominant involvement of the female sex and a "recognition age" of, as a rule, between 40 and 60, the main clinical symptom for the meningiomas of the posterior cranial fossa are hydrocephalic headaches, for the meningiomas of the base of the skull visual disturbances and exophthalmus, while the supratentorial meningiomas indicate their presence by focal or generalized attacks of convulsions with or without previous unilateral paralyses. For the early diagnosis of the condition, a consideration of changes in the bones of the skull is of importance.

REFERENCES

1. ALLEGRE, G., GOUTELLE, A., DECHAUME, I. P., DERUTY, R., RAVON, R.: Les méningeomes du bord libre de la tente. Neurochirurgie, Paris 16, 656 - 575 (1970).

2. CARTERI, H., NORI, H.: Meningiomata. Riv. Anat. Path. 22, 726 - 735 (1962).

3. COLLOMB, H., GIRARD, P. L., DUMAS, M. et al.: Méningeomes intracraniens (35 cas chez le noir senegalais). Bull. Soc. med. afr. noir lang. franc. 16, 534 - 541 (1971).

4. CUSHING, H., EISENHARDT, L. E.: Meningiomas. Thomas 1938.

5. EHLERS, N., MALMROS, R.: The suprasellar meningioma. A review of the literature and presentation of a series of 31 cases. Acta ophthal. (Kbh) supl. 121, 74.

6. ESSBACH, H.: Die Meningeome. Ergebn. d. allgem. Path. und path. Anat. 36 (1943).

7. FRIEDEMANN, G.: Zum röntgenologischen Nachweis der Olfactoriusmeningeome im Übersichtsbild. Zbl. Neurochirurgie 18, 206 - 211 (1958).

8. KAJIKAWA, H., IKEDA, I., ISHIKAWA, S.: A retrospective analysis of plain skull films and angiograms in 50 cases of supratentorial Meningeomas. Brain Nerve (Tokyo) 25, 693 - 698 (1973).

9. KENDALL, B., SHAH, S.: Investigations of meningiomas of cerebellar convexities. Neuroradiology, 162 - 176 (1972).

10. KUNFT, H. P., BINGAS, B., VOGT, U.: Die Meningeome der Keilbeinflügel. Zbl. Neurochirurgie 24, 171 - 188 (1964).

11. LINDGREN, E.: Röntgenologie. Hb. der Neurochirurgie Bd. 2, 51 - 62 (1954).

12. SCHÜRMANN, K.: Neurochirurgische Aufgaben in der Orbita. Arch. Oto-Rhino-Laryng. 207, 253 - 282 (1974).

13. STENDER, A.: Über das Meningeom des Keilbeinrückens. Z. ges. Neurol. u. Psych. 147, 244 - 262 (1933).

14. SYNOWITZ, H. I., SIEDSCHLAG, W. D., FELDMANN, H.: Zur Diagnosestellung von Meningeomen mit primären Augensymptomen. Dtsch. Ges. wesen 27, 1519 . 1521 (1972).

15. SZAROMA, H.: Meningeomas in plain radiograms of the skull. Neurol. Neurochirurg. Pol. 23, 571 - 574 (1973).

16. TÖNNIS, W., SCHÜRMANN, K.: Meningeome der Keilbeinflügel. Zbl. Neurochirurg. 11, 1 - 13 (1951).

17. ZÜLCH, K. J.: Die Hirngeschwülste. Leipzig: J. Ambrosius Barth 1951.

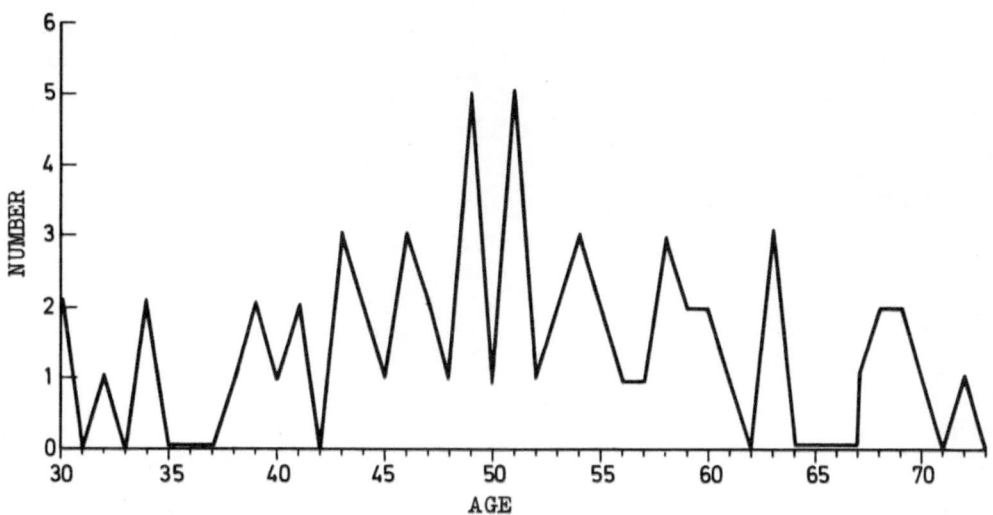

Fig. 1

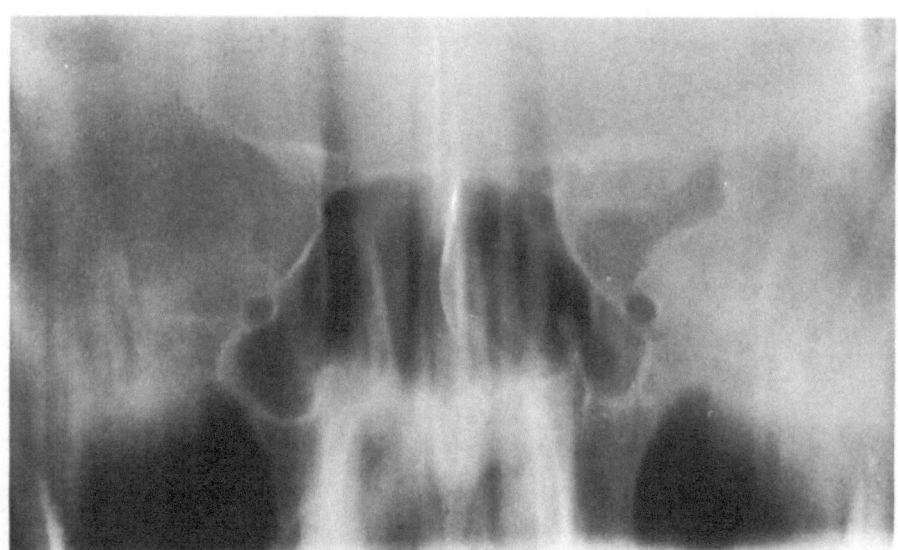

Fig. 2. Hyperostosis of the left lesser sphenoid wing

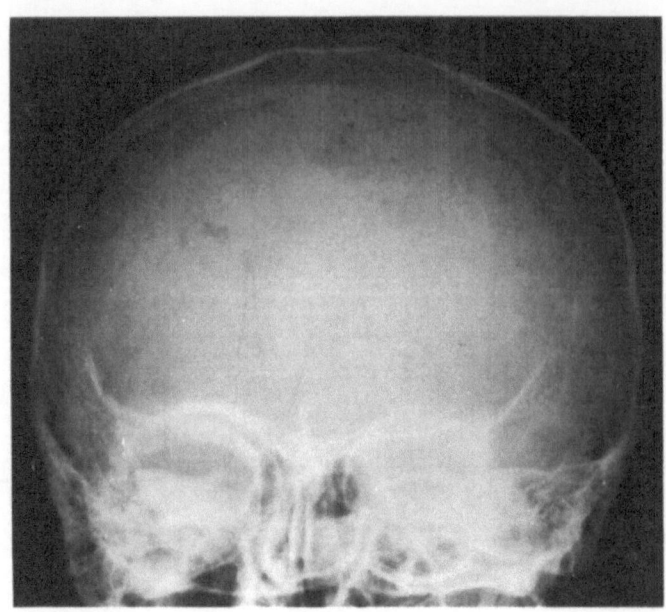

Fig. 3.
Hyperotosis of the
right orbit-roof

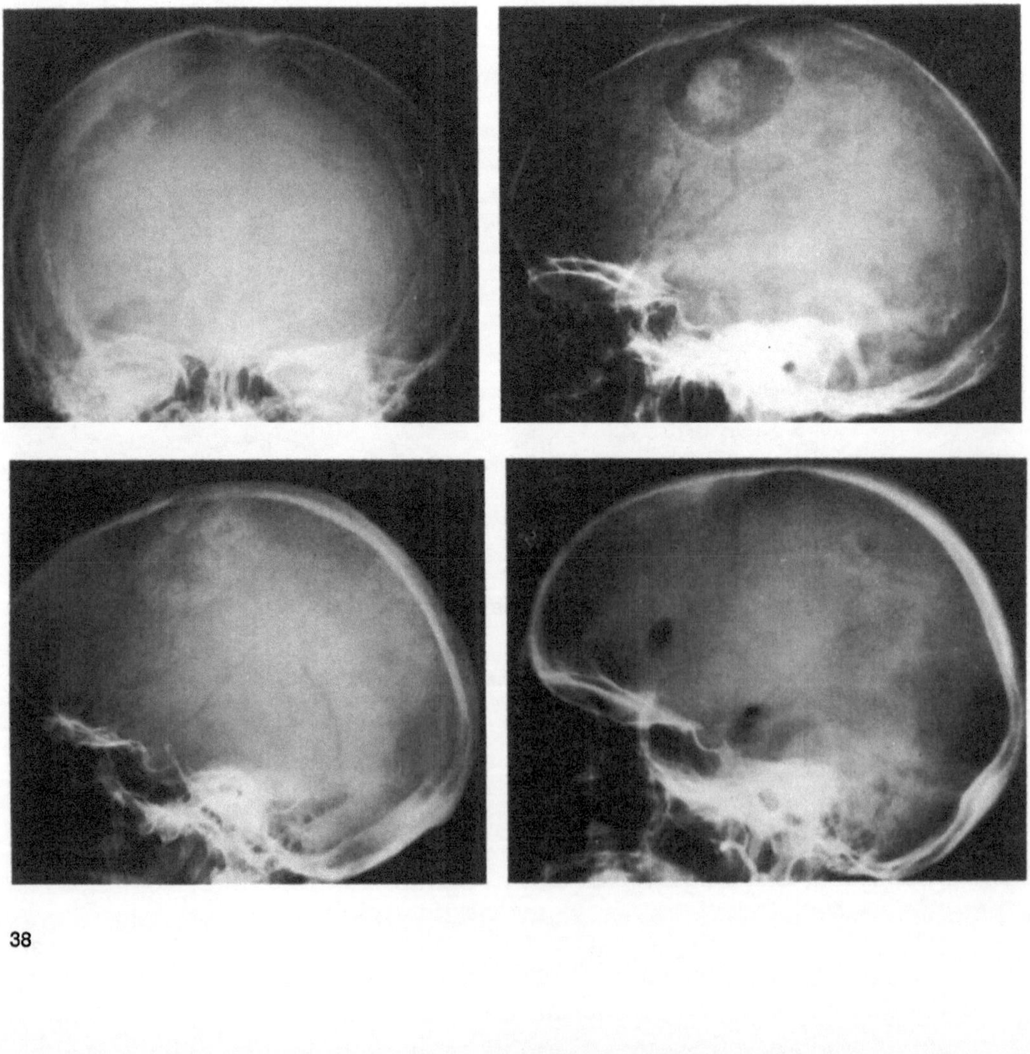

Fig. 4.
Hyperostosis in
convexity
meningiomas

▽

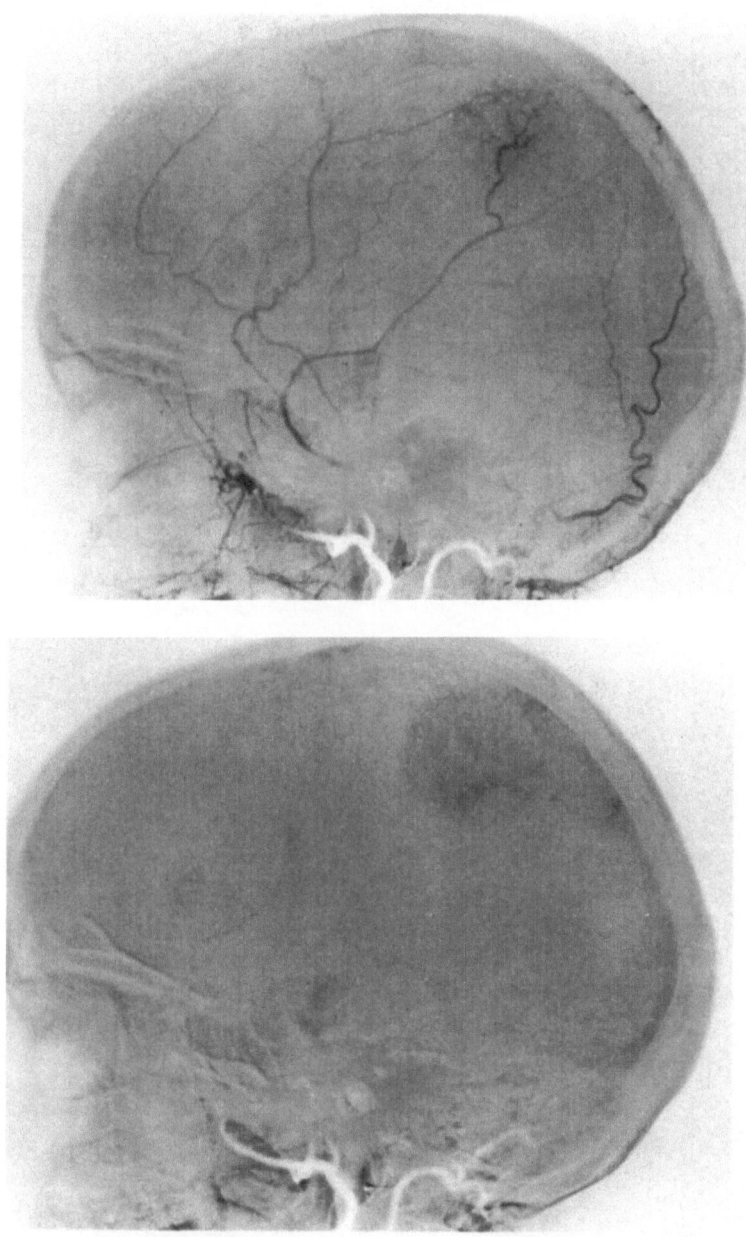

Fig. 5. Subtraction picture of a convexity meningioma

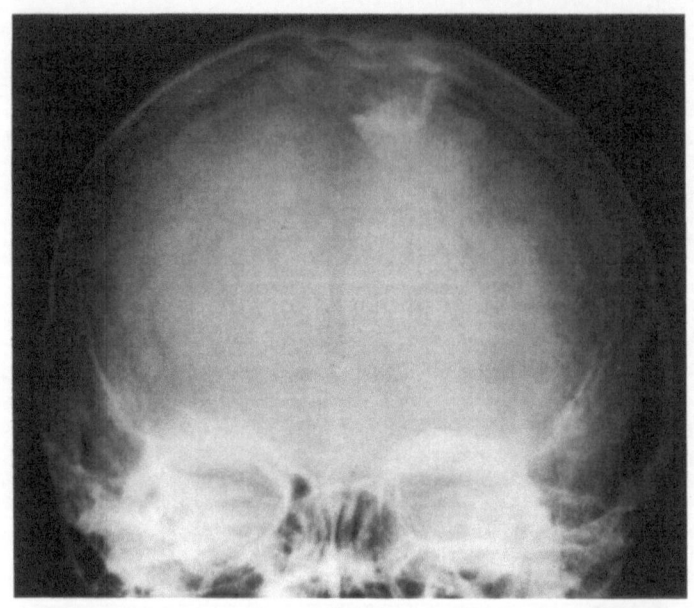

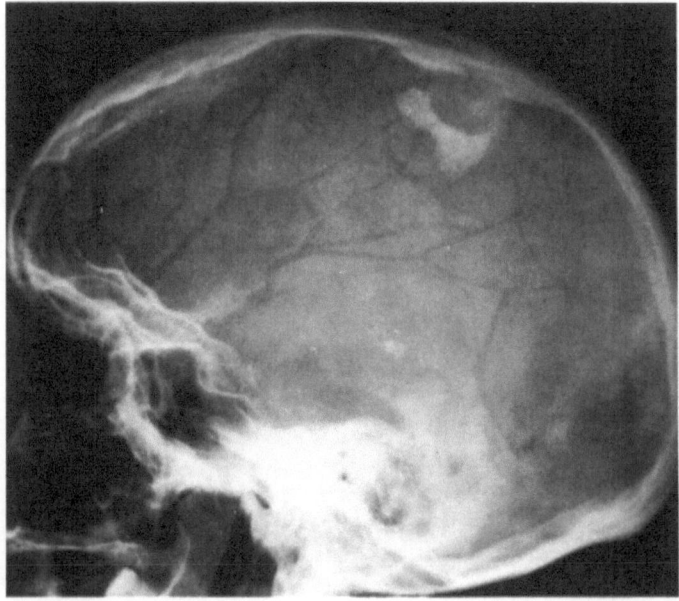

Fig. 6. Calcification of a parasagittal meningioma

The Clinical Picture of the Meningiomas from the Neurosurgical Viewpoint

W. KLUG

Exactly 120 years ago, i. e. in the year 1854, the publishing house of H. Laupp, Tübingen, brought out the HANDBUCH DER PRAKTISCHEN CHIRURGIE FÜR ÄRZTE UND WUNDÄRZTE by Victor Bruns, which included the part dealing with DIE CHIRURGISCHEN KRANKHEITEN UND VERLETZUNGEN DES GEHIRNS UND SEINER UMHÜLLUNGEN. On page 616 is found the following sentence: "Viel seltener entstehen Krebse primär in der harten Hirnhaut, und zwar dann gewöhnlich in Form von discreten rundlichen Geschwülsten, sowohl an dem das Schädelgewölbe, als an dem die Schädelbasis überziehenden Theile der harten Hirnhaut, zuweilen in mehrfacher nur ausnahmsweise noch gleichzeitig neben Krebsgeschwülsten in anderen entfernten Körpertheilen." ("Cancers arise only very rarely in the dura mater and when they do, then only in the form of discrete rounded tumors, both in the parts of the dura covering the vault and in the parts covering the base of the skull. Occasionally, they arise in groups simultaneously at various points of the dura, but only exceptionally simultaneously with cancerous tumors in other, distant parts of the body."). He then proceeds to describe an observation made by the French anatomist friend of Dupuytren and personal physician of Talleyrand, JEAN C CRUVEILHIER, and taken from his book "ANATOMIE PATHOLOGIQUE DU CORPS HUMAIN", which undoubtedly represents a parasagittal meningioma. This illustration was likewise reproduced by VICTOR BRUNS, 1854, on the plates in his work, and will be found on the two inside pages of our Programme.

Thus we have already arrived at the central topic of today: The most benign and possibly most rewarding cerebral tumor in terms of operation and prognosis, on the one hand, and the one that makes the utmost demands on the surgeon, on the other, if, for technical reasons, we are unable to remove it completely or, if we can, we nevertheless lose the battle postoperatively. On the one hand we have the clinically verified benignancy, on the other the recognition of the limits of our skill and ability. The provision of separate neuro-radiological departments which are capable of yielding a considerable amount of diagnostic information, is becoming increasingly important. The increasing use of the microscope also constitutes an enrichment and improvement in surgical possibilities. These two factors signify a great advance, but no breakthrough, so that we cannot be satisfied with them alone.

Consequently, this topic was deliberately included in the Congress programme. Only the multiplicity of individual experiences gained with a large number of patients can be a determining and orienting principle for us all. Each one of us will have a definite opinion of himself and of his abilities, but this will always be subjective in character, and might well be judged otherwise by others.

Who is not aware of the difficulty that can arise with suprasellar processes or olfactory meningiomas if the branches of the anterior cerebral artery and the optic nerve have become enclosed by the tumor or the hypothalamic region has become involved; who is not aware of the risks that attend the operation of large, basally localized, lateral sphenoidal bone tumors with their parts that creep along the base and which have grown round both the internal carotid artery and its branches, and is virtually obscuring even the oculomotor nerve.

Everyone of us can tell of the difficulties which are caused us to a high degree by the meningiomas localized in the centre of the tentorium. In such a case the problems frequently begin with the decision as to the most expedient approach. The same applies to the tumors of the posterior cranial fossa area, and last but not least: which of us does not know the feeling of uneasiness when we are confronted with a parasagittal meningioma of the medial or posterior third part of the sinus with an extensive point of attachment in the sinus cross-section? Even the partial blocking of the longitudinal sinus lumen cannot always be clarified from the outset by sinography.

All these problems that occupy our thoughts in connection with the meningioma operation are scheduled to be outlined today, and it is hoped that the relevant questions will be answered. What one of us does not know can perhaps be explained by another. It is my opinion that at a Congress of experts it is better to examine the difficulties and problems that each of us has, in the scientific session, and if possible to clarify them, than to wait until evening to discuss them in small groups in a quasi-confidential manner. Each one of us can report on a series of successes - but also - on failures. With the dramatic increase in the perfection of diagnostic methods and the introduction of magnification and other improved techniques for surgery, pathological processes are now being tackled which, a few decades ago, had no chance of being ameliorated or cured. But at the same time the risks have also increased considerably.

Processes which we operate today are, in terms of nature, localisation and size, the same as 20 or 30 years ago. The difference, however, is the fact that many of the patients can now be saved who would have died then. That must be made clear to those who hold responsible positions in the field of reporting. In every case a surgical operation is an intervention which is attended by a small, moderately large or very great risk. No human being can be compared with another. Age, constitution, sex, weather influences, emotional state, and above all the relationship with the doctor treating the patient are the factors that determine to a large extent the prospects of success of any therapy.

Let us be grateful for the possibilities which experience and technology now offer us in the treatment of diseases that were formerly fatal. Let us make every effort to ensure that new advances in combination with improved technical methods will positively influence our performance. But let us also hope that we, and our critics, will try to gain and retain the confidence of our patients. It is only on this sound basis that we can conduct serious and heroic operations, which up to a few years ago were still in the realms of phantasy.

But let us return now to the topic under review.

Our special problems, the meningiomas, I have just mentioned. They are characterized by their localization and size. Up till now the questions dealing with the pre-operative phase have also remained unanswered. For instance, that of early detection.

We all know patients who, without any long case history, and with only transient neurological disturbances or impairments, quite suddenly
develop pareses, paroxysms, disturbances of speech, functional impairments of the cerebral nerves etc. We know that the person thus affected can change within the shortest period of time from a person doing
a full job of work to a helpless wreck. The diagnosis may reveal a
huge, space-occupying process which would seem to refute the previous
history with its paucity of symptoms. Or, perhaps, we find that arteriography, encephalography or scintigraphy hardly yield an indication or only a vague suspicion of a space-occupying process; we operate notwithstanding and find ourselves faced with a parasagittal meningioma, whose great or minute size, as the case may be, causes us
embarrassment. Has anything gone wrong here? Did the patient perhaps
withold important particulars about his case history, did the doctor
fail in his detailed questioning at the examination, were our diagnostic methods inadequate, or are all these possibilities involved?
We are acquainted with the insidiousness of parasagittal meningiomas
with their, in part, complete immobilization of the anterior cerebral
nerve, or with the minimal depression of the ventricular roof when
the cerebral ventricles are filled with air, and with the sometimes
scarcely encouraging findings of scintigraphy. We know about the difficulty that the ophthalmologist has when trying to differentiate between neuritis of the optic nerve and the effects of an olfactory meningioma. But we also know of the problems of the patients and their
relatives: the man who tells nothing but jokes or phantastical sto-
ries for the pleasure of the children he is looking after, his fellow-
workers who construe his behaviour as a personal idiosyncrasy, the
wife who thinks her husband has developed a jocular of facetious turn
of mind. But we are all aware of how uncritical those husbands are
whose wives, in contrast to former years, suddenly become listless
and lazy, spend half the day in bed, and finally set before them a
dish of rotten meat already redolent of carrion, this latter fact at
least causing them to become mobilized and active. It just happens to
be a fact that meningiomas have a certain "haut gout".

We have all encountered those cases, too, in which the increasing paresis of a foot or leg has led us up the garden path - to a suspicion
of spinal involvement. And, ladies and gentlemen, has not each of us
experienced how prejudiced we ourselves have been by the diagnosis
produced by the patient on admission or by the knowledge of previous-
ly-employed therapies or diagnoses in the case of a so-called genuine
epilepsy or M. S. How many false interpretations are due to this false
stamp! Might it not be possible, when there is a suspicion of an intracranial space-occupying process, for the points that lead the way to
the neuro-surgeon to be set earlier? The latter is practically never
the first medical man to treat the case. The referral is usually to
the internist or the neurologist. In other cases it is the ear, nose
and throat specialist. But even then, when the patient has finally
landed at our address, and when all tests have proved negative, one
should have reservations about stating that the patient is completely
organically sound as regards the brain.

It is my conviction that it is better initially not to make any diagnosis at all rather than a wrong "good" prognosis, and thus to induce
in the patient and his family doctor a feeling of security. Follow-up
tests should be repeated wherever there is the slightest suspicion,
thus permitting not only a cross-section but also a longitudinal section.

From the patient himself less will be frequently learnt than from his
relatives who are not questioned in his presence. This refers in par-

ticular to character changes, shortcomings in the household, and sexual disorders, but, does not exhaust our pre-operative questioning. The necessary preparation in the ward or even in the Intensive Care Unit is of major importance in cases of metabolic disturbances, imbalance in the water equilibrium, in the electrolytes, and their regulation by means of suitable measures prior to the operation. With regard to the operation itself, the surgeon will apply his own specific techniques, whenever he can look back on years of neurosurgical activity.

Nevertheless, the microscope should play a permanent and integral part. This reduction of blood pressure during the operation to vital values, the careful monitoring by the anaesthetist, the speed and care on the part of the surgeon, are essential preconditions. To conduct a replacement of the medial or posterior parts of the sinus, possibly by carrying out plastic surgery here, or perhaps by compelling the tumor to react in such a way that the longitudinal sinus becomes blocked with a view to enabling the now obliterated sinus to be resected in a subsequent operation - all these are matters that are up for discussion.

Every operating surgeon knows when there was a particularly difficult problem during the operation. Consequently, he will, if necessary, be able to react accordingly later. Everyone has also experienced operations, however, which, technically, have been unreservedly perfect, but which, despite good urinary output, react suddenly and with unexpected severity with a cerebral swelling. This supervision lies essentially in the hands of anaesthetist. And it is largely with him that questions of the postoperative treatment should be discussed. A more individual agreement and co-ordination, not only amongst the members of the surgical team, but also with respect to the juvenile or elderly, the male or female patient, appears to me to appropriate here. Priority thinking should rank far behind the joint talks that are meaningful for the patient.

And now let me make just one more point. There are very many examples on hand to show that coming face to face daily with seriously ill and very seriously ill patients not only has the effect of blunting the edge of humaness but may also become routine. We should not forget that the unconscious patient is also a human being, and that he, having regained consciousness, takes note of everything: his environment as well as the persons tending to him. His human dignity should be preserved also in death. It was for this reason that one of our nurses who had been on active service for many years in the I. C. U. was awarded the Federal Order of Merit, because she, in addition to her nursing skills, never forgot that the sick patient and the relatives were also human beings anxious about his health. In other words, over and beyond the purely factual and technical questions there are also those of interpersonal relationships. With this observation allow me to conclude this paper.

Eleven Cases of Multiple Meningiomas

W. ISCHEBECK, A. CASTRO, and I. KUSKE

Between the years 1948 and 1974 a total of 714 meningiomas were operated on at the Neurosurgical Clinics in Bochum-Langendreer and Düsseldorf. Among these 11, i. e. 1.5 %, were multiple meningiomas. Two
cases of multiple meningiomas associated with RECKLINGHAUSEN's disease
and one case with a metastizing meningioma is not included in this
case report.

A few characteristics of the individual cases are given below:

Cases 1 - 3

In one case three left frontoparietal convexity-meningiomas (125 g
and 2 x 25 g) were found; in another case two left parietal convexity
meningiomas (100 g and 25 g) were operated on and in a further case
an olfactory-meningioma as well as a completely separate falx-meningioma occured.

These three cases had the following in common: no recurrence, simultaneous development, histological structure of a fibromatous meningioma without signs of malignancy and the fact that all three patients
were female.

Case 4

This patient was initially operated on for a bilateral falx-meningioma
of the frontal sinus. Six years later when operated on because of a
recurrence, four tumors the largest of which had the size of an egg and
likewise situated in the fronto-parietal area were removed and showed
no signs of malignancy. We think that this case can be compared to the
first three cases in so far as the other tumors must have already existed at the time of the first operation.

Case 5

In this case a large left-sided meningioma of the sphenoid ridge was
operated on. Nine months later the patient died of severe pneumonia
and necropsy showed an additional meningioma of the cerebello-pontine
angle on the same side.

Cases 6 and 7

Of these two patients one was operated on four times within 14 years,
the other seven times within 9 years. In each case an increased number
of mitosis and an infiltrating growth were already found during the
first operation. It was not until the last operation that multiple
meningiomas became apparent. Both patients died very soon thereafter.

Case 8

The association between multiple meningiomas and RECKLINGHAUSEN's disease has often been stressed in literature. The following case of a female patient must be considered in this context. Initially a large olfactory-meningioma and many smaller meningiomas attached to the dura were removed. At the same time a single neurofibroma of the scalp was extirpated. Four years later a neurinoma appeared in the supraclavicular fossa. After another six years several meningiomas were removed from the left parieto-occipital region. No signs of neurofibromatosis have been found as yet.

Case 9

A 47-year-old female patient had a neurinoma of the cerebello-pontine angle removed. Seven years later cancer of the cervix was treated. Already at this time a right parieto-occipital metastasis was suspected. Extensive examination revealed no further signs of metastasis in other organs. Therefore craniotomy was performed. Surprisingly, three fibromatous meningiomas could be removed.

Case 10

A left parasagittal meningioma was removed in 1969 from a 60-year-old female patient. Except for a slight hemiparesis right-sided, the postoperative condition was satisfactory.

In 1973 we saw the patient again: four months previously Jacksonian fits had appeared. All subsequent examinations proved that there was no intracranial recurrence. The patient showed signs of a slowly-developing paraparesis of the legs. Some time previously an artificial left hip-joint had been implatend. The fact that this artificial joint was not functioning optimally, caused a short delay of the diagnosis of a thoracal intraspinal meningioma (T - 5). The tumor had no dural connection. Both the intracranial and the intraspinal tumors were of the arachnothelial type.

Case 11

In this case multiple meningiomas on the dura of the cerebellum had to be removed twice with an interval of nine years. One year after the last operation paraplegia developed accompanied by hypaesthesia below T 10. Further diagnostic and therapeutic interventions were not taken into consideration because the patient was older than 70 and in a bad condition. We can only presume with reserve that an intraspinal growth had developed.

We think that all these cases fulfil the conditions of multiple meningiomas of CUSHING and EISENHARDT. The causes for the development of mulitple meningiomas are not known yet. Independently of the relation between multiple meningiomas and RECKLINGHAUSEN's disease, we think that a systemic disease must be taken into consideration as a cause.

The two last cases bring about the discussion of whether surgery can be the cause of dissemination along the CSF pathways or through the blood stream (2, 3, 4, 5). It remains to be mentioned that nine of our patients were female and two were male; their age varied between 29 and 70 years.

Summary

Eleven cases of multiple meningiomas are reported. Among these there
are four cases of simultaneously occuring fibromatous meningiomas,
two cases of intracranial meningiomas with intraspinal dissemination,
two others with signs of malignancy, two cases presenting multiple
meningiomas and neurinomas, and one case with a meningioma of the
sphenoid ridge associated with a meningioma of the cerebello-pontile
angle. Attention is drawn to the problematic interpretation of the
causes of multiple meningiomas.

REFERENCES

1. CUSHING, H., EISENHARDT, L.: Meningiomas, their classification,
   regional behaviour, live history, and surgical end results.
   Springfield/Ill.: C. C. Thomas 1938.

2. HOFFMANN, G. T., EARLE, K. M.: Meningioma with malignant transformation and implantation in the subarachnoid space $\underline{17}$, 486 - 492
   (1960).

3. WAGA, S., MATSUDA, M., HANDA, H., MATSUSHIMA, M., ANDO, K.:
   Multiple meningiomas, report of four cases. J. Neurosurg. $\underline{37}$, 348 -
   351 (1972).

4. ZERVAS, N. T., SHINTANI, A., KALLAR, B., BERRY, R. G.: J. Neurosurg. $\underline{33}$, 216 - 220 (1970).

5. ZÜLCH, K. J.: Handbuch der Neurochirurgie, pathologische Anatomie
   der raumbeengenden intrakraniellen Prozesse. Berlin - Göttingen -
   Heidelberg: Springer 1956.

Multiple Meningiomas

H. ABTAHI

Multiple meningiomas aroused particular interest because of their not uniform etiology and for the diagnostic and therapeutic difficulties they are presenting. Their incidence is reported to be approximately 2 per cent of all meningiomas. In our series of 351 intracranial meningiomas multiple tumors were found in 12 cases i. e. in 3,4 per cent.

Three groups of cases could be distinguished:

1st group: comprises 5 patients in whom tumors were located close one to another. Three patients out of this group had only 2 tumors.

2nd group: includes 3 patients with multiple meningiomas combined with bilateral acoustic neurinomas and peripheral neurofibromas.

3rd group: comprises 4 patients in whom multiple meningiomas were found during the second or third operation for recurrence. Apart from the recurrence of original growth, multiple tumor nodules attached to the recurrent tumor or quite separate from it were found. Although their growth rate was different, the histological picture remained the same.

A typical example of a case belonging to the 3rd group is a 53 years old female in whom a right occipital meningioma of the falx was removed 13 years ago. 11 years later a local recurrence was removed, tumor attachment to the falx excised and coagulated. 6 months later the patient had to be operated on for the third time for a left sided occipital meningioma, attached to the wall of the sinus. Apart from that, another meningioma, attached to tentorium was found. 2 years later 3 more small meningiomas on the right side, located more ventrally, and separated from bed of the original tumor by a sheet of uninvaded lyophilised dura, which had been inserted during one of the previous operations, had to be removed.

Whereas the occurence of multiple meningiomas with and without neurofibromatosis (group 1 and 2) could be regarded as a sign of a systemic process, the development of multiple tumors following surgery, apart from being influenced by general predisposition, must be also dependent upon local factors modified by the operation, leading possibly to small metastases in the vicinity of the original tumor.

Larger meningiomas can be easily diagnosed by angiography and scintigraphy. Smaller ones remain often undetected preoperatively.

In a 35 years old patient (group 1) with spastic paraparesis and caudal cranial nerves involvement, angiography (Fig. 1) revealed bilateral falx meningiomas attached to the middle part of sagital sinus and bilateral tumors in the posterior fossa. The latter were, not as expected, neurinomas, but 3 separate small meningiomas.

A 19 years old patient (group 2) had 2 meningiomas involving the calvarium, bilateral acoustic neurinomas and probably a calcified intraventricular meningioma (Fig. 2). Operative mortality and morbidity are now improved due to better operative technique, magnification and bipolar coagulation. 12 patients of our series underwent a total of 22 operations for 62 tumors (including local recurrence in patients of group 3). 2 patients died. One in 1958, after removal of bilateral acoustic neurinomas, another - 63 years old - died in 1966 following operation for removal of recurrence of bilateral falx meningiomas combined with a tentorial meningioma. In the former case authopsy revealed multiple, clinically silent supratentorial meningiomas. 9 patients had good or satisfactory results following surgery. In 2 patients (Fig. 1 and 2) removal of the remaining tumors - falx meningiomas and acoustic neurinomas respectively, is planned.

The tendency to recurrence is particularly high in patients belonging to group 3, whereas it does not manifest itself in the first two groups of patients.

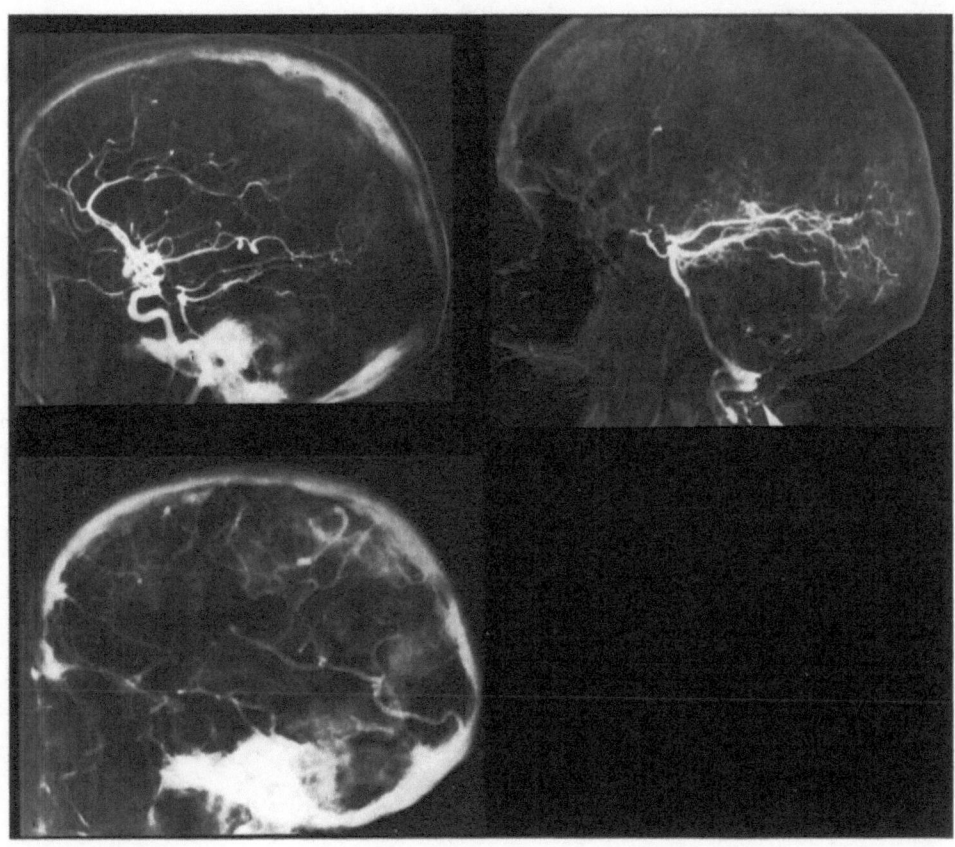

Fig. 1. 35 years-old female with bilateral falx meningiomas and bilateral tumors in the posterior fossa

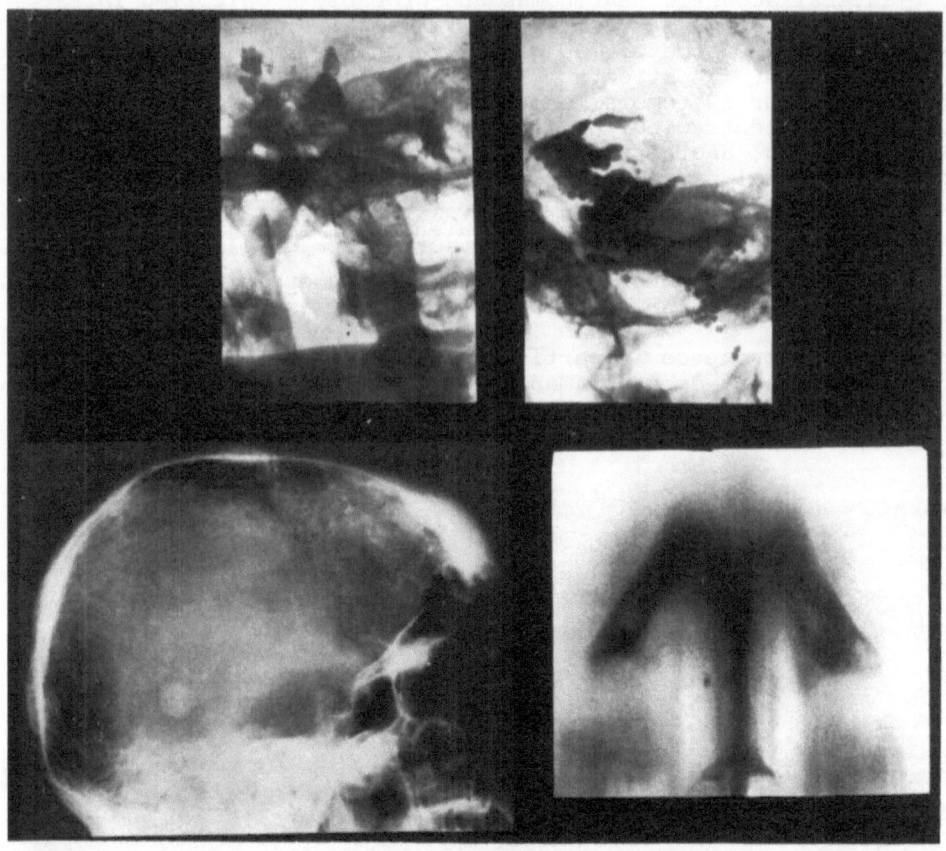

Fig. 2. 19 years-old patient with two meningiomas in the right frontal lobe and bilateral acoustic neurinomas and probably with an intraventricular calcified meningioma

Multiple Meningiomas

D. STÖWSAND

The incidence of multiple meningiomas among all meningiomas is about
1 - 2 % (2, 4, 7, 8). OLIVECRONA (6), in his monograph on parasagittal
meningiomas, states that multiple meningiomas are very rarely seen, so
that in practice they must not be considered. In our clinic, among 108
meningiomas which were operated on from 1964 - 1974, we observed one
patient with multiple meningiomas, on whom we are reporting in this
paper.

A 40-year-old man suffered from deafness of the right ear and blindness of the left eye with slowly progressive exophthalmos since about
ten years. He was admitted after several general convulsive seizures
had occured. Neurological examination demonstrated anosmia, deafness
and loss of vestibular function, peripheral facial paresis and choked
disc on the right as well as blindness with exophthalmos and paresis
of the 3rd cranial nerve on the left side. Conscience was clear. Plain
skull films showed calcifactions in the region of the left sphenoid
wing, in the middle of the anterior cranial fossa and above the right
petrous bone (Fig. 1) with destruction of its upper surface. Carotid
angiography demonstrated massive displacement of the anterior cerebral
artery to the left side (Fig. 2) and elevation of the anterior cerebral artery as well as a large frontal tumor stain (Fig. 3).

At craniotomy a right frontal falx meningioma of about 6 x 8 cm in
diameter, a small meningioma of the convexity and a meningioma of
the olfactory groove of 3 x 4 cm were removed. Histologically the
tumors were meningocytic meningiomas with fibroblastic components.
In the first two weeks following surgery the clinical course was
favourable. The patient then died suddenly from pulmonary embolism.

Autopsy revealed 59 circumscript intracranial meningiomas of typical
localization (several meningiomas of the falx, of the convexity, of
the tentorium, of the left sphenoid wing, of the posterior surface
of the petrous bone on both sides and a suprasellar meningioma (Fig. 4).
There were also several small spinal meningiomas in the thoracic
region.

The patient had no skin alterations (café au lait spots) or neurofibromas as found in RECKLINGHAUSEN's disease.

Although preoperative examinations had shown a multiple growth of tumors in our patient, operation seemed justified by raised intracranial
pressure and lack of signs of malignant tumor-growth.

Angiography had demonstrated a large frontal tumor, which could be
removed operatively. DANDY (3) has reported on a patient, from whom
one large and 15 smaller tumors were removed and who, 15 years later,
was "alive and well". In this patient many additional tumors had remained in the frontal and occipital regions.

The cause of multifocal origin of meningiomas is unknown. Our case should be classified in the group of multiple circumscript meningiomas, which can be distinguished from "diffuse meningiomatosis" with a carpet of more or less contiguous flat tumors (2). In some cases a clear distinction between these two forms seems not to be possible (9). In RECKLINGHAUSEN's disease, cases with multiple meningiomas are combined with neurofibromas and acoustic neurinomas (2).

In our case, which only had (meningocytic) meningiomas, it is without clinical meaning to speak of a "forme fruste" of RECKLINGHAUSEN's disease, as some authors do in such cases (1). Cases with multiple meningiomas such as our patient are extremely rare in the literature (5, 9).

Summary

A large frontal meningioma of the falx, a meningioma of the olfactory groove and a small meningioma of the convexity were surgically removed in a 40-year-old man. The clinical course was favorable during the first two weeks, the patient dying suddenly from pulmonary embolism. Autopsy showed 59 circumscript intracranial meningiomas of typical localization and several thoracic spinal meningiomas. Pathogenesis of multiple growth of meningiomas and therapeutical problems in these cases are discussed.

REFERENCES

1. BODECHTEL, G.: Zur Klinik der zentralen Formen der Neurofibromatose. Arch. f. Psych. u. z. Neurol. 185, 326 - 344 (1950).

2. CUSHING, H., EISENHARDT, L.: Meningiomas. Their Classification, Regional Behaviour, Life History and Surgical End-Results. Springfield/Ill.: C. C. Thomas 1938.

3. DANDY, W. E.: in LEWIS, D.: Practice of Surgery, Vol. 12, pp. 505 - 506. Hagerstown/Md.: W. E. Prior 1953.

4. FRAZIER, C. H., ALPERS, B. J.: Meningeal fibroblastomas of the cerebrum: a clinico-pathologic analysis of 75 cases. Arch. Neurol. Psychiat. 29, 935 - 989 (1933).

5. HOSOI, K.: Meningiomas with special reference to the multiple intracranial type. Amer. J. Path. 6, 245 - 260 (1930).

6. OLIVECRONA, H.: Die parasagittalen Meningeome. Leipzig: Georg Thieme 1934.

7. TAREN, J. A.: In: KAHN, E. A., CROSBY, E. C., SCHNEIDER, E. C.: Correlative Neurosurgery. pp. 82 - 83. Springfield/Ill.: C. C. Thomas 1969.

8. VESTERGAARD, E.: Multiple intracranial meningiomas. Acta Psychiat. Neurol. (Kbh.) 19, 389 - 411 (1944).

9. WAGA, S., MATSUDA, M., HANDA, H., MATSUSHIMA, M., ANDO, K.: Multiple meningiomas. J. Neurosurg. 37, 348 - 351 (1972).

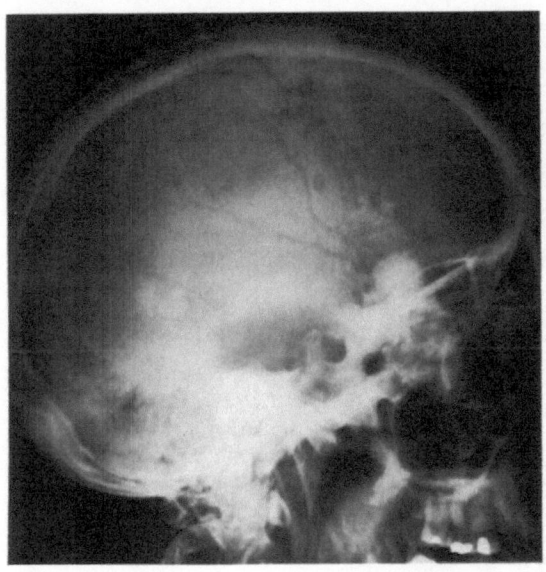

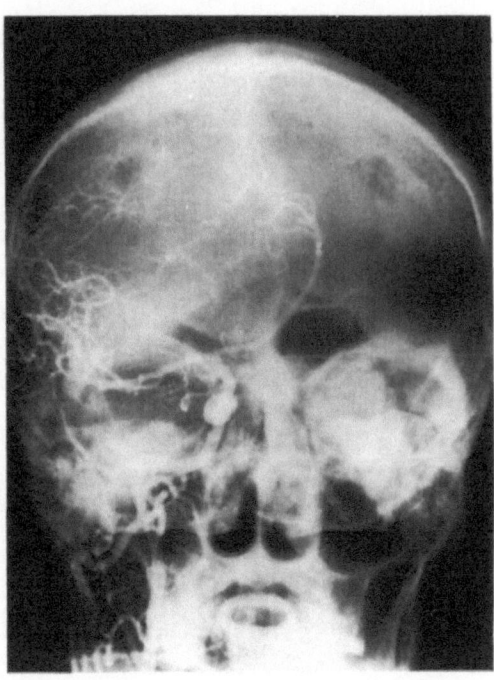

Fig. 1. Plain skull film with calfications in the anterior cranial fossa above the petrous bone

Fig. 2. Right carotid angiography showing massive displacement of the anterior cerebral artery to the left

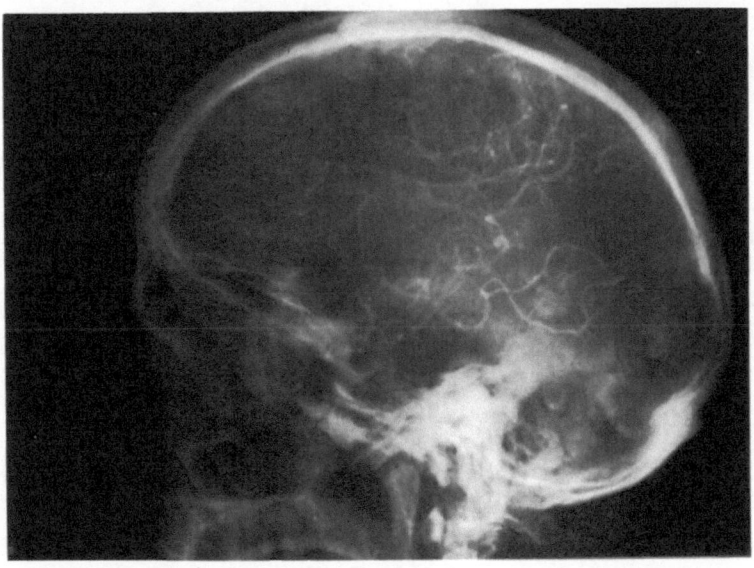

Fig. 3. In the lateral view right angiography demonstrates a large tumor stain in the frontal region

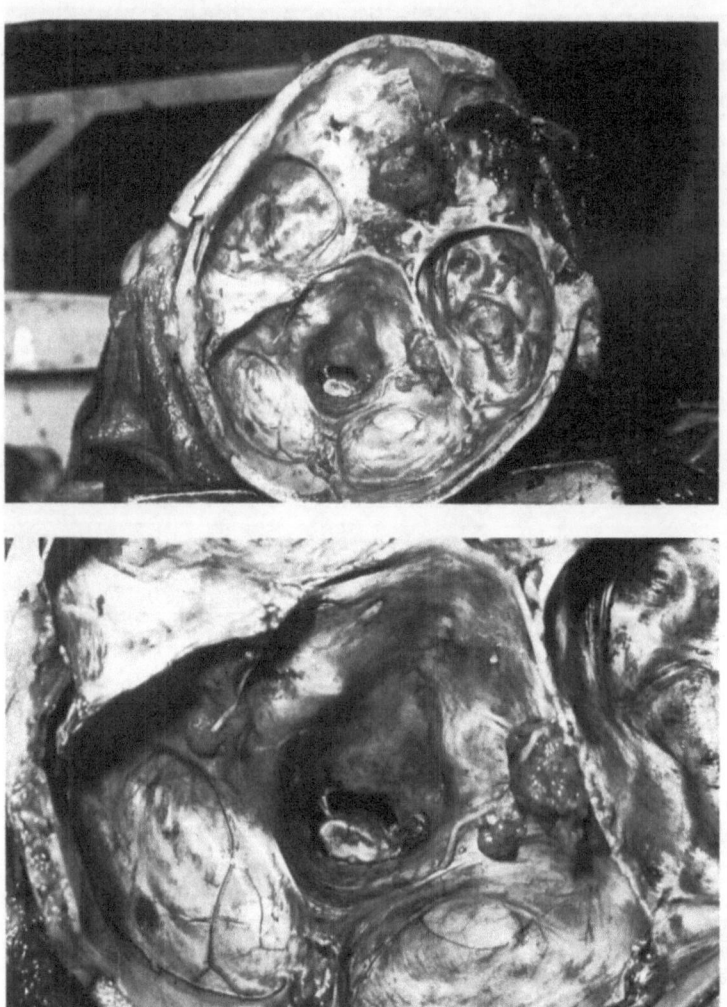

Fig. 4. Autopsy showing a suprasellar meningioma and several meningiomas of the petrous bone on both sides

The Suprasellar Meningioma

W. Krenkel and R. A. Frowein

The suprasellar meningioma is definded as a tumor, which originating
from the tuberculum sellae in the presellar area, and, developing between the two optic nerves, pushes the chiasm backwards and upwards.
The classic syndrome consists of a bitemporal hemianopia with primary
optic atrophy and a normal sella in an otherwise healthy middle-aged
person (2). Beside this more common type GUIOT and his collaborators
(7) have pointed out a type which starts from the diaphragma or dorsum sellae and has a tendency to develop retrosellarly.

The suprasellar meningiomata amount to between 9 and 11 % of all meningiomata in the extensive statistics (2, 3, 4, 6, 10, 14). They occur most frequently of all meningiomata in women, the relation between female and male patients being usually 3 : 1; with our own patients 38 : 8 or 4,75 : 1.

Taking into consideration 233 cases from the literature, the onset of
the symptoms shows a peak between the age of 35 and 45 (Fig. 1),
whereas with our own patients the average age on admission was 47
years for women and 49 years for men.

The rather long periods of time between the onset of the symptoms and
the operation are primarily due to the monosymptomatic course, consisting of failing visions. In these cases the average evolution time
takes about twice as long (52 months) as in cases with other primary
symptoms (25 months).

2/3 of all patients complain of failing visions in one eye as first
symptom, and almost one half of them had already turned blind on one
eye before the operation (22 out of 46 patients). Ophthalmologically
an unilateral deterioration of vision is ambigous; for many years the
diagnosis will remain that of an inflammatory or vascular process until the second eye is also affected (Fig. 2). In women, the onset or
increase of symptoms may occur during pregnancy; the symptoms may
even diminish after delivery; with our own patients there was such a
coincidence in 5 out of 14 women und 40 years of age.

But the difficulties of diagnosis are not confined to the ophthalmological side. There are 4 cases where we ourselves have to admit
errors. A 31-year-old female patient underwent surgery under the diagnosis of "arachnitis"; the suprasellar meningioma was an unexpected
finding. In a 61-year-old female patient a meningioma was first not
considered likely because of the normal brain scan. Only one year
later the tumor was discovered and successfully removed, this time
the brain scan being positive. A 35-year-old female patient presented
greater difficulties: there were additional paraesthesias and disturbances of sensibility on her trunk, so that the first diagnosis was
encephalomyelitis disseminata. A progressing deterioration of vision

finally lead to the discovery of the suprasellar meningioma. 4 years later the patient underwent surgery in another neurosurgical clinic for an intramedullary cyst in the spinal cord. Finally we wish to mention a case, which has already been published from the neuro-pathological side (11). After having undergone surgery for a suprasellar meningioma, there developed a CUSHING-syndrome in a 46-year-old female patient, which lead to various operations (extirpation of the suprarenal glands, implantation of radioactive yttrium). 2 years after the craniotomy necropsy revealed a pituitary adenoma as well as recurrence of a meningioma which had not been discovered.

Of the additional diagnostic measures radiography of the skull and isotope scanning are of only limited value; in 45 % of the cases the radiography of the skull was considered normal before surgery. The typical hyperostosis of the planum sphenoidale or the tuberculum sellae with a blistered enlargement of the bone structure was only described in 9 % of the cases. There existed a suprasellar calcification in 6 - 7 % (8, 12). A secondary decalcification of the dorsum sellae was the most frequent abnormal finding in our cases (16 out of 44). For isotope-diagnosis, too, the suprasellar meningioma is one of the most difficult localizations; only in half of the examinations (6 out of 12) there was definitely positive finding.

In the carotid angiogram most of the suprasellar meningiomata lead to typical elevation of the anterior cerebral artery; in 45 % of the cases additional tumor vessels could be pointed out. In 12 % angiography appeared normal. The variant of the retrosellar tumor should be mentioned here again. Here we find a lengthing of the carotid siphon and an elevation of the first part of the A. cerebri media. The pneumoncephalo-tomography may be called the safest diagnostic measure; a filling defect or obliteration of the chiasmatic cistern could be seen in every one of the examined cases, and the retrosellar extent, too, could exactly be defined.

The usual surgical approach of the tumor is by a right frontal craniotomy; controlled hyperventilation and the use of the operating microscope are indispensable operative aids; it may be helpful to cut a functionless optic nerve. The size of the tumor is reduced by using a small diathermic loop; it is then removed at the earliest possible moment through coagulation at the point of origin. In cases of a very large tumor a partial resection of the frontal lobe might exceptionally become necessary.

The surgical results (Table 1) of most of the authors (1, 2, 3, 4, 5, 6, 9, 10, 13) - the table takes into consideration - reports only on a larger number of patients reflect the surgical difficulties, which arise from the neighbourhood of the large vessels and the hypothalamus. With only a few exceptions, the operative lethality is 20 - 35 %. The size of the tumor is of significant influence; CUSHING (2) still thought that suprasellar meningiomata with more than 20 g of weight were inoperable. Also the age of the patient at the time of the operation is essential for the prognostic judgement. Among our patients the number of the more than 50-year-olds was about twice as high as the numbers given in the literature.

The majority of fatalities is caused by a failure of central regulation or by lesions of the large arteries, the primary lethality being 19,5 %. Four patients died later on from infection or pituitary insufficiency, bringing the clinical lethality to 28 %.

Table 1. The operative mortality in suprasellar meningiomata. A review of literature

Authors	year	n	†	%
Guillaumat + Vincent	1937	22	8	36
Cushing + Eisenhardt	1938	24	3	13
Grant + Hedges	1956	30	6	20
Cassinari + Bernasconi	1957	31	7	23
Weber	1965	44	17	38
Olivecrona	1967	64	14	22
Fusek + Kunc	1969	47	16	34
Jane + Mc Kissock	1962	small 17	0	0
		large 32	14	42
Ehlers + Malmros	1973	small 13	1	8
		large 18	2	11
Present series	1974	small 13	1	8
		large 33	12	36
	age - 50 y.	27	5	15
	age > 50 y.	19	8	42

We are familiar with the history of the 32 surviving patients (Table 2). 3 patients died from a recurrence, this share of 9 % corresponding with the more extensive statistics (CUSHING (2) - 9,5 %; JANE and McKISSOCK (9) - 11 %; OLIVECRONA (10) - 8 %; EHLERS and MALMROS (3) - 7 %). 4 more patients died of other non-cerebral reasons. Of the other 25 patients who have been operated on, 15 are fully able to work; restrictions in the ability to work are primarily caused by blindness.

Table 2. Late results of 46 suprasellar meningiomata

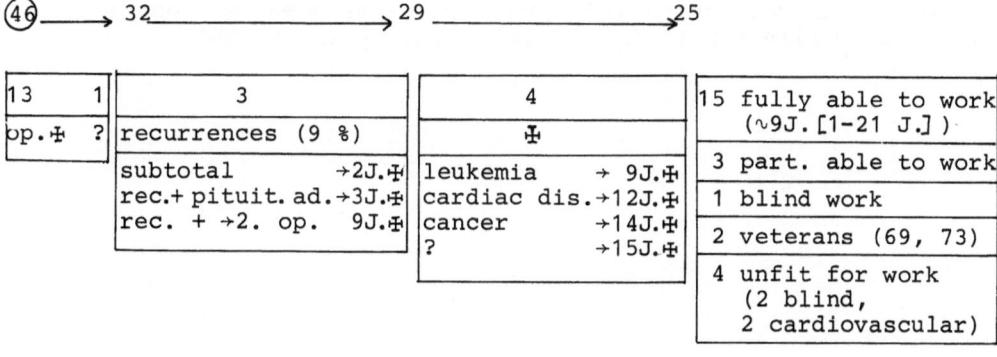

There can be no doubt that the results need to be improved. This can be achieved by admitting the patients earlier to the clinic, by using pneumoencephalo-tomography, which is essential for diagnosis, by using modern anaesthesiological and surgical equipment, and last not least - by having an experienced neurosurgeon and his team.

REFERENCES

1. CASSINARI, V., BERNASCONI, V.: Considerazioni clinico-radiologico su 35 casi di meningioma del tubercule della sella. Acta Neurol., Napoli 12, 648 - 669 (1957).

2. CUSHING, H., EISENHARDT, L.: Meningiomas: Their Classification, Regional Behaviour, Life History and Surgical End Results. Springfield/Ill.: C. C. Thomas 1938.

3. EHLERS, N., MALMROS, R.: The suprasellar Meningioma. Acta ophthalmologica, Copenhag., Suppl. 121, 1973.

4. FUSEK, I., KUNC, Z.: Causes of unsuccessful surgical treatment of suprasellar meningiomas. Cesk. Neurol. 32, 279 - 283 (1969).

5. GRANT, F. C., HEDGES, T. R.: Ocular findings in meningiomas of the tuberculum sellae. Arch. Ophthal., Chicago 56, 163 - 170 (1956).

6. GUILLAUMAT, L.: Les méningiomes supra-sellaires. Paris: Thèse 1937.

7. GUIOT, G., MONTRIEUL, B., GOUTELLE, A., COMOY, J., LANGIE, S.: Méningiomes supra-sellaires rétro-chiasmatiques. Neuro-Chirurgie 16, 273 - 285 (1970).

8. LOMBARDI, G.: Radiology in Neuro-Ophthalmology. Baltimore: Williams and Wilkins Co. 1967.

9. JANE, J. A., McKISSOCK, W.: Importance of failing vision in early diagnosis of suprasellar meningiomas. Brit. med. J. 2, 5 - 7 (1962).

10. OLIVECRONA, H.: The surgical treatment of intracranial tumors. In: Handbuch der Neurochirurgie. Bd. IV/4. (Hrsg. H. OLIVECRONA, W. JÖNNIS). Berlin - Heidelberg - New York: Springer 1967.

11. PROBST, A.: Kombination eines Cushing-Syndroms, Hypophysenadenoms und suprasellären Meningeoms - Fallbericht. Zbl. Neurochir. 32, 75 - 82 (1971).

12. TUCKER, R. L., HOLMANN, C. B., McCARTY, C. S., DOCKERTY, M. B.: The Roentgenologic Manifestations of Meningiomas in the Region of the Tuberculum Sellae. Radiology 72, 348 - 355 (1959).

13. WEBER, G.: Symptomatologie und Chirurgie der sellären und suprasellären Tumoren. Ophthalmologica 149, 326 - 342 (1965).

14. ZÜLCH, K. J.: Biologie und Pathologie der Hirngeschwülste. In: Handbuch der Neurochirurgie. (Hrsg. H. OLIVECRONA, W. TÖNNIS). Bd. III. Berlin - Heidelberg - New York: Springer 1956.

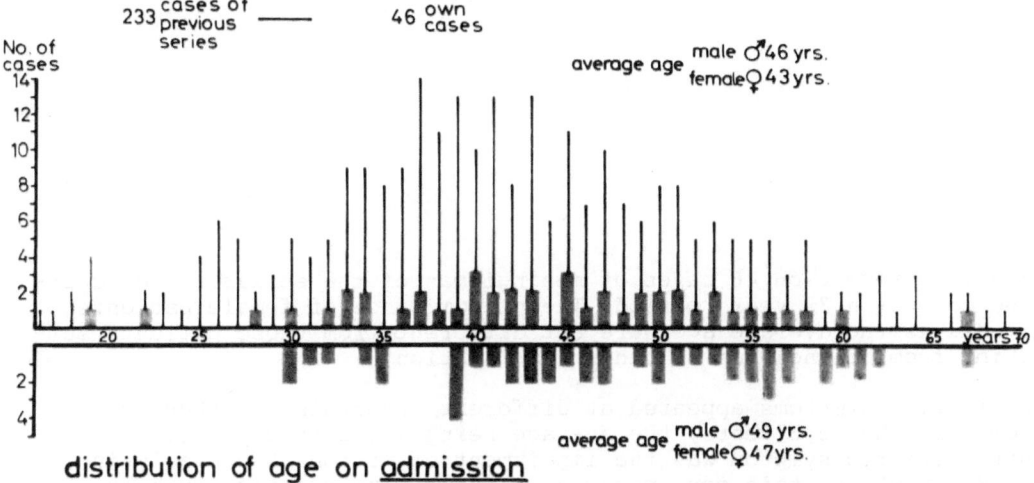

Fig. 1. The distribution of the age at onset of symptomes (233 cases of previous series and 46 cases of the present series) and on admission (only for own cases)

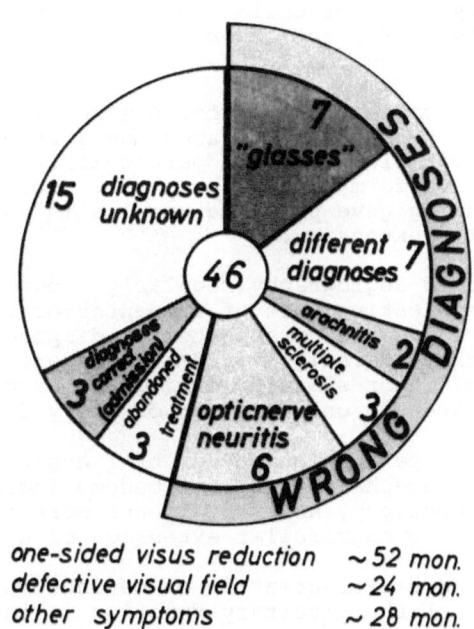

Fig. 2. Diagnostic errors in 46 own cases. A misleading diagnosis is known in 25 cases

Meningiomas of the Sellar Region

E. HALVES and H. VOGT

This is a report on 46 cases of meningiomas of the sellar region operated on over a 30 years period. The predominance of female patients
as well as the average age were not different from those patients suffering from meningiomas of other localization.

The initial symptoms appeared at different intervals and they ranged
from 2 months to 8 years, the average being 1 1/2 to 2 years. The
characteristic symptom was the impairment of vision. Especially in
the early stage, this may appear as being a non-specific compression-
syndrome of the optic nerve. This frequently lead to diagnoses such
as disseminated sclerosis, cerebral atrophy, or carotid artery stenosis. Consequently, most patients underwent surgical treatment at an
advanced stage of the disease.

On admission, 22 patients suffered from unilateral amaurosis and temporal hemianopia on the other eye. Such late symptoms as well as the
early signs of unilateral visual field impairment, which are characteristic for optic nerve compression, are suggestive for the presence
of a meningioma of the sellar region.

In 29 cases pathological changes in the sellar area could be seen on
plain X-rays. In 20 cases the area of attachment of the meningioma
was visible. This was particularly true with presellar tumors which
tend to form hyperostosis that could be verified at surgery. Brain
scanning gave positive results in cases of tumors with large suprasellar extension.

Carotid angiography regularly showed upward stretching of the pre-
communicating part of the anterior cerebral arteries, and frequently
elevation and dorsoposterior displacement of the supraclinoidal part
of the internal carotid and the anterior cerebral arteries was noticeable. Tumor-staining during the precapillary phase of the angiogram
was seen in only one out of every 8 meningiomas.

Due to perfection of cerebral angiographic techniques, conventional
pneumencephalography has become increasingly obsolete. Pneumoencepha-
lotomography, however, is apt more than any other technique, to out-
line the suprasellar extension of a tumor.

In the differentiation of meningiomas from pituitary adenomas, analysis of the pituitary function is indispensible, particularly determination of pituitary hormones following intravenous administration
of synthetic thyrotropin releasing hormone (TRH) and luteinizing
hormone releasing hormone (LH-RH).

Total surgical removal of meningiomas of the sellar region may be
achieved only, if separation of the tumor from the basal vessels and

the optic nerve is possible. In 30 patients total removal of a parasellar meningioma was possible. Dural attachment was at the tuberculum sellae (17 cases) and at the sphenoid plane (4 cases). The remaining tumors involved the dura of the sellar area circularly. This
was especially true in the cases presenting a large suprasellar mass.
A number of presellar meningiomas could not be distinguished from the
so called "Olfactory Meningioma".

Microscopic examination of the tumors showed no signs of malignancy.
No serious operative complications occured. During the immediate
post-operative period, however, there were 4 fatalaties due to intracranial hemorrhage following frontal lobe resection, and frontal brain
softening due to intraoperative ligation of one anterior cerebral artery.

Transitory psycho-syndroma was observed frequently. Hyperthermia,
diabetes insipidus and epileptic fits complicated the post-operative
course in a number of cases. In 19 patients the post-operative course
was uneventful.

Comparing preoperative with post-operative ophthalmologic findings,
there appeared to be no dependence on age or duration of the disease.
On the whole, a certain improvement of visual acuity and visual fields
was achieved by surgery, with the exception of cases of a recurrence
of the meningioma, and of cases of tumors adhesive to the optic nerve.
There was only one case of "real" recurrence of a meningioma following
removal. The interval was 2 years.

Summary

Early diagnosis appears to be the condition for successful surgical
treatment of meningiomas of the sellar region. Complications of surgical treatment are rare and the rates of lethality and recurrence
are small.

Microsurgery of Suprasellar Meningiomas

W. TH. KOOS, G. KLETTER, H. SCHUSTER, and A. PERNECZKY

Since 1940 73 patients with suprasellar meningiomas have undergone
surgery at the Neurosurgical Clinic of the University of Vienna Medical School. Of these, 54 were female and 19 male. Prior to the introduction of microsurgery in 1970 56 patients had been submitted to
conventional surgical procedures. After 1970 surgery for suprasellar
meningiomas was invariably done with the help of the surgical microscope. Conventional procedures such as practiced before 1970 were
associated with a mortality of 19 %, while microsurgical techniques
employed since 1970 reduced the mortality rate to 9 %, i. e., we only
lost 1 patient.

It is beyond the scope of the present paper to discuss the clinical
signs and symptoms of suprasellar meningiomas, which are well known.

On the basis of our material we should, however, like to review the
growth patterns of suprasellar meningiomas. Meningiomas generally
tend to displace and engulf existent anatomical structures. This tendency sets clear-cut limits to a radical macroscopic extirpation of
these tumors, if vital structures are to be preserved.

Table 1 shows that about two thirds of the tumors extend in the parasellar area with preferential growth on one side. This accounts for
the typical clinical picture characterized by optic nerve damage,
which may progress to complete blindness of one eye with temporary
hemianopsia of the other. In about 50 % of the cases the chiasm is
found to be elevated by the tumor and displaced dorsally, with tumor
growth extending occipitalwards beyond the level of the dorsum sellae
(Fig. 1).

Along this route of extension the tumor must necessarily establish
contact with the pituitary stalk and/or the infundibulum. CUSHING's
often quoted classification of suprasellar meningiomas in 4 growth
stages (1917) suggests that the tumor, while advancing occipitalwards
between the optic chiasm and the dorsum sellae, would come into contact with the infundibulum in the midline (Figs. 2 a, b). Progressing,
retrosellar tumor growth, as observed in the majority of our cases,
would, then, be expected to produce pituitary on hypothalamic disturbances (CUSHING III and IV). Nevertheless, neurosurgeons know that
endocrinologic changes are extremely rare in suprasellar meningiomas.
In our material we found only 4 cases of endocrinologic disturbances.
In 2 of these the sella turcica had been destroyed by exceptionally
extensive endosellar tumor masses. In another case the tumor had extended towards retrosellar and entered the lumen of the third ventricle. Finally, in 1 patient the tumor had demonstrably advanced far
into the hypothalamic region. Since endocrinologic disturbances were
absent in all other cases with extensive retrosellar tumor growth,
we particularly concentrated on the relationship of the tumor to the

Table 1. Suprasellar meningiomas, growth pattern. Tumor types A - D demonstrate parasellar growth (large numbers); the small numbers indicate the frequency of tumor growth in a sagittal plane

frontal section	ante- sellar	retro- sellar	intra- sellar	total	%
A	14	17	3	19	26
B	4	5	1	16	22
C	4	9	2	12	16
D	7	16	5	26	36
total	29	47	11	73	100

infundibulum in all microsurgical interventions for suprasellar meningiomas. Figs. 3 and 4 show the extirpation of extensive suprasellar meningiomas under the surgical microscope. Removal of the parasellar and retrosellar tumor masses exposed the infundibulum which had been laterally displaced, and had come to lie underneath the optic nerve. While extirpating the retrosellar portion of the tumor particular attention was paid to preserving the small vessels originating from the carotid and posterior communicating arteries and running towards the hypothalamus.

Careful removal of the tumor tissue invariably shows these vessels to be displaced by the tumor. Nevertheless, they are always found to be outside the tumor capsule, and can be well differentiated from the true tumor vessels (Figs. 5 a, b). In pituitary adenomas and craniopharyngiomas the pathogenesis involved accounts for the close topical relationship between infundibulum and tumor and the resulting functional deficits. In suprasellar meningiomas a different pathogenetic process is apparently at work, which explains why the infundibulum and its function are preserved in spite of extensive tumor growth.

REFERENCE

CUSHING, H., EISENHARDT, L.: Meningiomas. Their classification, regional behaviour, life history and surgical end results, pp. 224 - 249. Springfield/Ill.: C. Thomas 1938.

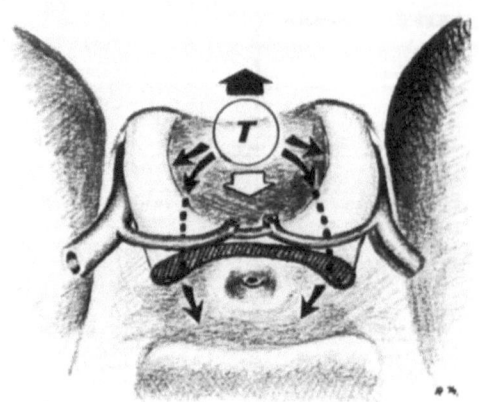

Fig. 1. Schematic demonstration of the direction of growth of suprasellar meningiomas (arrows). Displacement of the optic chiasm posteriorly and the optic nerves (and internal carotid arteries) laterally. Note the para-infundibular growth pattern in cases of a retrosellar tumor extension

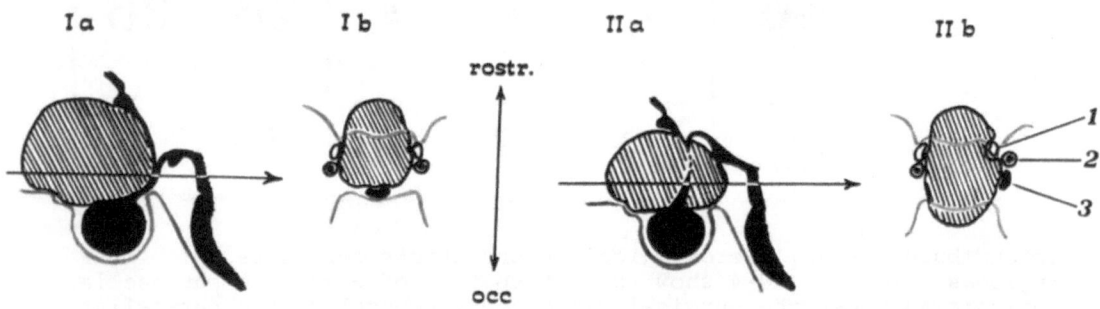

Fig. 2. Schematic drawing demonstrating the relationship of large suprasellar meningiomas to the infundibulum.

Sagittal section (I a) and horizontal section (I b) of a stage III meningioma according to CUSHING and EISENHARDT. The infundibulum is displaced posteriorly and shown in a midline position. -

II a and b: Topographic relations of large suprasellar meningiomas with retrosellar growth as observed by the authors during microsurgical tumor removal. 1 = optic nerve, partially surrounded by tumor; 2 = internal carotid artery; 3 = infundibulum, laterally displaced (!)

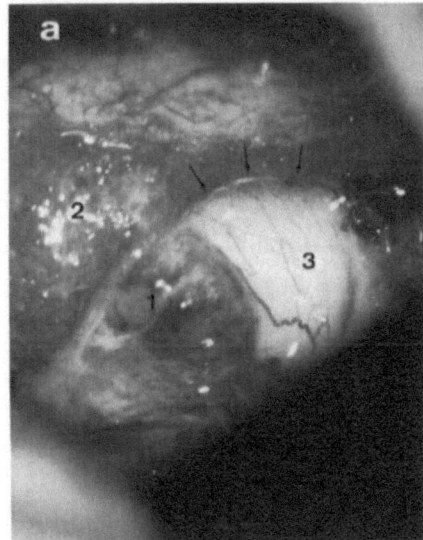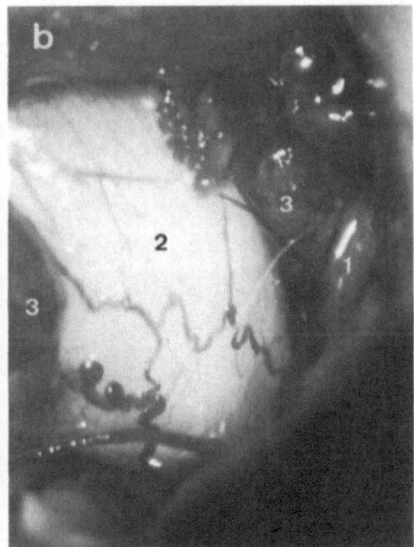

Fig. 3 a - d. Suprasellar meningioma originating from the tuberculum sellae and sulcus chiasmatis and growing para-, retro- and anterosellarly. Operation photograph; situation after right frontal craniotomy and retraction of the right frontal lobe

a) The main portion of the tumor is located in the supra-, retro- and parasellar regions (1); the tumor also covers the sphenoid planum (2). The right optic nerve (3) is extremely flattened by the underlying tumor and forms a thin ischaemic band arching upwards and laterally; at the site of entrance of the optic nerve into the optic canal (black arrows) the nerve is squeezed against the upper circumference of the canal entrance (despite preoperative blindness the patient regained vision following tumor removal and optic nerve decompression)

b) Same situs, higher magnification. Arterial branches arising from the internal carotid artery (1) and the anterior cerebral artery supply the optic nerve (2) as well as the tumor (3)

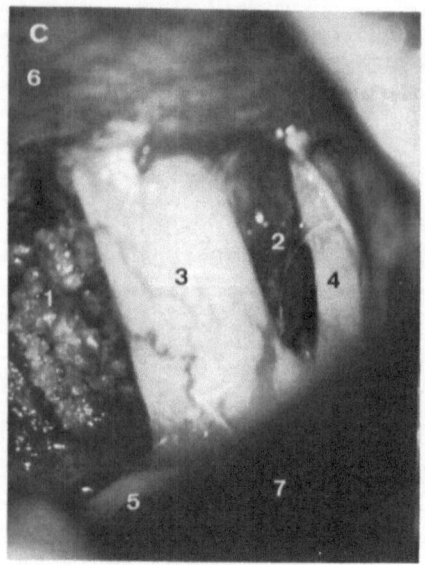
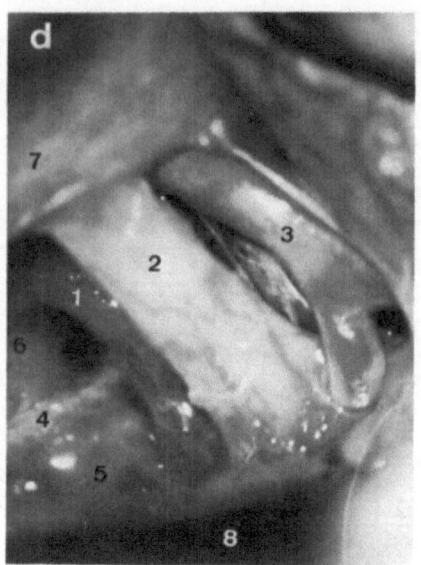

Fig. 3.

c) Situation after partial removal of the suprasellar tumor portion (1). 2 = parasellar extension of the tumor; 3 = right optic nerve partially decompressed; 4 = right internal carotid artery laterally displaced; 5 = right anterior cerebral artery; 6 = sphenoid planum; 7 = retracted right frontal lobe

d) Situation after total removal of the tumor. The laterally displaced infundibulum (pituitary stalk) (1) can be seen emerging from under the optic chism and disappearing into the sellar diaphragm; the infundibulum is covered by the right optic nerve (2). 3 = right internal carotid artery; 4 = dorsum sellae; 5 = arachnoid covering the interpeduncular cistern; 6 = diaphragma sellae; 7 = sphenoid planum; 8 = retracted right frontal lobe

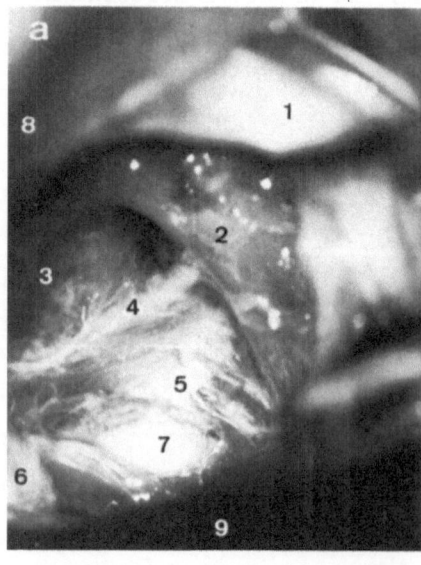
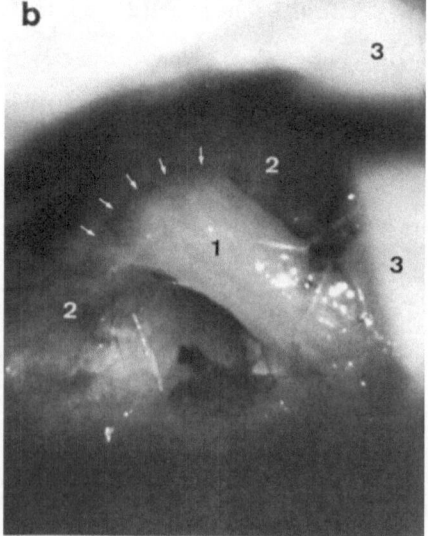

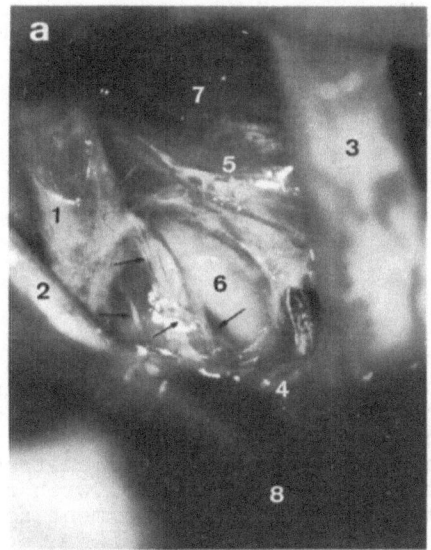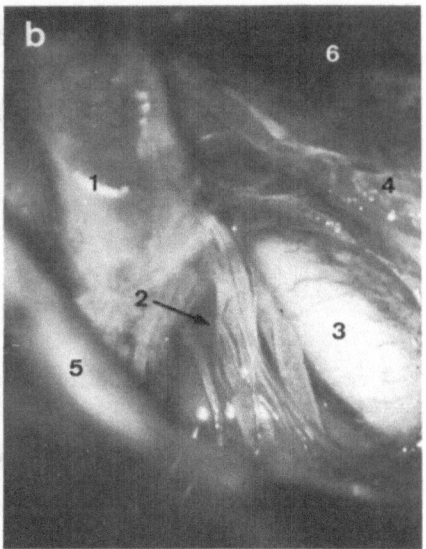

Fig. 5 a - b. Same case as in Figs. 3 and 4

a) Situation after total removal of tumor. The left internal carotid artery (1) and the left optic nerve (2) are brought into view. 3 = right optic nerve; 4 = optic chiasm; 5 = dorsum sellae. In the retrosellar region small arteries (arrows) originating from the internal carotid artery and the posterior communicating artery supply the infundibulum and the hypothalamic structures. These vessels are displaced by the tumor and can be distinguished clearly from arteries supplying the tumor. 6 = left oculomotor nerve; 7 = sellar diaphragm; 8 = retracted frontal lobe

b) Magnified section of Fig. 5 a. demonstrating the above mentioned vital arteries which supply the infundibulum and the hypothalamus. 1 = left internal carotid artery; 2 = left posterior communicating artery; 3 = left oculomotor nerve; 4 = dorsum sellae; 5 = left optic nerve; 6 = sellar diaphragm

◁ Fig. 4 a - b. Same case as in Fig. 3

a) Situation after total removal of tumor. The right optic nerve (1) is retracted laterally and the infundibulum (pituitary stalk) which was displaced to the right side by the tumor is brought into view (2). 3 = sellar diaphragm; 4 = dorsum sellae; retrosellar arachnoid tissue covering the interpeduncular cistern; 6 = left internal carotid artery; 7 = left oculomotor nerve; 8 = sphenoid planum; 9 = retracted right frontal lobe

b) Magnified section of Fig. 4 a. Site of entrance (small arrows) of the pituitary stalk (1) into the sellar diaphragm (2). 3 = right optic nerve

Diagnostical and Clinical Appearence of the Sphenoidal Ridge Meningioma en Plaque

E. W. KIENECKER, K. PISCOL, H. ARTMANN, and M. SHAABAN

The meningiomas en plaque of the sphenoidal wing still present diagnostic problems of differentiating between systemic lesions of the bone and monostotical lesions destructive of the sphenoidal ridge and adjoining skull. In addition to these diagnostic difficulties the meningiomas en plaque present therapeutical problems, with respect to the necessity for surgical treatment and the right moment for operative measures.

We would like to present the diagnostic features and discuss the therapy of meningiomas en plaque of the sphenoid wing, illustrated by five cases, three of being recurrent tumors (Table 1). The period of observation was from January 1st, 1971 to July 31st, 1974. Two additional cases were from the Department for Neurosurgery, University of Heidelberg [PISCOL and WULTZINGER (10)].

Table 1. Table of meningiomas en plaque of the sphenoidal ridge treated between January 1st, 1971 and July 31st, 1974

Patient	Initial symptoms	Indication for operation	Results
1. M.L. ♀ 40 years	exophthalmos right	visual acuity exophthalmos	+++(reop.)
2. M.K. ♀ 54 years	left nasal perimetric visual loss exophthalmos	perimetric visual loss exophthalmos	++ (reop.)
3. E.S. ♀ 41 years	exophthalmos right	exophthalmos headaches	+++(reop.)
4. H.G. ♀ 53 years	pressing headaches deformation of the left temporal fossa	headaches deformation	+++
5. A.H. o 72 years	deformation of the right temporal fossa	no operation	slowly growing deformity

Considering sex preference and age distribution, the meningiomas en plaque appear to behave as the globular meningiomas (8). The literature report on a total of 94 meningiomas en plaque of the sphenoidal ridge. 97 % of these cores are female and 3 % male patient (1, 2, 5, 8, 11, 14). Due to lack of information the age distribution cannot be exactly determinated. To divide the global meningiomas of the sphenoid wing region in a medial and a lateral subgroup [TÖNNIES and SCHÜRMANN (15)] does not appear possible, as there is expansive growth of the tumors and as the number of cases is small.

The patients with a meningioma en plaque of the sphenoidal wing complain about deformation in the temporal fossa, pressing, unilateral frontal headaches, exophthalmos and ipsilateral, perimetric visual loss in the nasal part, less frequently in the central part. Depending on the extent of the occlusion of the orbital foramina, visual acuity, ophthalmoplegia and lack of corneal reflex is found (14). When exophthalmos is more pronounced, there are complaints of double vision. The deformation of the temporal fossa may be of such extent that it presents not only a cosmetic problem, but also make special ophthalmological remedy necessary. Detailed descriptions on the meningioma en plaque are given by 1, 2, 3, 4, 5, 6, 7, 8, 10, 11, 14, 16, 17. The fact that the initial symptoms almost always proceed with visual disturbances explains why the patient calls on the ophthalmologist first of all.

Radiological examination is the method of choice in the diagnosis of the meningioma en plaque of the sphenoid wing. Plain skull X-rays show either a circumscribed or diffuse, mostly homogenous, more rarely clouded involvement of the sphenoid wing structures. These changes generally spread to adjoining bones, particularly the temporal bone. The adjacant sinuses of the nasal cavity are often involved. A meningioma en plaque can be expected, the more widespread there is a deterioration of the bone.

The value of angiography and encephalography in cases of meningiomas en plaque of the sphenoid wing is to exclude presence of an intradural braincompressing tumor. In none of our cases of meningiomas en plaque there was an intradural mass. On the other hand one case of olfactory meningioma could be angiographically differentiated from sphenoid wing meningioma en plaque. In this case the plain roentgenographs were suggestive for a meningioma en plaque of the sphenoid wing as there was massive infiltration of the bone as well as reactive hyperostosis of the medial part of the orbit, the orbital roof, the sphenoidal wings and the adjoining paranasal sinuses.

Orbital phlebography is valuable in cases of the sphenoid wing meningioma en plaque invading the orbit. Obstruction to the flow of the contrast through the retrobulbar, or IIIrd segment, of the superior ophthalmic vein as well as displacement of the vein are suggestive for the presence of intraorbital extension of the tumor. A detailed description of technique and findings are given by PISCOL and PENZHOLZ (9).

Scintigraphy appears to be of greatest importance in the diagnosis of localization and nature of the tumor. With sequencescintigraphy using the scintillationcamera, statements of considerable reliability can be made in the presence of global meningiomas (12). With the meningioma en plaque, however, our own experience is still very limited. According to observations by STERN (14) as well as in our own experience, it appears that meningiomas en plaque manifest themselves in the same way. In all our cases positive scintigraphic results were obtained. We were able to make a definite classification of our own five cases, as they show the typical accumulation of the nucleiotid, as global meningiomas do. The meningiomas en plaque accumulate the highest amount of radioactivity in rather a short time following application. The activity then increases only little and slowly. Cerebral scintigraphy using the scintillationcamera is suitable for pre- or postoperative control, as it is diagnostically reliable and as it presents practically no hazard to the patient (13).

The meningioma en plaque must be differentiated from other lesions of the skull presenting similar X-ray changes of the bone. Systemic le-

sions of the bone, such as ostitis deformans PAGET, fibrous dysplasia
JAFFE-LICHTENSTEIN, osteopetrosis ALBERS-SCHOENBERG and ostitis fi-
brosa castica von RECKLINGHAUSEN as well as acute disease of the bone
must be taken into consideration. Systemic lesions of the bone manifest themselves polyostotically and they may be diagnosed by appropriate radiological examination. Monoostotic lesions are less easy to
identify. The fact that PAGET disease is mostly found among male patients and the meningiomas mainly among females may be of some help.
The fibrous bone dysplasia is a special group of the ALBRIGHT SYNDROME
and it may be differentiated by anomalies of pigmentation as well by
signs of mal development. Osteomas are not found outside the sphenoidal wing proper, and metastatic neoplasms are usually characterized by
dramatic progression.

Operation on a meningioma en plaque of the sphenoidal ridge is indicated when there are a quick progression in the destruction of the
bone, neurologic symptoms and lasting, agonizing headaches. Cosmetic
problems may influence the decision for surgical treatment. Unfortunately, total removal is rarely possible. In our clinic, three cases
with progressive exophthalmos along with other ophthalmological disorders, as well as one case with a pronounced deformity of the temporal fossa, accompanied by agonizing headaches, underwent surgical
treatment. Only one case who had no complaints except for a slowly
growing deformity in the temporal fossa was not surgically treated.
In this case advanced age of the patient definitely influenced the
decision against surgical treatment.

The results differ greatly. Three cases had to be reoperated on for
recurrence of exophthalmos. Postoperative follow-up of the patients
did not show a tendency to greater extension of the tumor up to today.
None patient is suffering from headaches or other neurological symptoms. In one case the cosmetic result was not sufficient.

Summary

This report deals with the initial and clinical symptoms, diagnosis
and therapy of the sphenoidal ridge meningioma en plaque. The peculiarities of this tumor with respect to growth, expansion and histological appearance are discussed.

Clinical diagnosis, including differential-diagnostic problems, radiological appearance scintigraphic and sequencescintigraphic examination
are analyzed with respect to the possibilities and limitations of the
various techniques are discussed. Our own investigations are compared
with the experience from the world literature. A comment is given
with respect to possibilities of surgical treatment and prognosis.

REFERENCES

1. CASTELLANO, F., GUIDETTI, B., OLIVECRONA, H.: Pterional Meningiomas "En Plaque". J. Neurosurg. 9, 188 - 196 (1952).

2. CUSHING, H., EISENHARDT, L.: Meningiomas: Their Classification,
   Regional Behaviour, Life History, and Surgical End Results.
   Springfield/Ill.: C. Thomas 1938.

3. GERLACH, J., SIMON, G.: Die Beteiligung der Schädelknochen bei
   Geschwülsten der Orbita. In: Handbuch der Neurochirurgie, Bd.IV/1
   (Hrsg. H. OLIVECRONA, W. TÖNNIES), S. 249 - 262. Berlin - Göttin-
   gen - Heidelberg: Springer 1960.

4. KRAYENBÜHL, H., YASARGIL, M. G.: Die zerebrale Angiographie. Stuttgart: Georg Thieme 1965.

5. KUNFT, H.-D., BINGAS, B., VOGT, M.: Die Meningeome der Keilbein-flügel. Zbl. Neurochirur. 24, 171 - 188 (1964).

6. LINDGREN, E.: Roentgenologie. In: Handbuch der Neurochirurgie, Bd. II (Hrsg. H. OLIVECRONA, W. TÖNNIES). Berlin - Göttingen - Heidelberg: Springer 1954.

7. LOEPP, W., LORENZ, R.: Röntgendiagnostik des Schädels. Stuttgart: Georg Thieme 1971.

8. OLIVECRONA, H.: The Meningiomas. In: Handbuch der Neurochirurgie, Bd. IV/4 (Hrsg. H. OLIVECRONA, W. TÖNNIES), S. 125 - 191. Berlin - Heidelberg - New York: Springer 1967.

9. PISCOL, K., PENZHOLZ, H.: Die Bedeutung der retrograden Phlebo-graphie für die Diagnostik intra- und retroorbitaler Prozesse. Dtsch. med. Wschr. 95, 161 - 164 (1970).

10. PISCOL, K., WULTZINGER, H.: Das Meningeom en plaque des Keilbein-flügels. Personal communication.

11. POPPEN, J. L., HORRAX, G.: The Surgical Treatment of Hyperostoting Meningiomas of the Sphenoidal Ridge. Surg. Gynec. Obstct. 71, 222 - 230 (1940).

12. SAUER, J., FIEBACH, O., OTTO, H., LÖHR, E., STRÖTGES, M. W., BET-TAG, W.: Comparative Studies of Cerebral Scintigraphy, Angiography and Encephalography for Detection of Meningiomas. Neuroradiology 2, 102 - 106 (1971).

13. SCHENK, P., PENZHOLZ, H., PIETROWSKI, W., TORNOW, W.: Kamera-szintigraphie bei Hirntumoren. S. 119 - 126. 1-tes Heidelberger Symposium über Kameraszintigraphie 1968.

14. STERN, W. E.: Meningiomas in the Cranio-Orbital Junction. J. Neu-rosurg. 38, 428 - 437 (1973).

15. TÖNNIES, W., SCHÜRMANN, K.: Meningeome der Keilbeinflügel. Zbl. Neurochir. 11, 1 - 13 (1951).

16. TÖNNIES, W.: Diagnostik der intrakraniellen Geschwülste. In: Handbuch der Neurochirurgie, Bd. IV/3 (Hrsg. H. OLIVECRONA, W. TÖNNIES). Berlin - Göttingen - Heidelberg: Springer 1962.

17. WENDE, F., SCHULZE, A., MARZ, P.: Die neuroradiologische Diagno-stik der Meningeome. Radiologe 9, 26 (1969).

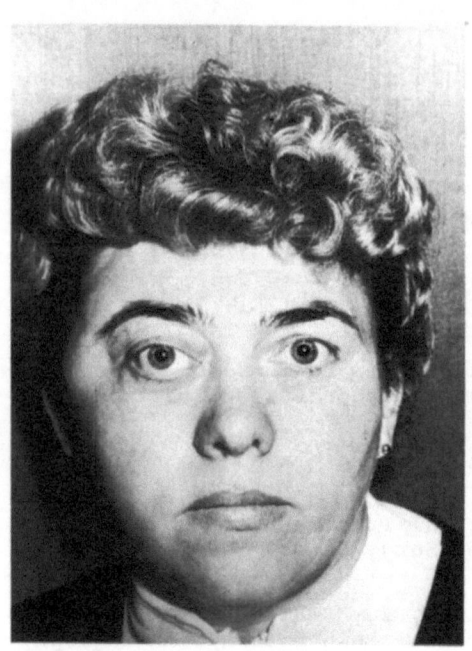

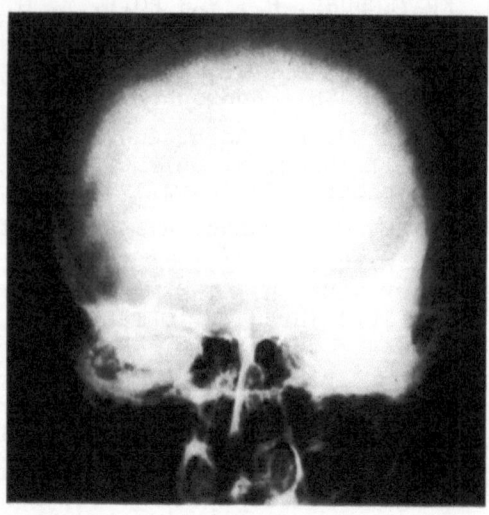

Fig. 1. 40-years old patient with strong deformation of the right temporal fossa due to a meningioma en plaque of the lateral sphenoidal ridge

Fig. 2. Roentgenograph of a meningioma en plaque with massive hyperostotic involvement of the left sphenoidal wing and the adjoining bone structures

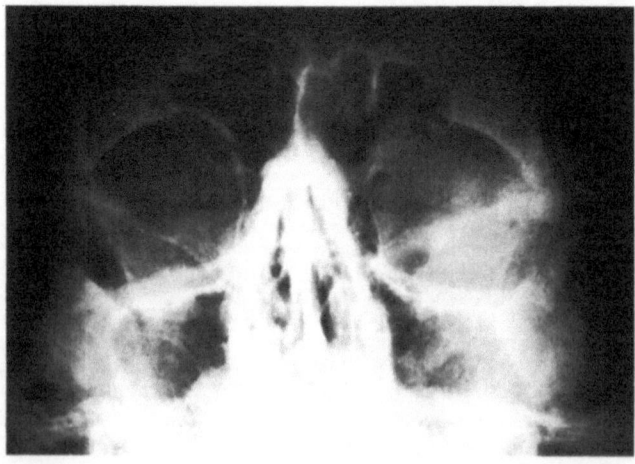

Fig. 3. Roentgenograph of the sinuses of the nasal cavity showing, on its left side, a diffuse homogenous involvement of the sphenoidal region and surrounding structures

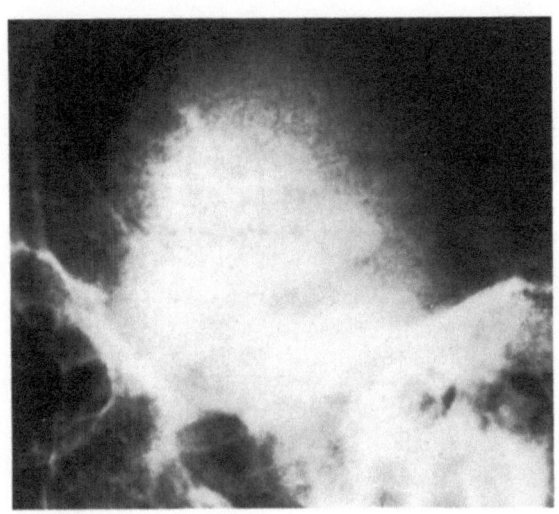

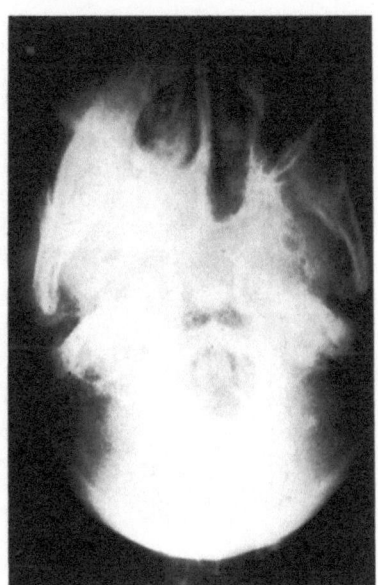

Fig. 4. Contact roentgenograph of hyperostotic reaction of the left temporal fossa caused by a meningioma en plaque of the sphenoidal ridge

Fig. 5. Roentgenograph of the base of the skull. Meningioma en plaque of the sphenoidal wing has invaded the right paranasal sinuses and adjacent structures

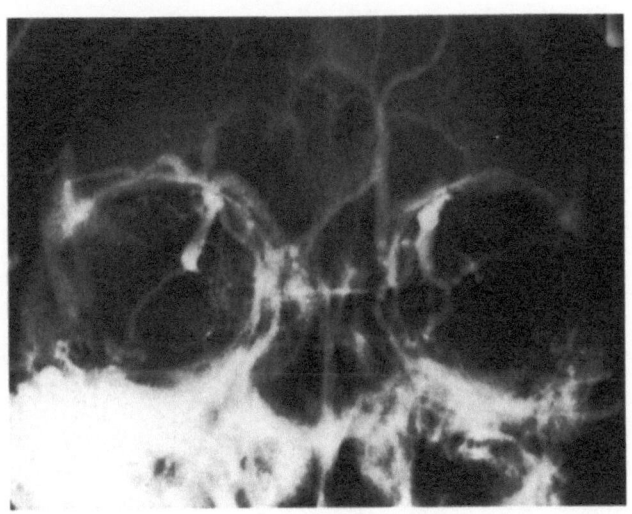

Fig. 6. Orbital veinography showing the displacement of the IIIrd segment. Note: stop of the contrast medium at the 2nd intersegmental angle of the right ophthalmic superior vein caused by a meningioma en plaque invading the right orbit

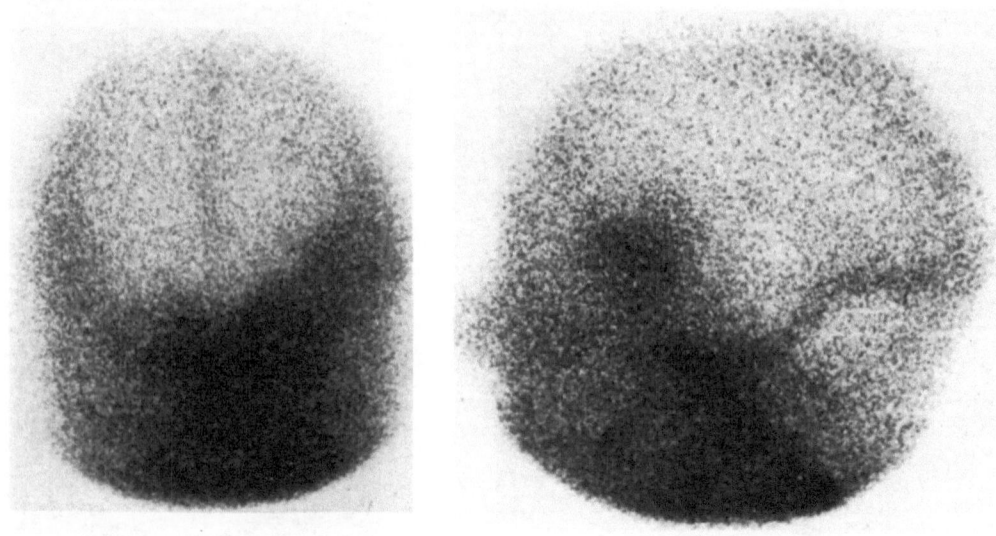

Fig. 7. Scintigraphy obtained from the scintillationcamera of a meningioma en plaque of the left sphenoidal wing, taken shortly following
application of the Tc-nucleotid
a) frontal view
b) lateral view

Problems in the Treatment of Basal Meningiomas

H. ARNOLD

Basal meningiomas represent a rather heterogenous group. Postoperative mortality depends on location and size of the tumor; generally it is rather high. Relapses are frequent. Microsurgical techniques and the development of better methods for repair of skull base defects have allowed neurosurgical procedures to be more radical. Radical tumor removal, however, still remains a problem. It is obvious, that meningiomas with close topographical relationship to carotid arteries or cavernous sinus present special difficulties in treatment.

Among a total of 231 basal meningiomas operated from 1949 - 1973 we selected a group of 64 tumors, which either had surrounded the carotid arteries partially or totally, or had invaded the cavernous sinus or its wall (cf. Table 1). This group includes meningiomas of the sellar region, of the deep or clinoidal third of the sphenoidal ridge, of the floor of the middle fossa, of the cavum Meckeli, of the pyramid, of the pontine angle, and of the clivus. Except for a few cases, all tumors originated from more than one of these structures.

Table 1. Number of medial meningiomas out of all basal meningiomas operated on from 1949 - 1973

Tumor site	Basal meningioma operations 1949 - 1973		"Medial" meningiomas 1949 - 1973
Olfactory groove	27		-
Optic sheath	3		-
Suprasellar region	33		6
Orbita roof	15		-
Sphenoidal ridge	99		
en globe		64	
en plaque		35	25
floor of the middle fossa cavum Meckeli, tentorial edge	25		19
Clivus	3		3
Pontine angle tentorium (basal, subtentorial)	26		11
Together	231		64

The operative results are discouraging (cf. Table 2). Of 47 patients
being operated upon in the years 1949 - 1968, 25 died postoperatively. From 1969 - 1973 there were 5 postoperative fatalities out of 17
cases. - Postoperative fatality means death in our department or in
an other hospital from any cause whatsoever following surgery, not
regarding the time elapsed between operation and death. Thus, of the
47 cases with "medial" meningiomas, only 18 were alive 5 years after
operation, 8 of them had recurrence of the tumor. Only 4 patients
were able to work and were selfsupporting.

Table 2. Operative mortality and five-year-results of "medial" meningiomas

	1949 - 1968	1969 - 1973
"Medial" meningiomas	47	17
Postoperative fatalities	25	5
Death within 5 years after operation	4	
Alive 5 years or more after operation	18	
Recurrences	8	
No evidence of reccurence	10	
Selfsupporting	4	

One question to be answered is whether or not our surgical technique
is to be held responsible for this disappointing outcome. A statistical survey of our entire case material of basal meningiomas (cf. Table 3), however, did not show any significant difference to other
follow-up studies (CUSHING and EISENHARDT, OLIVECRONA, TÖNNIES).

Table 3. Operative mortality and five-year-results of all basal meningiomas operated on from 1949 - -968

	1949 - 1968
Basal meningiomas	175
Postoperative fatalities	33 (18,9 %)
Death within 5 years after operation	27 (15,4 %)
Alive 5 years or more	115 (65,7 %)
Selfsupporting	49 (28,0 %)

Of a total of 175 patients, about 2/3 (115 patients) survived surgery
for 5 years or more.

If we separate the 47 "medial" meningiomas, the data of which are
summarized in Table 2, from our 175 cases we find a mortality rate of
6,3 % only for the remaining 128 patients (cf. Table 4). Of this group
75 % are alive 5 years following operation, half of them being able
to work.

Table 4. Operative results of basal meningiomas without topographical relationship to the carotid artery or the sinus cavernosus

	1949 - 1968
Basal meningiomas without "medial" tumors	128
Postoperative fatalities	8 (6,3 %)
Death within 5 years after operation	23 (18,0 %)
Alive 5 years or more after operation	97 (75,7 %)
Selfsupporting	45 (35,1 %)

Comparing these 128 cases with the 47 patients suffering from "medial" meningiomas the following conclusions can be drawn:

"Medial" meningiomas represent only 1/4 of the total group of basal meningiomas, however they account for 2/3 of the total postoperative mortality. Thus medial meningiomas are considered to be of extremely high operative risk. There are two principal ways to achieve improvement of their prognosis:

1. Better surgical technique. Introduction of microsurgery already reduced operative mortality in "medial meningiomas from 50 % to 30 % within the recent 5 years (cf. Table 2). This difference, however, is not significant due to the small number of operated cases.

2. Better separation of groups to be operated on or not. Reviewing the operations in 64 patients with "medial" meningiomas it was observed, that only 34 patients were operated on because of increased intracranial pressure, while 30 patients were operated on because of local symptoms, almost always cranial nerve palsy. 15 patients had meningiomas en plaque out of which 10 cases ended fatally after quite extensive but never radical operations.

Table 5. Indication for surgery in 64 "medial" meningiomas

Kind of Meningioma	Intracranial pressure	Focal neurological symptoms
En globe	34 (+ 17)	15 (+ 7)
En plaque	0	15 (+ 10)

Our impression is, that the decision to operate in the latter group should be done more carefully. Regarding the slow growth of meningiomas and present therapeutic possibilities, which rarely allow radical neurosurgical procedures in "medial" meningiomas en plaque, we conclude, that it is better not to operate on these patients in the first place, or to interrupt a procedure, once a situation has been surgically cleared. The diagnosis of a histologically benign meningioma is not in itself an indication for an operative procedure.

REFERENCES

1. CUSHING, H., EISENHARDT, L.: Meningiomas - their classification, regional behaviour, life history and surgical end results. N. Y. 1938, reprinted 1962.

2. OLIVECRONA, H.: The surgical treatment of intracranial tumors. In: Handbuch der Neurochirurgie, Bd. IV/4 (Hrsg. H. OLIVECRONA, W. TÖNNIS). Berlin - Göttingen - Heidelberg: Springer 1967.

3. TÖNNIS, W.: Diagnostik der intrakraniellen Geschwülste. Handbuch der Neurochirurgie, Bd. IV/3 (Hrsg. H. OLIVECRONA, W. TÖNNIS). Berlin - Göttingen - Heidelberg: Springer 1962.

"Micromeningiomas" of Cavum Meckeli

D. KIRCHHOFF

Introduction

Meningiomas of the cavum MECKELI were first described by CUSHING in 1920 and remained a rarity in the neurosurgical literature (2, 4, 6, 11, 15, 21, 27, 28). They produced so called symptomatic trigeminal neuralgia with a constant facial pain and less frequently, typical tic douloureux. There often is a sensory loss of the Vth nerve and usually the IIIrd, IVth and VIth cranial nerves are affected, sometimes the VIIth and the VIIIth nerves are involved (1, 2, 5, 7, 9, 15, 16, 22, 23, 26). "Micromeningiomas" which are limited to the cavum MECKELI are infrequent and can cause considerable diagnostic and therapeutic problems because their symptoms are difficult to differentiate from idiopathic trigeminal neuralgia.

The aim of this report is to present two cases of such tumors and to discuss the diagnostic and therapeutic problems.

Case Report

Case 1 - F. A. Case History 216/67:

62 old female patient, was admitted with a history of 2 episodes of episcleritis within the last two years, connected with constant burning and stabing pain of the left eye and orbita. She was symptomfree after subsidence of corneal inflammation. Two weeks after the last episode she started to complain about intermittent pain in the first division of the trigeminal nerve which had a character of tic douloureux and could be provoked by touching or pressing the left side of her face or by chewing and swallowing. Neurological examination, apart from revealing hyperaesthesia in the first division of the trigeminal nerve, was normal. Routine skull X-rays showed moderate ellargement and decalcification of the sella. Electroencephalography (EEG) revealed dysrhythmic waves in the right (contralateral) temporoparietal region. Special X-rays of the petrous bone, cerebral angiography and cerebro spinal fluid (CSF) examination were all normal. Local infiltration of the supra- and infra-orbital nerves and electrocoagulation of the GASSERIAN ganglion produce no sensory deficit and no pain relief. Exposure of the ganglion through the temporal extradural approach revealed a double, beansized meningioma, expanding diffusely between the nerve fibres (Fig. 1 b). The tumor and the ganglion were excised.

Case 2 - O. M. Case History 2913/60:

63 years old female patient, was admitted with a 6 years history of typical neuralgia of the third division on the right side. She had 3 electrocoagulations of the GASSERIAN ganglion in the past which re-

sulted in 1 1/2, 1 and 1/2 years pain free intervals respectively.
However, she has had no sensory loss in the face. Following the recurrence of pain after the last coagulation, two alcohol injections
were performed with no effect upon the pain. Complete anaesthesia in
the territory of the medial part of the third division was produced.
Because of recurrence of pain, this time also in the second division,
she was admitted to our department. Skull X-rays, EEG and CSF examination were normal. The neurological examination apart from the above
cited sensory loss, was entirely normal. The GASSERIAN ganglion was
exposed through the right temporal extradural approach. This revealed
the presence of a small meningioma of the cavum MECKELI which compressed the root, ganglion and its divisions against the petrous bone.
The tumor and the ganglion were excised.

Comment

In our series of 351 intracranial meningiomas, including one case of
a large meningioma of cavum MECKELI, we were able to find, only two
cases of so called "micromeningiomas". The incidence of these tumors
in patients presenting trigeminal neuralgia is also small. In our
series of 550 patients with trigeminal pain, there were 60 patients
with symptomatic neuralgia, out of this number, 20 proved to have an
intracranial space occupying lesion. Three of them were the above
mentioned meningiomas.

Literature data confirm the rarity of occurence of "micromeningiomas"
and the fact that they are usually discovered by coincidence (3, 4,
9, 12, 14, 15, 18). In a patient described by SACHS (19, 20) sensory
trigeminal loss followed one year after history of trigeminal neuralgia; in RAPPOPORTS (17) case, after 15 years history of trigeminal
neuralgia, sensory loss, facial weakness and ocular muscle paresis
developed. In the case reported by TÖNNIS (26) a small bone defect
of the petrous was found. Younger age of the patients, type of localization of the pain can sometimes direct the diagnosis towards symptomatic neuralgia.

The analysis of 9 adequately described cases in the literature (1, 4,
8, 10, 12, 13, 15, 18, 24, 26) to which we added our two own cases,
showed that 6 patients were younger than 50 years, two were aged between 50 and 60, and 3 were over 60 years old. Both sexes were equally
affected. 8 patients and probably another two mentioned by OLIVECRONA
(15) presented with a typical tic douloureux but in four of them
neuralgia changed gradually into a constant facial pain. 3 patients
exhibited atypical trigeminal neuralgia from the onset of their symptoms. Slight hyperaesthesia was recorded in two cases. None of the
patients reported had deficiency of the cranial nerves with the onset
of pain.

In 6 cases the pain was localized in the third trigeminal division
only, in the second and third division in 2 cases, in the first division, in the first and second, and in all three divisions in one
case respectively. No additional diagnostic criteria can be drawn
from the length of the history. It varied between 3 months and 6 years.
The anamnesis in cases of large meningiomas of cavum MECKELI is also
not longer and RAPPOPORTS case with 15 years history is an exception.
There were no abnormalities in the additional investigations which
were performed in these cases (25).

Apart from the above mentioned clinical data which could suggest
atypical or so called symptomatic neuralgia there are additional

Table 1. Cases of "micromeningiomas". In most cases these were casual findings
A Skull X-rays; B Angiography; C Encephalography; D Electroencephalography (EEG)

Author year of public.	Sex	Age	Symptom begin	pain typical	pain atypical	Localization	V Deficit	Other deficits	Auxillary examinations A B C D	Operation for	Histology	Casual findings
Frazier, C, H. 1918	o	53	3 M.	-	+	1. + 2. left	-	-	- - - -	Pain	Endothelioma	Yes
Love, J.G. et al. 1942	o	66	5 Years	+	-	2. + 3. right	-	-	- N - N	Pain	Meningioma	Yes
Rappoport, F. et al. 1932	o	40	16 years	-	+	3. left	After 15 years all 3 left	3, 6, 7 left after 15 years	+ N - N	Tumor	Meningioma	-
Mehta, D. S. et al. 1971	o	26	2 Years	+	-	3. right	-	-	- N N N	Pain	Cholestatoma	Yes
Sachs, B. et al. 1913	o	37	1 Year	-	+	2. + 3. left	After 1 year hypest. 2. + 3.	-	N - - -	Tumor	Meningioma	-
Verbrugghen, A. 1952	o	49	3 M.	+	-	3. left	-	-	N - - -	Pain	Meningioma	Yes
Olivecrona, H. 2 patients; 1959												Yes
Stammers, F.A.R. 1930	o	52	4 Years	+	+	1. + 2. + 3. right	-	-	N - - -	Pain	Meningioma	Yes
Russel, E. C. 1925	o	55	1,6 Years	+	+	3. left	-	-	N - - -	Pain	Endothelioma	Yes
Tönnis, W. 1961	o	22	1 Year	+	+	3. left	-	-	+ - - -	Tumor	Meningioma	-
Kirchhoff, D. 1974	o	63	6 Years	+	-	3. right	-	-	N - - -	Pain	Meningioma	Yes
	o	62	2 Years	+	+	1. left	Hyper-esthesia 1. left	-	+ N N +	Pain	Meningioma	Yes

factors which point to that diagnosis and which, after we have retrospectively analyzed our two cases, might have been of importance.
Failure to produce sensory deficit of one of our cases following three
electrocoagulations and two alcohol injections, should have suggested
a process localized laterally from the ganglion. Short lasting pain
relief without sensory loss and progressive involvement of other divisions of the trigeminal nerve are also of importance and should
evoke the suspicion of cavum MECKELI tumor.

X-ray changes by "micromeningiomas" of cavum MECKELI were described
only in one case published by TÖNNIS (26). One could presume that
routine tomography (25) of the petrous bone could have revealed discrete compressive lesions.

As far as treatment is concerned even a suspicion of a compressive
lesion of the cavum MECKELI should be an indication for exploration.

Summary

"Micromeningiomas" of the cavum MECKELI are an extreme rarity and
present, clinically, as typical trigeminal neuralgia over many years.
They are usually discovered by coincidence. The analysis of cases
described in the literature, to which two own cases are added, suggests
that changing character of the trigeminal pain, a progressive spreading of pain to another division as well as failure to produce anaesthesia by technically correct electrocoagulation should indicate the
possibility of the presence of a space occupying lesion located in
cavum MECKELI.

REFERENCES

1. ver BRUGGHEN, A.: Paragasserian Tumors. J. Neurosurg. 9, 451 -
   460 (1952).

2. CUSHING, H.: Meningiomas. New York: Hafner 1962.

3. FORTUNA, A., GAMBACORTA, D.: Cylindroma in the region of the
   Gasserian ganglion. J. Neurosurg. 34, 427 - 431 (1971).

4. FRAZIER, C. H.: An operable Tumor involving the Gasserian ganglion. Amer. J. med. Sci. 156, 483 - 490 (1918).

5. GIANI, R.: Über einen Fall von Endotheliom des Ganglion Gasseri.
   Mitt. Grenzgeb. Med. Chir. 19, 457 - 485 (1908).

6. HASSLER, R., WALKER, A. E. (eds.): Trigeminal Neuralgia. Stuttgart: Georg Thieme 1970.

7. HELLSTEIN, M.: Ein Fall von Ganglion Gasseri Tumor. Dtsch. Z.
   Nervenheilk. 52, 290 - 305 (1914).

8. HOFMEISTER, MEYER, E.: Operierter Tumor des Ganglion Gasseri.
   Arch. f. klin. Chir. 65, 206 - 222 (1902).

9. JACOBY, W.: Die Geschwülste des Ganglion Gasseri. Bruns Beitr.
   z. klin. Chir. 202, 160 - 189 (1961).

10. KREBS, M. E., RAPPOPORT, M. F., DAVID, M.: Méningeome de la gaine
    du Trigumeau. Rev. neurol. 6, 700 - 713 (1932).

11. LOEW, F., TÖNNIS, W.: Klinik und Behandlung der Neurinome des
    Nervus trigeminus. Zbl. Neurochir. 14, 32 - 41 (1954).

12. LOVE, J. G.: Trigeminal neuralgia and tumors of the Gasserian
    ganglion. Staff meetings of the Mayo Clinic 17, 490 - 496 (1942).

13. MEHTA, D. S., MALIK, G. B., PATH, M. C., DAR, J.: Trigeminal neu-
    ralgia due to cholesteatoma of MECKEL's cave. J. Neurosurg. 34,
    572 - 574 (1971).

14. MINGAZZINI, G.: Ein Fall von Meningeom des medianen Teiles der
    Schädelbasis. J. Psychol. Neurol. 37, 208 - 222 (1928).

15. OLIVECRONA, H.: The surgical treatment of intracranial tumors. In:
    Handbuch der Neurochirurgie (Hrsg. H. OLIVECRONA, W. TÖNNIS) Bd.
    IV/4, Berlin - Göttingen - Heidelberg: Springer 1967.

16. RAND, C. W.: Tumor of the left Gasserian ganglion. Surg. gynec.
    Obstet. 40, 49 , 54 (1925).

17. RAPPOPORT, F., DAVID, M.: Méningeome de la gaine du trigumeau.
    Ablation. Guérison. Discussion du diagnostic et des indications
    opératoires dans les cas d'atteinte organique de la cinquième
    paire. Rev. neurol. 2, 700 - 713 (1932).

18. RUSSEL, E. C.: Two primary tumors of the Gasserian ganglion.
    J. A. M. A. 84, 413 - 415 (1925).

19. SACHS, B., BERG, A. A.: Operative Heilung einer Geschwulst des
    Ganglion Gasseri. Berliner klin. Wschr. 80, 1395 - 1396 (1918).

20. SACHS, E.: Tumors of the Gasserian ganglion. Ann. Surg. 66, 152 -
    159 (1917).

21. SEEGER, W.: Trigeminusneuralgie bei raumfordernden intrakraniel-
    len Prozessen. Zbl. Neurochir. 23, 152 - 165 (1973).

22. SHELDEN, W. D.: Tumors involving the Gasserian ganglion. J.A.M.A.
    77, 700 - 705 (1921).

23. SPILLER, W. G.: Tumor of the Gasserian ganglion. Amer. J. med.
    Sci. 86, 712 - 725 (1908).

24. STAMMERS, F. A. R.: A study of tumors and inflammations of the
    Gasserian ganglion. Brit. J. Surg. 18, 125 - 153 (1930).

25. TÄNZER, A., DIECKMANN, H.: Die Bedeutung der Tomographie im Be-
    reich der Schädelbasis für die Tumordiagnostik. Dtsch. Z. Nerven-
    heilk. 178, 1 - 20 (1958).

26. TÖNNIS, W.: Die Trigeminusneuralgie in ihrer symptomatischen Be-
    deutung. Zbl. Neurochir. 21, 152 - 157 (1961).

27. UMBACH, W.: Differentialdiagnose und Therapie der Gesichtsneural-
    gien. Stuttgart: Georg Thieme 1960.

28. WEBER, E.: Zur Problematik der Trigeminus-Neuralgie. Nervenarzt
    31, 88 - 91 (1960).

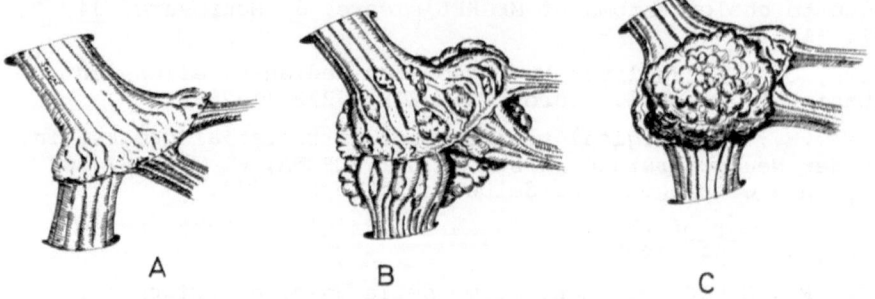

Fig. 1. A Normal ganglion Gasseri
        B The meningioma (our first case) grows through the "loose"
          fibres of the ganglion
        C The tumor adhere on the ganglion Gasseri, which is com-
          pressed against the petrous bone (our second case)

Meningioma of the Middle Cranial Fossa and Epidermoid of the Clivus and Cerebellopontine Angle in the Same Patient

G. Thomalske and W. Galow

Introduction

Multiple tumors of the CNS in humans more frequently occur than generally accepted. Most often tumors of the CNS are found with neoplasms outside the CNS (2, 5, 10, 11, 12, 17, 19, 34, 35, 40, 42).

Less often tumors of the same histological type are found in the CNS (14, 16, 23, 25, 27, 30, 32, 37, 38, 41) and even more rarely histologically different neoplasms of the CNS occur in the same patient.

Our knowledge of the literature points to the following sequence in decreasing frequency of the different combinations of mulitple CNS-tumors:

1. Combination of a benign with a malignant neoplasm (1, 1 a, 3, 6, 7, 8, 13, 15, 18, 18 a, 20, 22, 24, 26, 28, 31 a, 35, 39, 42).

2. Double occurrence of malignant tumors of different histological type (4, 16 a, 28, 33, 36) - and finally

3. Combination of two benign tumor types (9, 21, 29, 38 a).

The combination of a meningioma with an epidermoid has not been reported in the literature (31, 42, 43). That is the reason to report our case:

Case Report

Medical history of this female patient aged 38 1/2 years at the time of operation was negative except for tonsillectomy and operation for gastric ulcer perforation. Two sons aged 4 and 13 years. Two years before hospital admission progressive gait disturbance, vertigo, pricking pain in the left orbital region. 1 1/2 years before admission she developed tinnitus followed by progressive impairment of hearing on the left. Two months before admission to the hospital patient was no longer able to leave her house because of marked gait disturbance: Tendency to fall to the left with double vision and tic douloureux on the left.

Findings on Admission

Psychical State: Conscious, well orientated. Suffers from aspontaneity, affective lability and irritability.

General Physical Findings: Good general condition without particularities besides scar after gastric ulcer operation.

Neurological Findings

Nystagmus, no papilledema, deafness on the left; possible slight diminution of left corneal reflex, hypesthesia in the left trigeminal region, left symptomatic V-Neuralgia, right mimic facial paresis, pronounced cerebellar ataxia with gait deviation and tendency to fall to the left; left ataxia of extremities.

E. N. T. Findings: Left deafness. Changing findings on vestibular exploration: Virgorous spontaneous nystagmus, more to the right at straight gaze. Left labyrinth seems to react still to caloric excitation.

CSF: 2/3 lymphocytes, 5/3 segmented cells, 19,4 mg % total protein, normal normo-mastix reaction. -

Laboratory Findings: Normal.

EEG: Normal

ECG: Regular sinus rhythm, indifferent type, slight disturbance of repolarisation.

X-Ray Findings: Skull in 3 planes and chest-X-ray: Without abnormality.

STENVERS and tomogram of petrous bones: Questionable decalcification of the tip of left petrous bone and of left tuberculum jugulare.

Left Carotid Angiogram (Via Femoral Catheter)[1]: Space occupying lesion medial to the left occipital and temporal lobe and displacing the left posterior cerebral artery upwards (Fig. 1). -

Left Vertebral Angiogram: Displacement of basilar artery and cerebellar post. inf. artery indicating left-sided, more rostrally located infratentorial space occupying lesion (Fig. 2).

Pneumencephalogram[2]: Big, lobulated extracerebral and possibly partially intracerebral space occupying lesion extending from lateral parts of IVth ventricle through cerebellopontine angle up to the supra-tentorial region, displacing the temporal lobe laterally and upwards (Figs. 2, 4 and 5).

Operation, June 4th, 1973

Left temporo-occipital craniotomy. Strong tension of dura mater. Resection of lower parts of the temporal lobe down from T3 extending 8 cm back from the tip of temporal lobe uncovers a *Meningioma*, 4 x 3 x 3 cm in size arising from the tip of the petrous bone and reaching to the free edge of tentorium cerebelli. Total removal. Lobulated, nacreous masses, typical of *Epidermoid* appear in the tentorial incisure.

Incision of the tentorium cerebelli and successive removal of the epidermoid masses, extending far caudally on the clivus and contralaterally beyond right N. VIII. Under control of operation microscope, con-

---

[1]Zentrum der Radiologie, Prof. Dr. A. GEBAUER, Klinikum der Johann-Wolfgang-Goethe Universität Frankfurt/Main.

[2]Neuroradiologische Abteilung, Zentrum der Radiologie, Prof. Dr. H. HACKER, Klinikum der Johann-Wolfgang-Goethe-Universität Frankfurt/M.

siderable amount material was removed, especially from the clivus and left cerebello-pontine angle. Parts of the thin capsule of the tumor had to be left on the brain stem surface in order to prevent damage to superficial brain stem vessels. Decompression was effected by left lateral ventricle drainage.

Histology[3]

1. Fibromatous meningioma with many collagenous fibers.
2. Epidermoid cyst.

Postoperative Course: Patient awoke immediately after surgery. Slight bulbar speech, swallowing disturbance, tic douloureux triggered by swallowing.

First days feeding by gastric tube. Primary healing. No hyperpyrexia. Oral feeding from 10th day postop.

Began to walk from 12th day postop.

CSF Examination (June 28th, 1973): 16/3 lymphocytes, 4/3 segmented cells, 20,0 mg % total protein.

EEG 4 Weeks Postop: No general disturbance. Local anomalies over the left temporal region with slow waves in theta and rarely in delta frequency, moderately activated by hyperventilation with appearance of some dispersed sharp waves. Anomalies limited to operated region.

Discharge from Hospital: 5 weeks postop.

Findings 1 Year Postop: Subjectively well. Slightly unsteady gait with tendency to walk to the left. Plays again piano. No more V-neuralgia. No fits. (Medication: 5 x 1 Tegretol and 1 x Valium 5 in the evening).

Neurologically: Fine nystagmus on looking to the right and coarse nystagmus on looking to the left. Latent heterophory, double vision on downward gaze.

Hypesthesia in left V-area. V-motor function intact. Right mimic VII-paresis. Left deafness. Soft tissues in trepanation defect without tension. Slight ataxia of left extremities. Abdominal reflexes absent.

EEG: General non-specific changes and theta and rare delta in the left parieto-temporal region with some sharps in phasic opposition. Slight activation by hyperpnea with minimal diffusion to the contra-lateral side.

In comparison with last the EEG record slight diminution of irritative character of anomalies.

Summary

Report on a 38 1/2 year old female patient with a meningioma of the middle cranial fossa and an epidermoid of the clivus and cerebello-pontine angle.

The operation consisted of total removal of the meningioma and sub-total removal of the epidermoid leaving a portion of that part of the

---

[3]Max-Planck-Institut für Hirnforschung, Prof. Dr. W. KRÜCKE, Frank-
  furt/Main.

capsule attached to the brain stem. Description of pre- and postoperative course. Summary of bibliography of multiple CNS-tumors.

REFERENCES

1. ADAM-FALKIEWICZ, St.: Zwei Geschwülste verschiedenen Baues und von verschiedener Entstehungszeit im gleichen Gehirn. Polska Gaz. lek. 867, 1936.

1a. BANERJEE, A. K., BLACKWOOD, W.: A Subfrontal Tumor with the Features of Plasmocytoma and Meningioma. Acta Neuropath. (Berlin) 18, 84 (1971).

2. BANKL, H., GRUNERT, V., SUNDER-PLASSMANN, M.: Endokrine Polyadenomatose kombiniert mit einem Tentoriummeningeom. Wiener klin. Wschr. 82, 257 - 259 (1970).

3. BRIHAYE, J., DANIS, P., DROCHMANS, P.: Tumeur cérébrale multiple avec syndrome de Foster Kennedy: Gliomes du corps calleux et du lobe temporal, meningiome du nerf optique. Acta neurol. et psychiatr. belg. 51, 35 - 55 (1951).

4. BASTIAN, F. O., PARKER Jr., J. C.: A Rare Combination of Multicentric Gliomas: A Problem of Interpretation. Am. J. Clin. Pathol. 54, 839 - 844 (1970).

5. BAUGHMAN, F. A. Jr., LIST, C. F., WILLIAMS, J. R., MULDOON, J. P., SEGARRA, J. M., VOLKEL, J. S.: The Glioma-Polyposis Syndrome. New Engl. J. Med. 281, 1345 - 1346 (1969).

6. BELZA, J.: Double Midline Intracranial Tumors of Vestigial Origin: Contiguous Intrasellar Chordoma and Suprasellar Craniopharyngioma. Case Report. J. Neurosurg. 25, 199 - 204 (1966).

7. BINGAS, B., BRUNNGRABER, C.: Das gleichzeitige Vorkommen von Meningeom und Glioblastom. Zbl. Neurochir. 24, 271 - 275 (1964).

8. BOUCHARD, G.: Mehrfachtumoren in Hypophyse, Schläfenlappen und Lunge. In: BUSHE, K.-A. (ed.): Fortschritte auf dem Gebiet der Neurochirurgie, S. 272 - 276. Stuttgart: Hippokrates 1970.

9. BOUDIN, G., et al.: Les tumeurs multiples du système nerveux au cours de la maladie de Recklinghausen. A propos d'une observation anatomo-clinique avec adénome chromophobe de l'hypophyse. Presse Med. 78, 1427 (1970).

10. CHAPMAN, R. C., KEMP, V. E., TALIAFERRO, I.: Pheochromocytoma Associated with Multiple Neurofibromatosis and Intracranial Hemangioma. Amer. J. Med. 26, 883 - 890 (1959).

11. CHAPMAN, R. C., DIAZ-PEREZ, R.: Pheochromocytoma Associated with Cerebellar Hemangioblastoma - Familial Occurrence. J. Amer. med. Ass. 182, 1014 - 1017 (1962).

12. COLEY, G. M., OTIS, R. D., CLARK, W. E.: Multiple Primary Tumors Including Bilateral Breast Cancers in a Man with Klinefelter's Syndrome - Cancer 27, 1476 - 1481 (1971).

13. COOPER, D. R.: Contiguous Meningioma and Astrocytoma in Brain. N. Y. J. Med. 69, 969 - 972 (1969).

14. COURVILLE, C. B.: Multiple Primary Tumors of the Brain. Review of the Literature and Report of 21 Cases. Amer. J. Cancer Res. 26, 703 - 731 (1936).

15. COURVILLE, C. B.: Primary Intracranial Tumors of Multicentric Origin. Bull. Los Angeles Neurol. Soc. 2, 26 - 30 (1937).

16. COURVILLE, C. B.: Multiple Gliomas of Right Frontal Lobe. Bull. Los Angeles Neurol. Soc. 1, 62 - 64 (1936).

16a. COURVILLE, C., EDMONDSON, H. A.: Relationship of Cranial Two Subjacent Cerebral Tumors; Report of a Case of Fibrosarkoma Eroding Frontal Bone Associated with Underlying Glioblastoma Multiforme. Bull. Los Angeles Neurol. Soc. 18, 103 - 109 (1953).

17. FARNSWORTH, J.: Regressing Melanoma Metastasizing to an Oligodendroglioma. Pathology 4, 253 - 7 (1972).

18. FEIRING, E. H., DAVIDOFF, L. M.: Two Tumors Meningioma and Glioblastoma Multiforme, in One Patient. J. Neurosurg. 4, 283 (1947).

18a. FENYES, G., KEPES, J.: Über das gemeinsame Vorkommen von Meningeomen und Geschwülsten anderen Types im Gehirn. Zbl. Neurochir. 16, 251 - 260 (1956).

19. FILIPPOVA, L. A.: Case of Chronic Lympholeukosis Complicated by Meningioma, Kidney Adenoma and Hypernephroid Carcinoma. ARKH Patol. 35, 72 - 4 (1973).

20. FISHER, R. G.: Intracranial Meningioma Followed by a Malignant Glioma: Case Report. J. Neurosurg. 29, 83 - 86 (1968).

21. HOFFMAN, E. P., SHELDEN, C. H., MILLER, A., KOEHLER, A. L.: Chromophobe Adenoma of Pituitary with Acromegaly and Acoustic Neurinoma Occurring in the Same Patient. A Case Report and Review of the Literature. Bull. Los Angeles Neurol. Soc. 38, 37 - 45 (1973).

22. HOSOI, K.: Meningiomas, with Special Reference to the Multiple Intracranial Type. Amer. J. Path. 6, 245 - 260 (1930).

23. JIMENEZ, J. P., GOREE, J. A., PARKER, Jr., J. C.: An Unusual Association of Multiple Meningiomas, Intracranial Aneurysm, and Cerebrovascular Atherosclerosis in Two Young Women. Am. J. Roentgenol. Radium Ther. Nucl. Med. 112, 281 - 8 (1971).

24. KIRSCHBAUM, W. R.: Intrasellar Meningioma and Multiple Cerebral Glioblastomas. J. Neuropath. 4, 370 (1945).

25. MACIAS SANCHEZ, R., SANCHEZ-CABRERA, J. M., DE LA CUEVY, H. C., ORDONEZ MARTINEZ, S.: Caso clinico. Neurofibromatosis Multiple Intracraneana y intrarraquidea. Arch. Invest. Med. (Mex.) 3, 55 - 62 (1972).

26. McCORMICK, W. F., MENEZES, A. H., GRINOD, J. R.: Meningioma Occurring in a Patient Treated for Medulloblastoma. J. Iowa Med. Soc. 62, 67 - 71 (1972).

27. MINAUF, M., SUMMER, K.: Primäre Melanoblastose der Leptomeningen. Wien. Z. Nervenheilkd. 30, 150 - 7 (1972).

28. NASTASI, G., FILIZZOLO, F., MORELLO, A.: Le neoplasie encefaliche multiple e di diversa linea germanativa. Acta Neurol. (Napoli) 27, 622 - 31 (1972).

29. PROBST, A.: Kombination eines Cushing-Syndroms, Hypophysenadenoms und suprasellären Meningeomes. Fallbericht. Zbl. Neurochir. 32, 75 (1971).

30. REGAN, T. J., FREIMAN, I. S.: Multiple Cerebral Gliomas in Multiple Sclerosis. J. Neurol. Neurosurg. Psychiatry 36, 523 - 8 (1973).

31. RUSSELL, D. S., RUBINSTEIN, L. J.: Pathology of Tumors of the Nervous System. 3. Auflage. London: Arnold 1971.

31a. SCHULZE, A.: Histologisch differente multiple Hirntumoren. Acta Neurochir., Suppl. VI, 219 - 226 (1959).

32. SEDZIMIR, C. B., FRAZER, A. K., ROBERTS, J. R.: Cranial and Spinal Meningiomas in a Pair of Identical Twin Boys. J. Neurol. Neurosurg. Psychiatry 36, 368 - 76 (1973).

33. SHUANGSHOTI, S.: Neoplasm of Mixed Mesenchymal and Neuroepithelial Origin: Liposarcomatous Meningioma Combined with Gliomas. J. Neurol. Neurosurg. Psychiat. 36, 377 - 382 (1973).

34. SKRZYPCZAK, J.: Neurofibromatosis Recklinghausen mit Phaeochromozytom des Nebennierenmarks und Großhirnspongioblastom. Dtsch. Gesundheitsw. 26, 2173 - 5 (1971).

35. SORENSON, B. F.: Multiple Primary Tumors of the Brain and Bowel. Case Report. J. Neurosurg. 36, 93 - 96 (1972).

36. STARODUBTSEV, A. I., IURCHENKO, P. T.: A Combination of Arachnoendothelioma and Glioblastoma Multiforme of the Braina. VOPR NEIROKHIR 34, 55 - 6 (1970).

37. WAGA, S., MATSUDA, M., HANDA, H., MATSUSHIMA, M., ANDO, K.: Multiple Meningiomas. Report of Four Cases. J. Neurosurg. 37, 348 - 51 (1972).

38. WAHL, R. W., DILLARD, S. H. Jr.: Multiple Ganglioneuromas of the Central Nervous System. Arch. Pathol. 94, 158 - 64 (1972).

38a. WILD, K. v., RUF, H.: Diagnostic Problems and Errors in Suprasellar Meningiomas. In: Modern Aspects of Neurosurgery, Vol. IV, p. 43 - 47. Amsterdam: Excerpta Medica 1972.

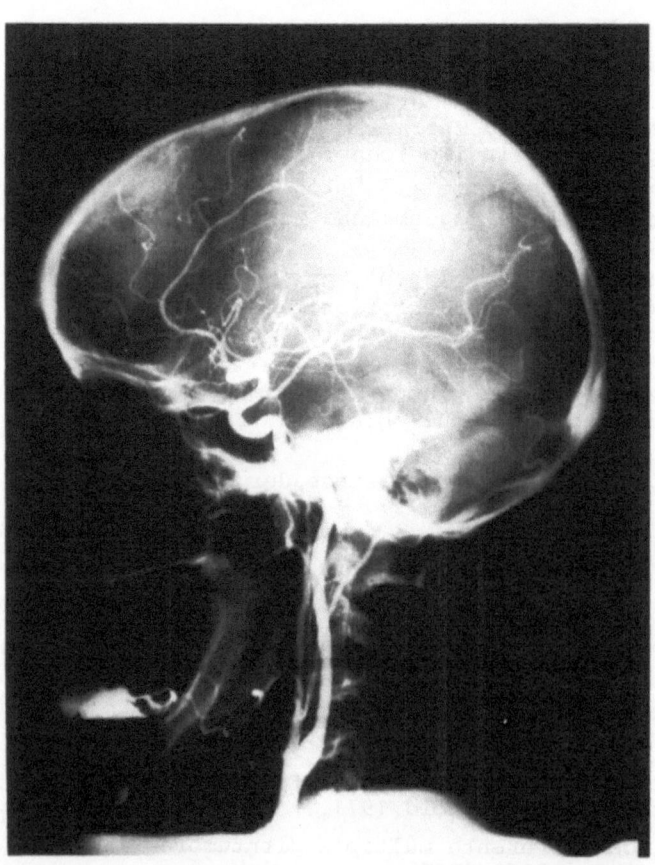

Fig. 1. Lateral view of left carotid angiogram showing lifted posterior cerebral artery

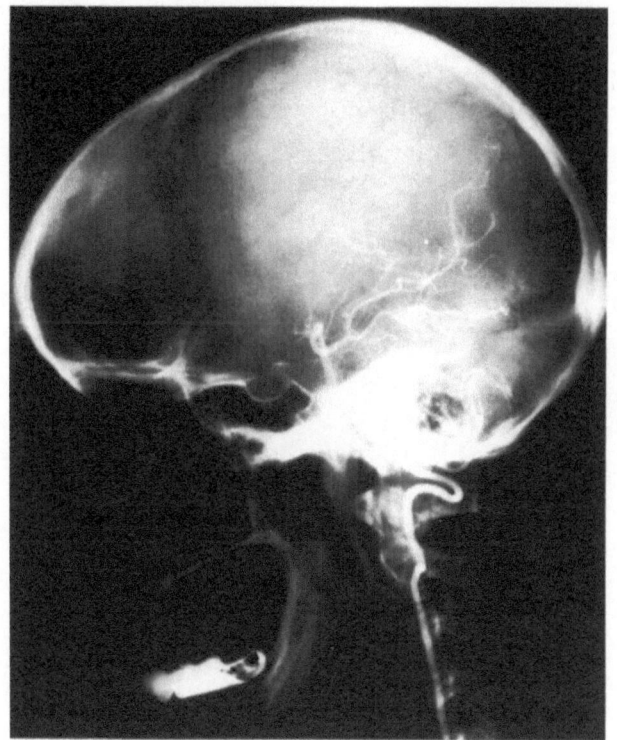

Fig. 2. Lateral view
of left vertebral
angiogram showing
upper part of basilar
artery displaced
backwards, cerebellar
posterior inf. artery
displaced downwards.
Normal course of
right posterior cere-
bral artery

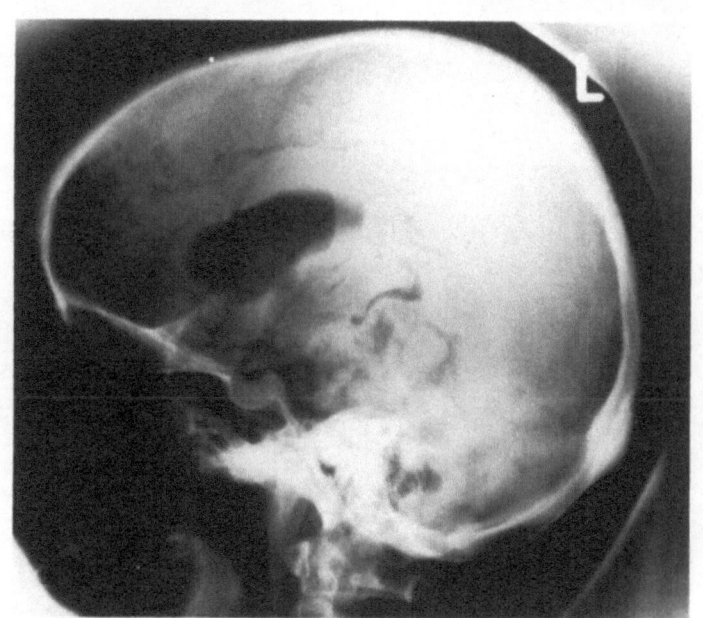

Fig. 3. Lateral view of PEG with upward displaced of ambient cistern
and typical lobulated air distribution around backwards displaced
brain stem

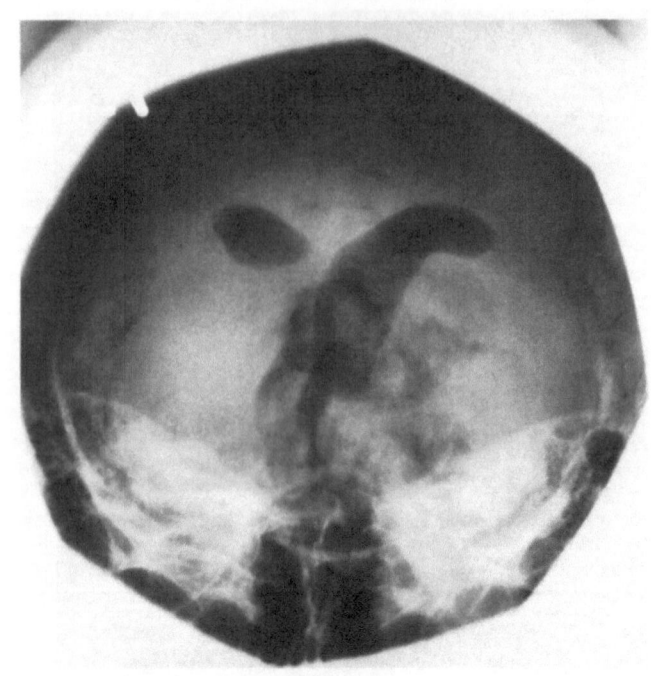

Fig. 4. A. p. oblique
view of PEG: Lobulated
design of retropyramidal
masses. Upper part of IV
ventricle, displaced to
the contralateral side

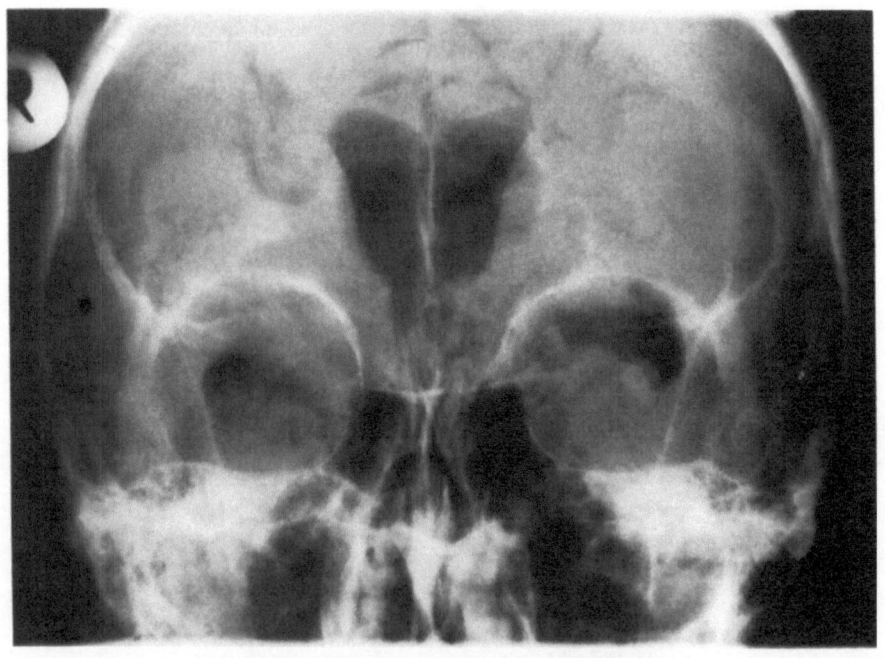

Fig. 5. A. p. view of PEG: Dilated left temporal horn, lifted upwards

Meningiomas of the Left (Dominant) Temporal Region – Catamneses

K. E. Richard

Temporal meningiomas of the dominant hemisphere require special attention, because the speech disorders that are typical of this localization in connection with other sequels, e. g. hemipareses, attacks and disorders of sight, prejudice the patient's lives completely and especially drastically.

Patients: Between 1951 and 1973, 116 patients with meningiomas in the temporal region received surgical treatment. The present study is based on the catamneses of 40 surviving patients out of a group of 64 patients with meningiomas of the dominant, mostly left-sided temporal region.

According to the well-known CUSHING classification, meningiomas in these patients were found (Fig. 1)

- on the temporal convexity: 4 patients
- on the outer third of the wing of sphenoid: 10 patients
- on the middle third of the wing of sphenoid: 7 patients
- on the inner third of the wing of sphenoid: 5 patients
- on the base of fossa media: 4 patients
- bone infiltrating, "en-plaque" like from
  temporal bone and roof of orbit: 10 patients

Facts about the present state of the patients were obtained either by O.P.D. follow-up examinations or by questionnaires sent to them.

Results (Fig. 2): At the time this compilation was done, which was at the end of August 1974, 32 (= 80 %) out of 40 patients were still alive. 3 patients (= 7,5 %) had died.

One patient, 62 years old, 11 years after her first operation and 1 year after operation of a recurrence; one patient, 41 years old, 1 year after partial extirpation of meningioma situated on the middle base of the skull with circumgrowth of A. carotis interna; one 73-year-old patient, 15 years after total resection of an "en plaque" meningioma of a carcinoma of the postate.

5 patients (= 12,5 %) gave no reply: two of these had been fully fit to work when having their last follow-up examination, two had been disabled and one 60-year-old patient had been completely unfit for work.

The average duration of all catamneses is 10.5 years with a maximum of 23 years and a minimum of 1 year.

13 patients (= 32 %) (Fig. 3) did not show any trouble or neurological sequels at the time of their last examination. These and 2 further patients with head-ache and abducens pareses, i. e. a total of 15 pa-

tients (= 37.5 %) were considered to be completely fit to work. 16 patients (= 40 %) were considered to be partially fit to work and 9 patients (= 22.5 %) were unfit for work.

13 patients had suffered from pre-operative *speech disorders* (Fig. 4).
In 7 patients these disturbances did not disappear completely, 6 of
them remained handicapped by further residual disturbances such as
brachial hemipareses, attacks, occulomotor pareses with double vision,
so that 5 of them remained unfit for work and only 2 were partially
fit to work. Meningiomas which had developed near the fissura Sylvii
caused persistent disorders of speech more frequently (5/14) than
"en globe" meningiomas of other localizations (2/16). No disorders
of speech were to be observed with mere "en plaque" meningiomas.

Pre-operative hemipareses that were strikingly frequent in our patients disappeared in only 50 % of the cases after operation. In connection with disorders of speech (4 patients), ocular muscle pareses
(2 patients), attacks (2 patients) or trigeminal neuralgia, they presented such a severe defective syndrome that these patients either
regained their working capacity only partially (4 patients) or remained unfit for work (4 patients).

7 patients remained more or less severely handicapped by *attacks*.
4 of these showed additional neurological sequels and remained unfit
for work.

Persistent *ocular muscle pareses* (mostly abducens pareses) with double
vision prejudiced the working capacity only in such cases where combined with further sequels.

Progressing *loss of vision* reduced the working capacity in 5 patients
with bone infiltrating sphenoid meningiomas considerably. 3 patients
remained unfit for work because of simultaneously occurring persistent
therapy-resistent facial neuralgias.

Discussion

Apart from the degree of tumor dependent brain lesions, catamnestic
results are dependent on

1st the extent of tumor resection, and
2nd the age of the patient at the time of operation.

1st: Extent of Tumor Resection: in 30 surviving patients with "en
globe" meningiomas the tumor had been totally extirpated macroscopically in 28 of the cases (= 90 %) (Fig. 5). Only 2 patients, whose A.
carotis at the base of the skull had been circumgrown by the meningioma, could not be completely relieved from the tumor. During the
time they survived, 5 and 1 year respectively, these patients remained disabled and unfit for work respectively. Bone infiltrating
"en plaque" meningiomas, however, could only be extirpated in 2 patients. Only these 2 patients regained their full working capacity.

In the number of patients of CUSHING (1) (Fig. 5) there is a considerably lower number of totally extirpated meningiomas of this localization. Surgical death rate of these patients was lower, but their
catamneses show a higher percentage of persistent disorders of speech
and, accordingly, a relatively higher number (= 50 %) of patients unfit for work.

2nd: The Age at the Time of Operation: This could be much lower in many patients, if diagnoses were found as soon as the first symptoms of brain tumor show (3). The localization-specific disorder of speech is of minor importance in this respect, as it is distinctly a late symptom.

Comparison of medium age levels at time of operation (Fig. 3) shows that those patients who regained their working capacity had, at the time of operation, been about 4 - 5 years younger than those who remained partially fit to work or completely unfit. As, on the other hand, brain tumor specific symptoms had shown much earlier in those patients, who remained unfit for work than in the ones, who regained their full or partial working capacity, diagnosis could have been found at a younger age of these patients. Especially in cases of bone infiltrating meningiomas, early diagnosis and extent of the possible tumor resection are closely linked, which was pointed out especially by GUIOT and co-workers (2) recently.

The chance of a complete prevention of specific defective syndromes of the dominant temporal lobe - disorders of speech with hemipareses or focal attacks, etc. - by early diagnosis and surgical treatment seems to be more limited; patients who recovered from the specific temporal lobe syndromes (N = 6) were more or less 15 years younger ($\bar{x}$ = 37 years) than those with persistent disorders of speech (N = 7; $\bar{x}$ = 52 years). Brain tumor symptoms in these patients would have allowed diagnosis only about 1.7 years earlier.

The age at the time of operation is, thus, a factor of decisive importance for the reversibility of temporal lobe syndromes. Complete reversibility can generally be expected only in patients with manifestation of the disease and operation at an early age.

Summary

Catamneses of 40 patients with meningiomas of the dominant temporal brain region out of a total of 116 patients with temporal meningiomas are being discussed. Reversibility of dominant temporal lobe specific defective syndromes as well as working capacity are closely linked with age of patient at the time of operation and extent of tumor resection.

REFERENCES

1. CUSHING, H.: Meningiomas, their classification, regional behaviour, life history, and surgical end results. Vo. I, pp. 298 - 387. Vol. II, pp. 338 - 403. New York: Hafner 1962.

2. GUIOT, G., TESSIER, P., GODON, A.: Faut-il opérer les méningeomes en plaque de l'arête sphénoidale? Min. Neurochir. 14, 293 - 304 (1970).

3. RICHARD, K. E., FROWEIN, R. A., FRIEDMANN, G.: Temporale Meningeome. Zbl. Neurochir. 29, 109 - 129 (1968).

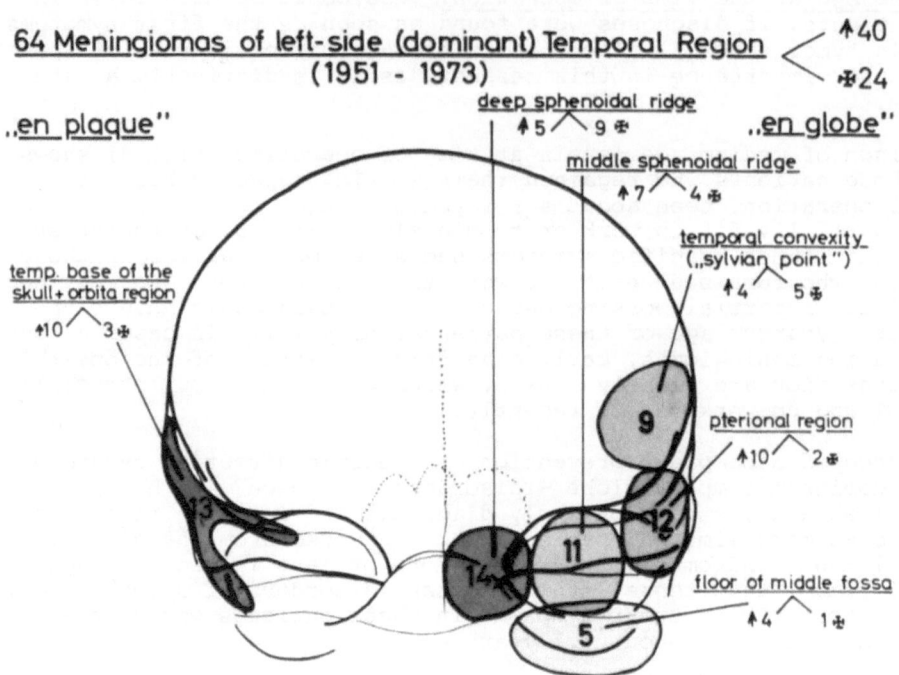

Fig. 1. Frequency and Distribution of 64 surviving (N = 40) and dead (N = 24) patients with meningiomas of the left dominant temporal region

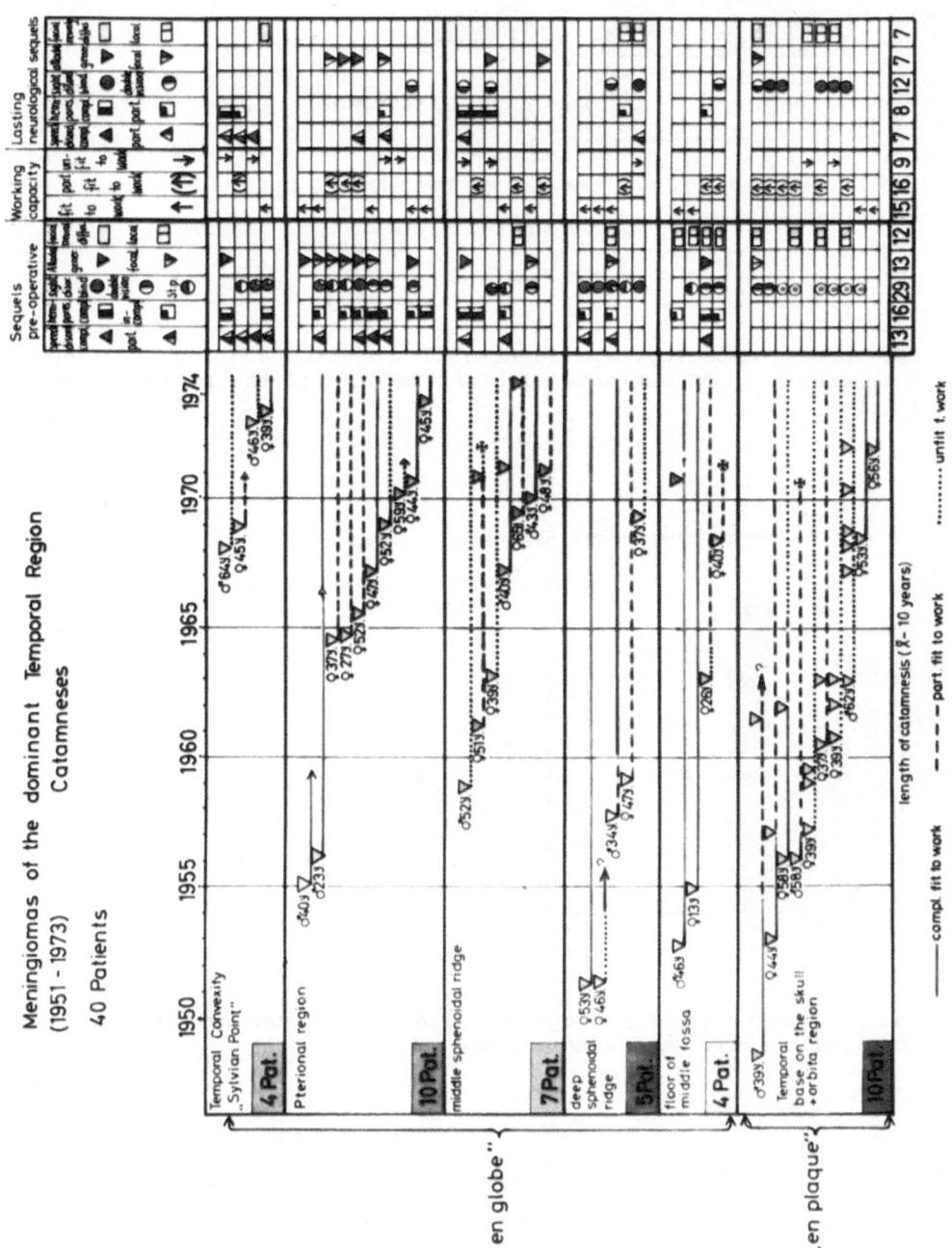

Fig. 2. Length of Catamnesis, pre-operative sequels, persistent defective syndromes and working capacity of 40 patients with meningiomas of the dominant temporal region

97

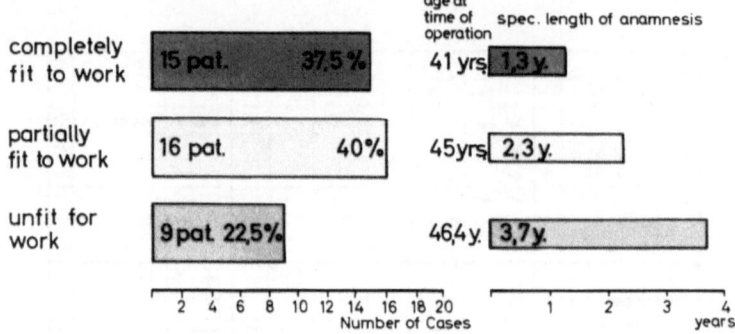

Fig. 3. Working capacity, age at time of operation and length of specific anamnesis in 40 patients with meningiomas of the dominant temporal lobe

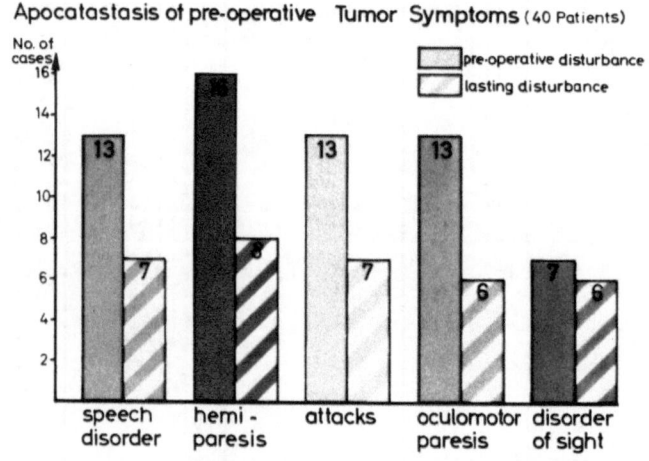

Fig. 4. Reversibility of pre-operative brain symptoms in 40 patients
with meningiomas of the dominant temporal lobe

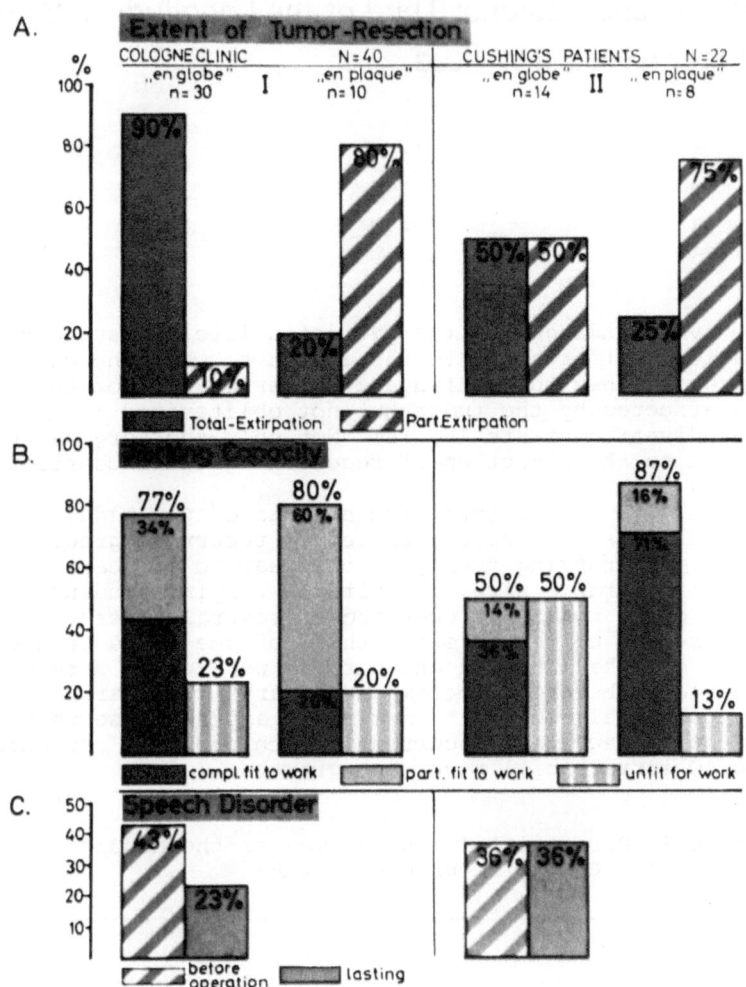

Fig. 5. Extent of tumor resection (A), working capacity (B) and relative frequency of persistent disorders of speech (C) in patients
with meningiomas of the dominant temporal region
 I. Own patients (N = 40)
II. CUSHING's patients (N = 22)

Recidivation and Possibilities of Surgery in Meningiomas of the Middle and Posterior Third of the Longitudinal Sinus

K. HARTMANN and W. KLUG

To avoid endangering the patient's life the surgeon must accept limitations with respect to the extent to which he can go when performing surgery, when the median and posterior part of the longitudinal sinus is affected by the tumor but not obliterated (1). The possibility of recidivation exists (6, 16). Not only the surgical procedure itself but also the detection of recurrent growths constitute problems (12).

Of the 112 parasagittal meningiomas of the middle and posterior sinus, in nine cases we have operated on recurrent growths (Table 1) after intervals ranging from just one year to 16 years. They were in part of considerable size, exhibited a varying tendency to grow, and in some cases had to be operated on several times (12, 13, 15, 16). In the region of the anterior third of the sinus we have seen no recurrent growths (15). In one patient we excised a recurrent growth in the galea before it became necessary, two years later, to remove an intracranial recurrent growth. In another case we had to operate twice on an intracranial recurrent growth, so that our experience extends to 10 intracranial recurrent growths.

Table 1. Parasagittal Meningiomas of the Middle and Posterior Sinus Thirds 112 Cases. Recurrent Growths

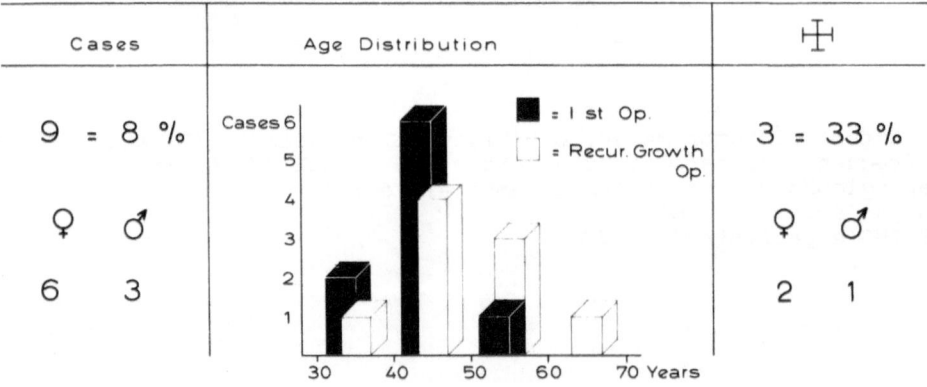

The ratio of 2 : 1 for the six females and three males affected reflects the distribution of all our 131 parasagittal meningiomas.

While in 2/3 of the cases (Table 2) no malignity was demonstrated histologically, transitional malignant forms were described for the three remaining cases (16). This concerned the case with the shortest interval, which was also clinically characterized by malignancy, but also concerned the case with the longest interval.

Table 2. Intervals Precedg. Recur. Growth Op. (= R)

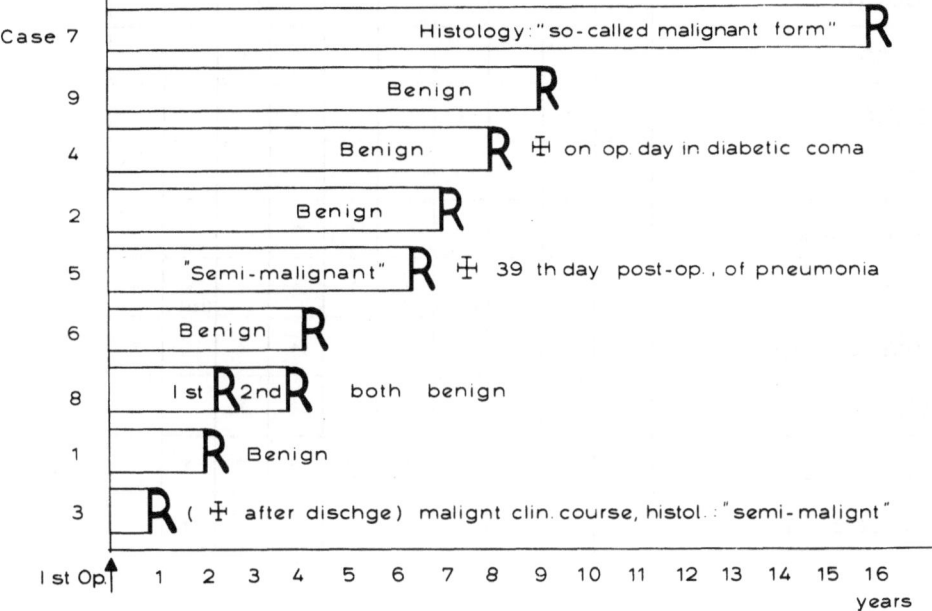

The recurrent growths (Table 3) manifested themselves principally by fits and pareses. The problems lie, however, in the evaluation of these clinical symptoms, which makes it difficult for the recurrent growths to be detected. Fits and pareses - partly of the apoplectic type - occurred in individual cases even years before the recidivation was detected (Table 4).

On the other hand, the diagnosis of "bloodflow disorders" or "adhesions" was made only a short while before the detection of the recurrent growth actually present. This happened to us in Case 9, a female, in whom Jacksonian attacks without loss of consciousness, followed by pareses 2 1/2 years after the first operation and 6 1/2 years before the recurrent growth was operated on, were interpreted as sequelae of bloodflow disorders, with the anterior cerebral artery in middle position and a slightly bowed downward displacement of the arteria pericallosa. Also, when the same patient came to be re-examined on account of increased frequency of fits - this time (seven years after the first operation and two years prior to the operation on the recurrent growth) with loss of cinsciousness - adhesions were assumed, the angiographic findings having remained unchanged. Presenting with symptoms of constant fits and increasing hemipareses, finally with headache, nausea, and hemianopia, the patient was operated on for recurrent growth after the midline echo, the anterior cerebral artery and the arteria pericallosa now revealed distinct displacements. It is worthy of note that nearly all patients with recurrent growths finally revealed mental disorders to a more or less marked degree (Table 3).

Table 3. Symptomatology of Recurrent Growths

Symptom \ Case	7 ♀ S.	9 ♀ V.	4 ♀ B.	2 ♂ D.	5 ♀ K.	6 ♀ R.	8 ♀ Sch.		1 ♂ B.	3 ♂ L.
Ext. bulging					+					+
Giddiness							+	+		
Headache		+		+		+	+			
Nausea		+								
Fits (U=Unconsciousness)	+	+U	+	+		+U	+			
Pareses	+	+	+	+(rest?)	+		+	+	+(rest?)	+
Sens. disturbances	+		+				+	+		+
Speech "	+	+		+			+	+		
Mental "	+	+	+	+	+	+	+	+	+	
Pappilloedema					(+)				(+)	+

Table 4. Course before Recur. Growth Op.
Occurrence of Fits and Pareses

F = Fits
F_U = With unconsciousness
P = Pareses

Years before Recur. Growth Op.

16 15 14 13 12 11 10 9 8 7 6 5 4 3 2 1 ↑ Rec. Gr. Op.

Case
1 st Op. ... P ... PFP   7
1 st Op. FP F FF F_U F_U PFP   9
1 st Op. PF ... FP   4
1 st Op. F ... FF   2
1 st Op. ... P   5
1 st Op. F F F_U F_U   6
1 st Op. FF R P   8
1 st Op.   1
1 st Op. P   3

The technical tests (Table 5) were found to have a varying value in the detection of recurrent growths. The strongest evidence was provided by angiography and, as far as such were conducted, scintigraphy (10) and filling of the cerebral ventricles with air. It was the objective findings resulting from this that set the signal for operation.

Table 5. Technical Tests for Detection of Recurrent Growths

Method \ Case	7 ♀ S.	9 ♀ V.	4 ♀ B.	2 ♂ D.	5 ♀ K.	6 ♀ R.	8 ♀ Sch.	1 ♂ B.	3 ♂ L.
Skull X-Ray	Ø	Ø	Ø	Ø	+	Ø	Ø	Ø	+
Echo -EG		+			Ø				
EEG	+	+	+	Ø	+	+ (rest?)	+ (rest?)	+	Ø
Scanning	+			+			(+)		
Angiography	+	+	+	+	+	+	+	+	+
Encephalograph				+					+

+ = pos. contribution Ø = no contribution

Electro-encephalography and echo-encephalography were able to provide indications and should be carried out as a routine measure in suspected cases.

In three operations on recurrent growths the sinus was found to be completely infiltrated by the tumor, so that it could be removed over a length of 15 cm (2, 3, 4, 8, 11). While one patient died of bronchopneumonia on the 39th postoperative day, a further patient was still psychologically disturbed on discharge and still had a paresis of an arm and a spastic paraparesis. He was a double amputee and wore legs protheses below the knee, and for this reason alone was handicapped in walking. In this case, however, as already mentioned, the clinical course of the disease was in any case malignant.

The tumor, which had penetrated through the bone into the galea, had invaded far into the depths on both sides of the falx and had infiltrated the roof of the sinus in its medial part over a length of 13 cm, but had not obliterated it. The surgeon had to be content with resecting the part of the roof affected and closing it with a suture. Eight months later it became necessary to remove the recurrent growth in the galea. When, two months later, an intracranial recurrent growth weighing 100 g was removed, the sinus was occluded and was removed over a length of 13 cm. At the time of his discharge recurrent growths were again detected in the galea and the patient's appearance reflected the fateful prognosis.

In the case of the third patient, 45 years old, it was possible in a second operation to remove the sinus that had been obliterated by the tumor over a length of 13 cm, together with a strip of the falx cerebri of 1 to 2 cm in width, while preserving the inferior sagittal sinus. At discharge, the postoperative hemiparesis was found to have receded well. Eight months after the operation the patient is doing well, walks freely without a stick, and has just spent her holidays in the mountains.

Our epicritical observations have induced us to develop surgical methods which cause the tumorous growth gradually to infiltrate the sinus. Then, after a collateral circulation has developped, the operating surgeon is in a position to proceed radically in a second operation and also to remove the sinus as the probable source of a recurrent growth without endangering the patient (2, 3, 4, 7).

To this end we surround the sinus that has been attacked by the tumor, but still perfused by blood, with a cuff of pedicled flaps derived from the falx and dura (Fig. 1).

The case of a cerebral metastasis of a cholangio-cellular hepatic carcinoma, which initially presented the appearance of a meningioma, enabled us - due to the rapid growth of the tumor - to obtain an immediate check on our procedure on the basis of the autopsy material. The tumor had destroyed the bone, infiltrated into the galea and attacked the sinus; but as the latter was still patent, it could not be resected.

The dura was now incised on both sides in a semi-circular manner and folded together over the sinus.

The pictures (Fig. 2) show schematically how this was done. Thus, the procedure followed was carried out in the expectation that the slow further growth of the tumor would lead to a gradual occlusion of the sinus and that an appropriate collateral circulation would develop. Three days after the operation a total paralysis of all the extremities occurred. But this initially alarming picture then improved very rapidly and the paralysis disappeared. Six months after the operation the patient died of cachexia with hepatic metastases and ascites.

Although the initially existing pareses had virtually disappeared, and had not reappeared until the end, at autopsy an occlusion of the superior sagittal sinus in its medial third was seen (Fig. 3) 15 cm from the frontal end, at one localized point. It was observed histoligically that the sinus had not been obliterated by the tumor tissue but by fibrous hyperplasia of its interior wall.

In our efforts to avoid an interruption of the sinal circulation (1, 5, 9, 14), as far as possible, in other cases we replaced the invaded sinus by a falx-dura cuff which was formed around a plastic tube which, for the duration of the operation, secured the venous drainage and was removed afterwards. A plastic tube - of the type we use for Redon drainage - was also employed in one case as a permanent implant to bridge the sinus defect.

With this report it was our intention to make a contribution to the plastic methods of sinus surgery for use in parasagittal meningiomas.

REFERENCES

1. BONNAL, J., BROTCHI, J., STEVENAERT, A., PETROV, V. T., MOUCHETTE, R.: L'ablation de la portion intrasinusale des méningiomes para-

sagittaux rolandiques, suivie de plastie du sinus longitudinal supérieur. Neuro-Chirurgie 17, 341 - 354 (1971).

2. DAVID, M., BISSERY, BRUN, M.: Sur un cas de méningiome de la faux opéré avec succès. Absence de troubles paralytiques après résection du sinus lognitudinal au niveau de l'abouchement des veines rolandiques. Rev. Neurol. 61, 725 - 730 (1934).

3. DAVID, M.: Traitement opératoire des méningiomes parasagittaux. In: Traité de technique chirurgicale 11, p. 752 - 754. Paris: Masson et Cie 1942 - 1944.

4. DAVID, M., POURPRE, H., LEPOIRE, J., DILENGE, D.: Les méningiomes parasagittaux. In: Encyclopédie Médicale. Neuro-Chirurgie, p. 374 - 376. Paris: Flammarion 1961.

5. DONAGHY, R. M. P., WALLMAN, L. J., FLANAGAN, M. J., NUMOTO, M.: Sagittal sinus repair. Technical note. J. Neurosurg. 38, 244 - 248 (1973).

6. GUILLAUME, J., BILLET, R., CARON, J. P., CUCCIA, D.: Les méningiomes. Etude clinique et chirurgicale. Paris: Presses Universitaires de France 1957.

7. HOESSLY, G. F., OLIVECRONA, H.: Report on 280 cases of verified parasagittal meningioma. J. Neurosurg. 12, 614 - 626 (1955).

8. JAEGER, R.: Observations on resection of the superior longitudinal sinus at and posterior to the rolandic venous inflow. J. Neurosurg. 8, 103 - 109 (1951).

9. KAPP, J. P., GIELCHINSKY, I., PETTY, C., McCLURE, C.: An internal shunt for use in the reconstruction of dural venous sinuses. Technical note. J. Neurosurg. 35, 351 - 354 (1971).

10. KUBA, J., KONTNY, V., KLAUS, E.: Hirnszintigramm in der Diagnostik von Rezidiven intrakranieller Raumforderungen. Fortschr. Röntenstr. 117/2, 173 - 178 (1972).

11. McCARTY, C. S.: Surgical techniques for removal of intracranial meningiomas. Clinical Neurosurgery 7, 100 - 111 (1961).

12. PAILLAS, J. E., SEDAN, R., RAKOTOBE, A., SALAMON, G., COMBALBERT, A.: Les récidives des méningiomes sus-tentoriels (à propos de 15 observations). Marseille Médical 102, 661 - 665 (1965).

13. RAY, B. S.: Surgery for recurrent meningiomas. Clinical Neurosurgery 10, 1 - 9 (1962).

14. RISH, B. L.: The repair of dural venous sinus wounds by autogenous venorrhaphy. J. Neurosurg. 35, 392 - 395 (1971).

15. SCHAFER, E. R.: Recidivhäufigkeit bei Meningeomen. Verlaufsbeobachtungen über 20 Jahre. Acta Neurochir. 13, 186 - 195 (1965).

16. SIMPSON, D.: The recurrence of intracranial meningiomas after surgical treatment. J. Neurol. Neurosurg. Psychiat. 20, 22 - 39 (1957).

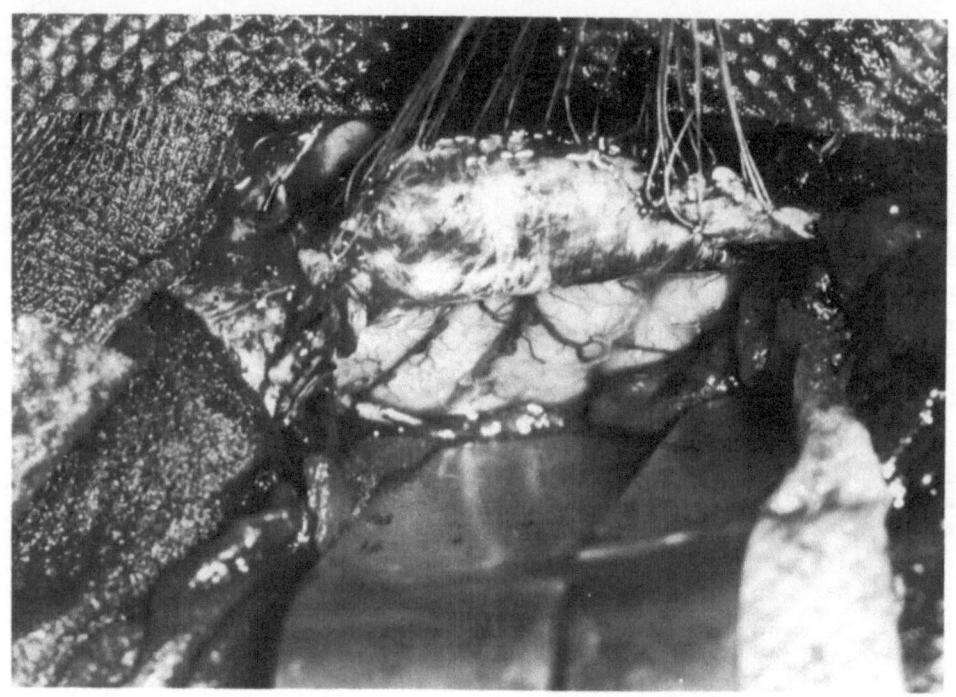

Fig. 1. A cuff of pedicled parts of the falx and dura embraces the superior sagittal sinus

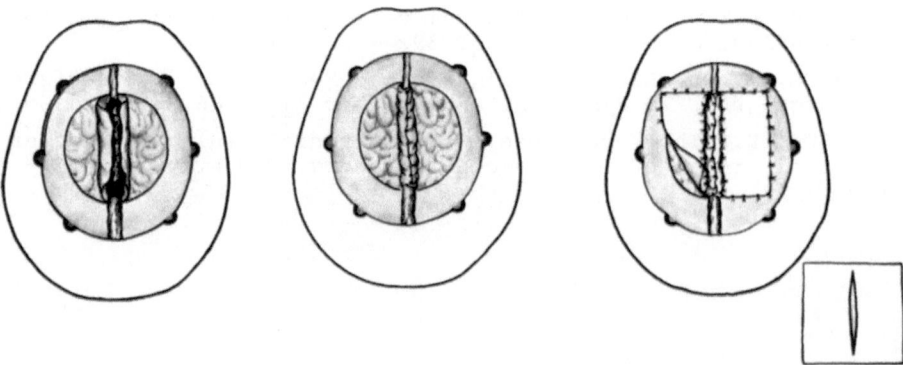

Fig. 2. Dura incised in a semicircular fashion on either side, folded together above the superior sagittal sinus and sutured to form a cuff. Plastic closure of the dura defect

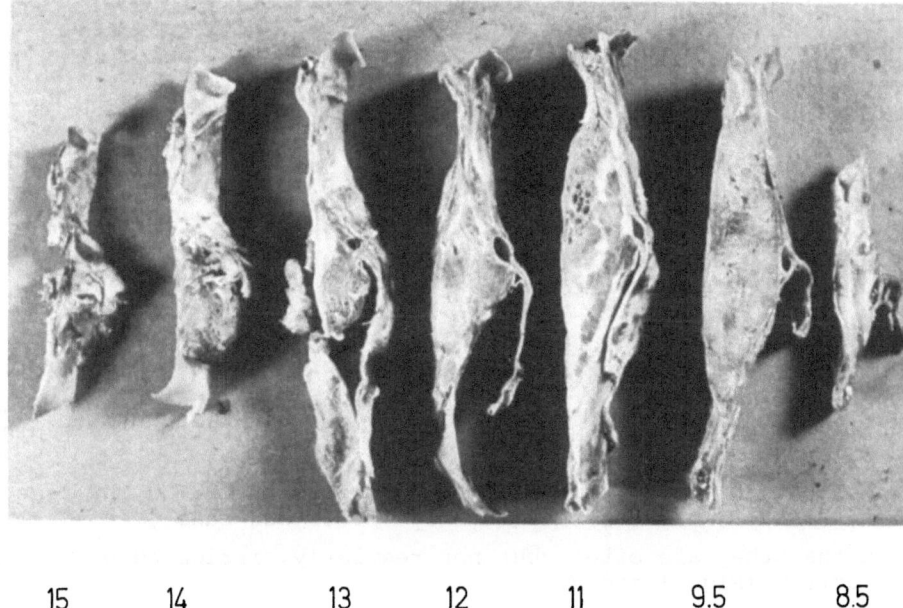

15   14   13   12   11   9.5   8.5

Fig. 3. Sections through the superior sagittal sinus surrounded by structures affected by the tumorous growth. At a distance of 15 cm from the frontal end, the sinus is closed

Tentorial Meningiomas

R. A. FROWEIN

Three facts are *well known* about the tentorial meningiomas (TM):

first that they are rare, since they represent only 4 % of all intracranial meningiomas, respectively about 18 % of cerebellar meningiomas (M),

second that they can grow "on iceberg" above and below the tentorium, which, however, was observed in only 1/5 of our cases,

third that they are often, but not regularly, irrigated by the tentorial artery (Fig. 1 and 2).

On the other hand, it is *less known*, at least for me, that wrong diagnosis (in our material) amounts to 16 %, the recurrences to 18 %, the prospect of full working capacity may be 11 %, and the lethality rate up to 19 - 36 % (Table 1).

The wrong diagnoses have different reasons, as shown by Prof. TÖNNIS' (10) patients treated in Würzburg, Berlin, Langendreer and Cologne, and by our patients, totalizing 45 cases (Table 2).

Age and Sex: 2/3 of the cases were female and 1/3 male. Age ranged from 30 to 60 years, the average being 48 years. There was one child, and four patients were more than 60 years of age.

Evolution amounted to 3 to 5 years on average, but in 13 % of the patients evolution was of a few months only, which led to the wrong diagnosis of a malignant tumor.

As regards the various clinical examinations, we observed that (Table 3):

- the *complaints* are unspecific in most cases.

As to the *neurological symptoms*, PETIT-DUTAILLIS and coll. (6) described the coincidence of cerebellar deficit with hemianopia as a special syndrome in 1953.

This syndrome was found rarely by BARROW and HARTER (1), but there is no doubt that it was the reason for one of our wrong diagnoses.

Altogether, the results of out-patient investigations, namely case history, neurological syndrome, X-rays and EEG are not specific for tentorial meningiomas.

This unfavourable situation was decidedly improved by *isotope diagnosis*: by application of As 74 and Cu 64, nearly all the results become positive; in 70 % of the cases there are strong concentrations in the tumor region and also in the cerebellar fossa. This good re-

Table 1.

Author (4)	Year	Number	Localization as to the tentorium			Course			Deaths without surgery
			supra	bilat	infra	alive	postop. deaths	%	
Cushing a. Eisenhardt	1938	15		1	14	11	3	27 %	1
Tönnis	1935	2		2		2			
Campbell a. Whitfield	1948	5							
D'Errico	1950	6							
Russel a. Bucy	1953	2				1	1		
Castellano a. Ruggiero	1953	21							
Markham at al.	1955	7	2	2	3	5	2		
Tristan a. Hodes	1958	8							
Barrow a. Harter	1962	25	8		16	17	7	29 %	
Sachs	1962								
Merli a. Carteri	1966	1	1			1			
Schechter et al.	1968	20	6	9	5				
Olivecrona	1967	21	10	11		16	5	20 %	
Smith, Ferry, Kempe	1969	3							
Allègre et al.	1970	4							
Lecuire, Dechaume et al.	1971	46				37	7	16 %	2
Tönnis, Frowein et al.	1971	45	24	8	13	25	20	44 %	2
		51 Op.				33	17	34 %	

Table 2. Forty-five tentorial meningiomas: duration of evolution, age at surgery, postoperative course

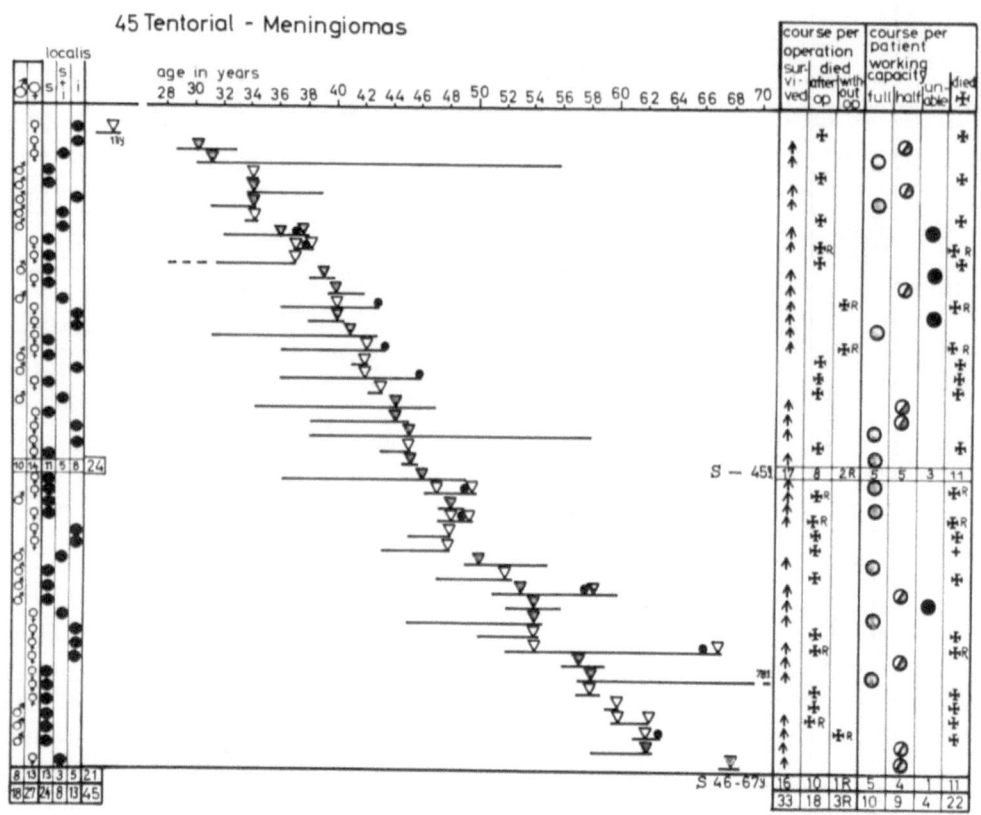

45 Tentorial - Meningiomas

Table 3. Diagnostic value of the several methods of examination

		Anamnesis	Symptomatology	Echo	EEG	isotope scan	x-ray	angiography	pneumoenceph.	diagnosis + operation	
specific for tentorial meningioma	s		○			⊗⊗⊗○○		○○○○○	○○	⊗⊗⊗○○	10
	i					○○○○○		○○○○○		⊗⊗○○	8
	s+i					○○○		○○		○○○	3
21 = 46%											
correct localisation	s	○○	⊗⊗⊗○○		⊗⊗⊗○○	○○○○	○	⊗⊗⊗○○	○○○	⊗⊗○○	8
	i	○○○	⊗⊗○○			○○○	○○○	○○	⊗○○○○	○○○○	4
	s+i	○	○○				○○	○○	○○○○	○○○○○	5
17 = 38%											
suspicion of tumor	s										
	i										
	s+i										
unspecific	s										
	i										
	s+i										
incorrect localisation	s										
	s+i										
incorrect histology	s										
	i										
	s+i										
wrong diagnosis	s										
	s+i										7 = 16%

sult, however, is certainly favored by the fact that the patients were investigated comparatively at a late stage and, therefore, with very large tumors. There is no proof that the small tumors will give the same excellent results (4).

Despite a positive scintigraphy, the surgeon needs the *arteriography* (Fig. 2). Displacement of vessels occurs only in the presence of tumors large enough. SCHECHTER and coll. (7) regard the curved elevation of the superior cerebellar artery as a specific sign of the TM on iceberg.

On the other hand, SMITH and coll. (8) destroyed the myth of the tentorial artery, not only because this vessel can be seen in about 60 % of the TM only, and is hypertrophied even more seldom, but also because it is not specific and appears also in angiomas, malignant gliomas, trigeminal and acoustic neurinomas, etc.

In earlier cases both carotid and vertebral arteriographies were not performed regularly as done nowadays. Consequently, a strong opacification, meningioma stain, may occur more often than in 50 % of the cases as has happened until present.

It has to be taken into consideration, however, that the larger portion of infratentorially but medially developped Ms appears superposed on the transverse sinus in the lateral projection of the arteriography because of the tentlike ascending tentorium.

Nowadays a complete diagnosis can be achieved by scintigraphy and arteriography. The wrong diagnosis and the non-detection of the TM practically belong to the time before the isotopes or are due to an inexcusable omission of scintigraphy.

Despite the complete scintigraphic and arteriographic diagnosis, a *pneumoencephalography* or ventriculography was also performed in 2/5 of our cases within the last few years. This was done in order to find out the best operative approach to the tumor. Besides, pneumencephalography demonstrated that half of these cases already showed a considerable hydrocephalus. This fact proves that the operation of the TM is the only, though limited chance.

However, the question of the most favorable *operative approach* was already cleared by CASTELLANO and RUGGIERO (1953) (2) based on OLIVE-CRONA's material (5) in the sense that the operation must not only be performed by the infratentorial but only or also from the supratentorial approach. Nevertheless, CUSHING (1938) (3) operated on all his 15 TM by the infratentorial route and also had lethality of 27 %, nearly the same result as OLIVECRONA. This might have been so because CUSHING operated on nearly all his TM in two steps.

Nowadays surgery in the sitting position works similarly and is improving with not too aged patients. Even this method, however, can hardly improve the high lethality of the medial M of the free edge of the tentorium, the so called "carrefour falco-tentoriel" (9). This localization is considered the most difficult, also in the statistic material of BARROW and HARTER (1).

In our cases the age of the patients was not decisive. *Operative-mortality* in patients over 45 years amounted to 53 %, in younger patients to 46 %.

All these diagnostic and operative technical difficulties are seen again in the unsatisfactory *catamnestic results*:

In our series only 10 out of 23 patients who survived the first operation achieved full working capacity; this means 22 % of all patients. In addition, 9 patients regained a limited working capacity. Accordingly, there are about 2/3 of the patients who returned to a job or to homework, but often after a long rehabilitation period.

The reasons for this are the serious defects such as hemianopia, pareses, mental disturbances, rarely epilepsy, but recurrences in 10 % of the cases. These disturbances were partly reversible, especially if the edema was venous in origin. This can, perhaps, be improved by carefully sparing the veins and by avoiding the errors committed by us.

REFERENCES

1. BARROW, H. J., HARTER, D. H.: Tentorial meningiomas. J. Neurol. Neurosurg. Psychiat. 25, 40 - 44 (1962).

2. CASTELLANO, F., RUGGIERO, G.: Meningiomas of the posterior fossa. Acta radiol. (Stockh.) Suppl. 104 (1953).

3. CUSHING, H., EISENHARDT, L.: Meningiomas. Springfield/Ill.: C. Thomas 1938.

4. FROWEIN, R. A., WILCKE, O.: Meningiomas. In: Handbook of Clinical Neurology (eds. VINKEN and BRUYN). Amsterdam: North Holland Publ. Comp. (in press).

5. OLIVECRONA, H.: The surgical treatment of intracranial tumors. In: Handbuch der Neurochirurgie, Bd. IV/4. Berlin - Heidelberg - New York: Springer 1967.

6. PETIT-DUTAILLIS, D., GUIOT, G., PERINO, A.: Méningiomes tentoriels perforants. Rev. Neurol. 89, 523 - 525 (1953).

7. SCHECHTER, M. M., ZINGESSER, L. H., ROSENBAUM, A.: Tentorial meningiomas. Amer. J. Roentgenol. 104, 123 - 131 (1968).

8. SMITH, D. R., FERRY, D. J., KEMPE, L. G.: The tentorial artery: Its diagnostic significance. Acta Neurochir. 21, 57 - 69 (1969).

9. TALLAIRACH, J., DAVID, M., FISCHGOLD, M., ABOULKER, J.: Falcotentoriographie et sinusographie basale. Presse Med. 59, 725 - 772 (1951).

10. TÖNNIS, W.: Die Behandlung der Meningiome des Tentoriums. Arch. klin. Chir. 183, 48 - 49 (1935).

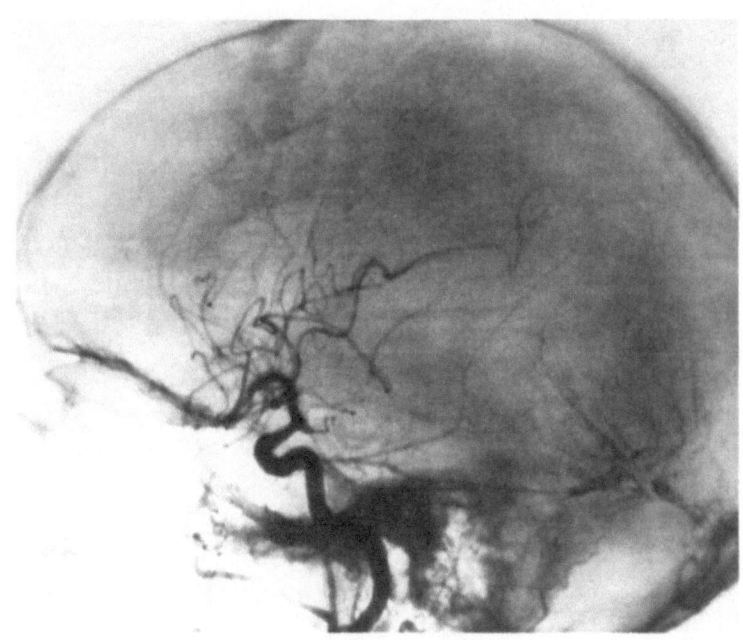

Fig. 1 a

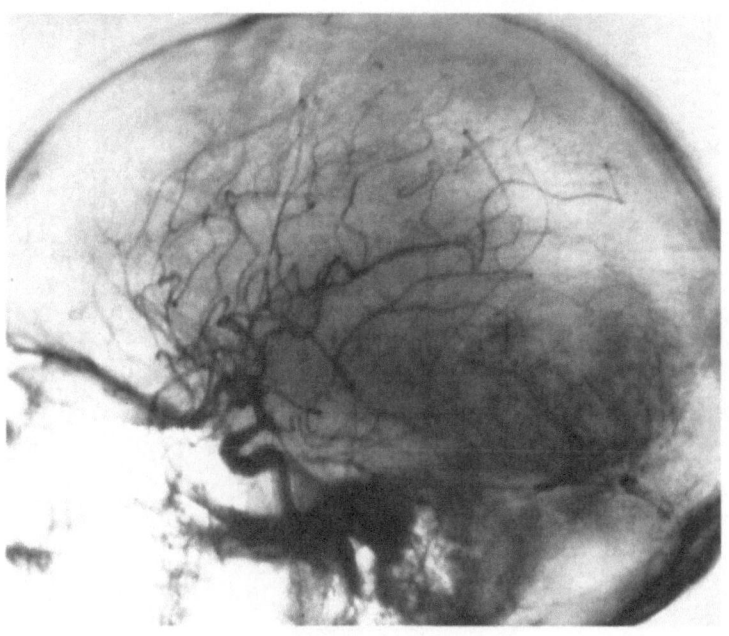

Fig. 1 b

Fig. 1 a - d. Lateral view of a left supratentorial meningioma on carotid arteriography; the tumor is partly irrigated by the tentorial artery

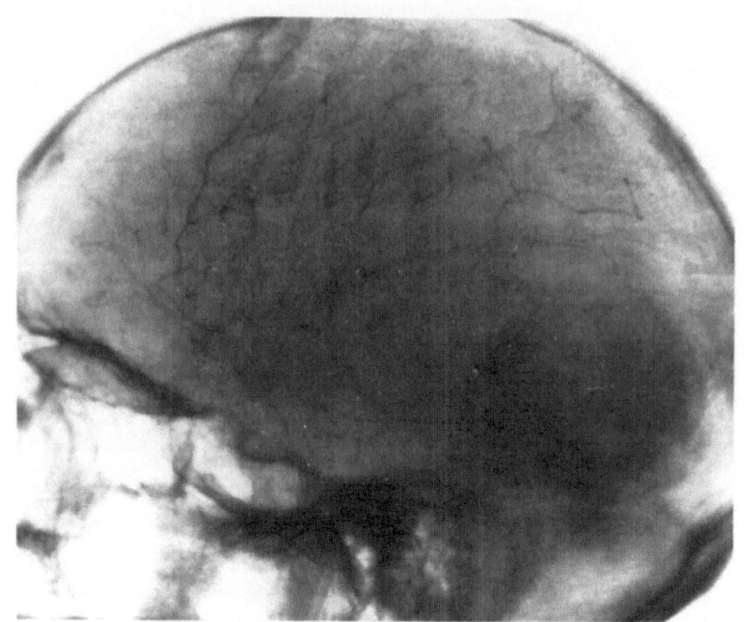

Fig. 1 c

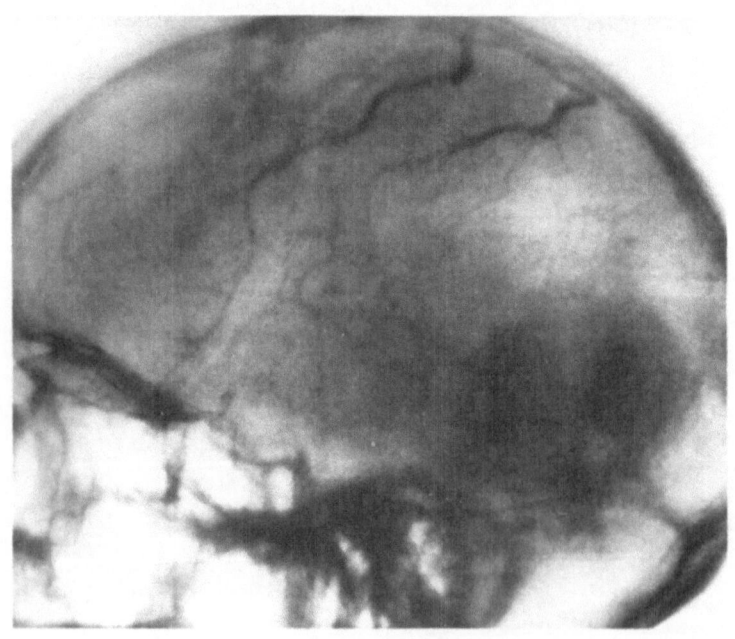

Fig. 1 d

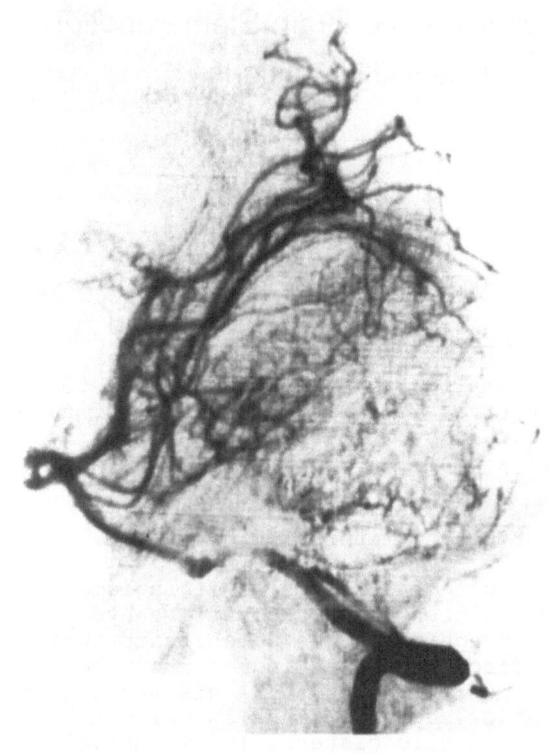

Fig. 2. Infratentorial meningioma: left lateral vertebral subtraction
arteriography

Meningiomas of the Posterior Fossa – Disturbances of CSF Circulation and Brain Stem Functions

R. KNÜPLING and E. C. FUCHS

Introduction

The complications which sometimes follow ventriculography, or postoperative edema in the presence of tumors of the posterior fossa may
be caused by disturbances in CSF circulation. RISA cisternography
(131 I-HSA) is a method for studying the dynamics of CSF circulation.

Material and Methods

In 29 out of 33 cases of meningioma of the posterior fossa, the tumor
had not been diagnosed until a hydrocephalus had developed. Pneumence-
phalographic studies demonstrate that disturbances of infratentorial
CSF circulation may induce a hydrocephalus even when no aqueduct occlusion is present. RISA cisternography indicates that CSF flow to the
superior sagittal sinus is delayed because the CSF passage through the
mesencephalic cisterns is extensively blocked at the level of the tentorial notch. For this reason, a pathological filling of the ventricular system occurs (Fig. 1). Even at this stage, CSF pressure is increased to the same extent within the infratentorial and the supratentorial space.

The expanding lesion within the posterior fossa eventually causes a
chronically progressing herniation, upwards through the foramen ten-
torii and later, in most cases, downwards through the foramen magnum.
Generally a discrete homolateral or bilateral hyperreflexia, more
pronounced in the hindlimbs, is an early sign of the ascending transtentorial herniation. This results from compression of the contralateral or of both cerebral peduncles against the clivus and the tentorial margin. Histological studies demonstrate the localized mesencephalic reactions in the region of the cerebral peduncles (edema, cellular reactions, demyelinization, gliosis) (Fig. 2) (3, 4). Clinically,
latency shifts of auditory evoked potentials (2) may appear later, as
a sign of compression of the mesencephalic tectum, which is primarily
protected by the anterior cerebellar lobe displaced rostrally. Disturbances of consciousness, the corneomandibular reflex and pathological
oculovestibular and oculocephalic reflexes (1, 5) indicate, at a later
stage, that edema affects the mesencephalic and pontine tegmentum as
a result of the progredient centripetal compression.

When the compensating supratentorial hypertension decreases during
ventriculography or by ventricular drainage in the stages of hydrocephalus or of midbrain compression, disturbances of consciousness
and vegetative dysregulations may occur as a result of an acute ascending transtentorial herniation. Tachyarrhythmia in the electro-
cardiogram should be interpreted in this way. We recorded disturbances
in consciousness and/or vegetative dysregulations in 8 out of 20 ven-

triculographies in both late stages. Moreover, pneumoventriculographic
visualization of the infratentorial CSF spaces was insufficient in
many cases during both late stages. Consequently, if we suspect an expansion in the posterior fossa, we prefer to localize the focus during
both late stages by homolateral angiography. Angiographic studies did
not cause any complication during both late stages, and demonstrated
satisfactorily the tumor expansion in all 11 cases (contralateral displacement of the chorioidal loop and/or rostral displacement of the
superior cerebellar artery and/or contrast staining). A dislocation
of the chorioidal loop of the inferior posterior cerebellar artery indicates the displacement of the fourth ventricle (Figs. 3 and 4).

In some patients CSF hypertension continued during the postoperative
phase. RISA cisternography demonstrates that this is a result of a
persisting CSF congestion at the level of the mesencephalic cisterns.
Postoperative perifocal edema may, in this way, cause a progressive
ascending herniation and a compression of the mesencephalic and pontine tegmentum. In the group of 11 patients with meningeomas of the
posterior fossa and with preoperative signs of midbrain compression,
the rate of postventriculographic and of postoperative complications
was especially high. In this stage, only 6 out of 11 patients survived the phase of the postoperative perifocal edema. In this stage,
only those patients survived who did not have a ventriculography or
who had it just before surgery. In this stage, furthermore, only
those patients survived the phase of the postoperative perifocal
edema, whose brain stem was bilaterally decompressed. In our experience, postoperative perifocal edema during both late stages may be
overcome best by bilateral suboccipital craniotomy, laminectomy of
the atlas and a duraplasty, or if adequate supplementary space is
provided by incision of the tentorium through a transtentorial approach (Table 1).

Table 1. Meningiomas of the posterior fossa

Stage	Lesion	Symptoms	Diagnostic Procedures	Treatment
I Focal				
II Expansive				
III Hyper-tensive	Mesencephalic cisterns	Hydrocephalus	Echo - EG (RISA) Angiography	Extirpation bilateral decompres-sion
IV Herniation	Basis mesencephali	Pyramidal signs		

Summary

Meningiomas of the posterior fossa manifest themselves, in most of
the cases, by disturbances of CSF circulation (hydrocephalus in the
echoencephalogram) or by signs of ascending transtentorial herniation
(homolateral or bilateral hyperreflexia more pronounced in the hindlimbs). During these stages we prefer homolateral angiography to localize the lesion, and bilateral suboccipital craniotomy, laminectomy
of the atlas and duraplasty to decompress the brain stem.

Key Words

Meningioma, posterior fossa, CSF circulation, brain stem functions,
bilateral decompression.

REFERENCES

1. ASINK, B. J. J.: Physiologic and clinical investigations into 4 brain stem reflexes.

2. GERULL, G., GIESEN, M., MROWINSKI, D., RUDOLPH, N.: Untersuchung eines frühen, von der Kopfhaut ableitbaren Potentials für die objektive Audiometrie.

3. KERNOHAN, J. W., WOLTMAN, H. W.: Incisura of the crus due to contralateral brain tumor. Arch. Neurol. Psychiat. (Chic.) 21, 274 - 287 (1929).

4. KNÜPLING, R., STOLTENBURG, G.: Tumors of the posterior fossa. Morphological signs of ascending transtentorial herniation (in print).

5. PLUM, F., POSNER, J. B.: The Diagnosis of Stupor and Coma. 2nd edition, pp. 120 - 139. Philadelphia: F. A. Davis Company.

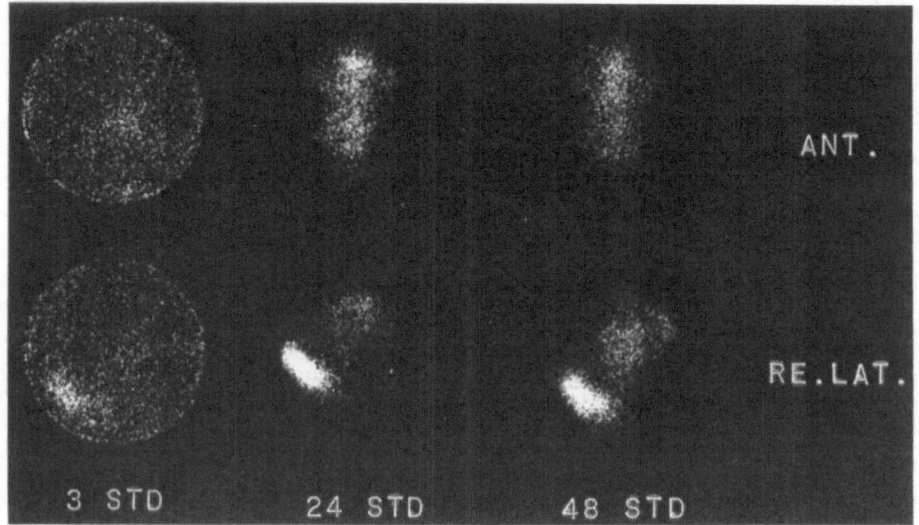

Fig. 1. The RISA cisternogram demonstrates CSF congestion at the level of the mesencephalic cisterns, pathologic reflux into the ventricular system and delayed CSF flow to the superior sagittal sinus

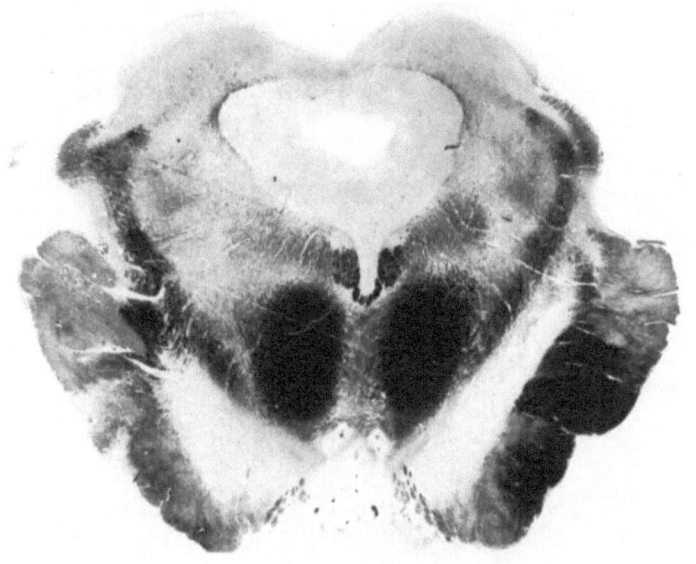

Fig. 2. Bilateral, localized demyelinization in the area of the cerebral peduncles (myelin sheath stain)

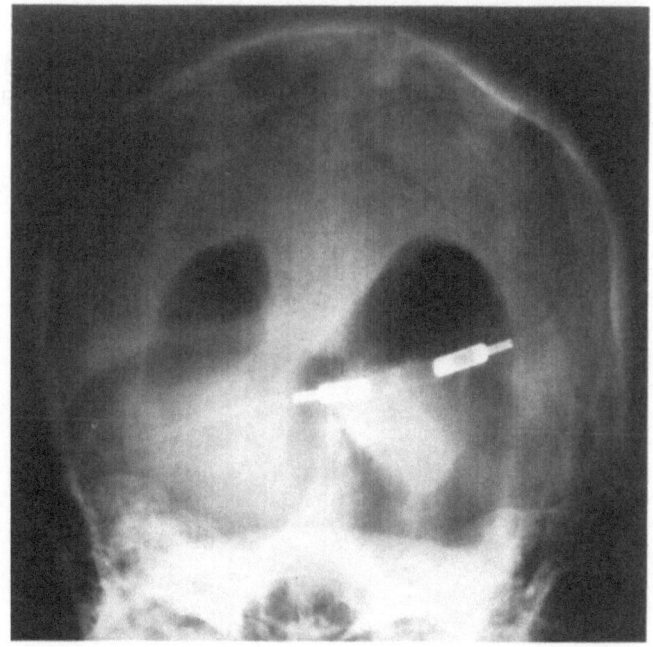

Fig. 3. Meningeoma of the posterior surface of the right petrous bone. Ventriculography: displacement of the fourth ventricle

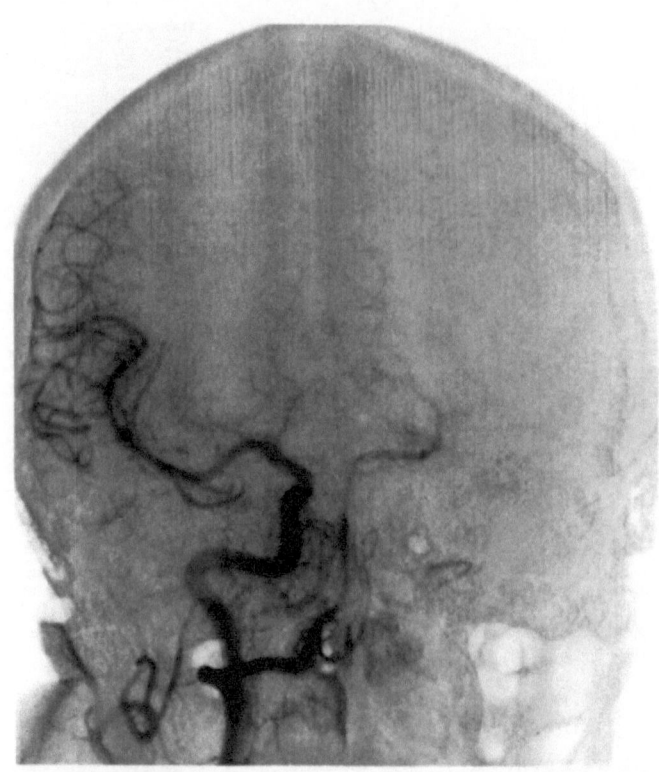

Fig. 4. The same case as in Fig. 3. Homolateral angiography: dislocation of the right choroidal loop indicating contralateral displacement of the fourth ventricle

Meningiomas in Childhood

G. PENDL

Introduction

Meningiomas are extremely rare in the pre-adolescent age group. If observed, they are noteworthy for their tremendous size and unusual location. The following is a report of 2 of the author's own cases. These were of special interest, since one of them was associated with von RECKLINGHAUSEN's disease, while the other occurred in combination with histiocytosis-x.

Case Reports

The two pediatric cases presented were selected from a total material of 45 intracranial and 10 spinal meningiomas seen in the past 4 years.

Case 1

From birth this 5-year-old boy had von RECKLINGHAUSEN's disease with peripheral facial palsy and café-au-lait spots. After endotracheal anesthesia for orchiopexy generalized convulsions occurred postoperatively. Postictal paresis of the left extremities with exaggerated reflexes persisted for 24 hours. The child was admitted to the neurosurgical department for papilledema, more pronounced in the right eye, and uncoordinated EEG with accentuation of dysrhythmic tracings on the right side.

On admission the patient was found to be fully oriented and alert. Clinical signs and symptoms other than congenital weakness of the buccal branch of the right facial nerve and choked disks bilaterally were absent. A Technetium brain scan revealed increased activity in a right central area of approximately 5 cm diameter (Fig. 1). On carotid angiography the anterior cerebral artery was found to lie in a midline position with discrete evidence of a poorly vascularized spherical tumor localizing in the central region. Two weeks following the onset of clinical symptoms the patient was subjected to surgery. On right parietal craniotomy dural tension was found to be normal without any evidence of straining. With the dura opened the gyri were seen to be flattened and the sulci effaced. Tumor tissue was not noticeable at the brain surface. The postcentral region showed increased consistency. Incision of the cortex produced a sharply demarcated tumor in a depth of 1.5 cm, which was dissected and piece-meal resected. A major arterial vessel, coursing up from the depth and apparently supplying the tumor tissue, was clipped. Exploration of the tumor cavity showed it to be 5 to 6 cm in diameter and surrounded by medullary tissue. There was obviously no communication between the tumor cavity and the ventricular system. Both intra-operatively and on subsequent histological examination the tumor was identified as a meningioma. Postoperative recovery was rapid. There were no neurological deficits, and anticonvulsive therapy was gradually withdrawn in the following months with the patient being followed up by EEG at regular intervals. One year postoperatively, the child goes to school, is making good progress and learns to swim.

Case 2

Since her first year of life this 16-year-old girl has been followed up at the pediatric department for histiocytosis (HAND-SCHÜLER-CHRISTIAN's disease) with manifestations in the bony skull, the floor of the sella, the vertebral column and the pelvic floor. On a routine follow-up she was found to have papilledema bilaterally. A Technetium brain scan revealed increased activity in a right fronto-parietal area the size of an apple (Fig. 2), far in excess of the activity usually associated with granuloma formation. The right carotid angiogram corroborated the extension of the space occupying process. The girl showed stunted growth and mental retardation. Neurological findings, however, were non-contributory. Surgical exposure of the space-occupying process revealed an extensive frontal meningioma localized at the falx. This was extirpated in toto together with portions of the falx. The presumptive diagnosis of meningioma of the falx was confirmed by histological evidence. The postoperative course was uneventful except for temporary left hemiparesis, which subsided after a few days. The patient was discharged 12 days postoperatively. Neurological findings were still negative 8 months postoperatively.

Discussion

Meningiomas account for about 2 to 3 percent of pre-adolescent neoplasms in major tumor collectives. In his critically reviewed and reclassified material of 1.375 tumors involving the central nervous systems JELLINGER (5) found 4 out of a total of 173 tumors in children up to the age of 16 years to be meningiomas (= 2.3 percent). In adults the ratio was 313 of a total of 1.202 (= 26 percent). MATSON (9) reported only 3 meningiomas among 750 tumors in children under age 14 years. The incidence of connatal meningiomas is still lower. JELLINGER and SUNDER-PLASSMANN (6) gathered 7 cases from the literature, but none in their own series of 56 connatal intracranial tumors.

The remarkable size of these tumors in children and the absence of gross neurological signs (see our case 2) is well documented by other workers (3, 7, 9, 14). Intracerebral meningiomas completely surrounded by brain tissue, such as our case 1, which do not have any contact with the brain surface, the dura mater or the ventricular system, are extremely rare (1, 2, 7). Meningiomas are rarely associated with von RECKLINGHAUSEN's disease, although the combination of these 2 pathologies is well established. A recent report (10) documents the possible combination of neurofibromatosis and juvenile xanthogranulomatosis. This is in agreement with our case 2, where an extensive meningioma of the falx was associated with histiocytosis-x. The considerably increased activity such as was shown on the brain scan in our case might have suggested a granuloma, since granulomas are occasionally visualized as a circumscribed area on the scan (12). A coexistence of the 2 pathologies in our case is probably accidental.

Both our cases were characterized by a relatively large size, such as is well established in the literature for pediatric meningiomas. Con-

sidering that one was fully intracranial, while the other presented
as a giant space-occupying process at the falx in association with
histiocytosis and was virtually asymptomatic, the designation of meningiomas as "chameleon among the brain tumors" (4, 8, 11, 13) appears
to be fully justified.

Summary

Of a total of 55 meningiomas only 2 affected children. Both presented
interesting aspects. Case 1, a 5-year-old boy, had a purely intracranial meningioma in the right parietal region. There was no communication with either cortex or dura mater and no evidence of a possible
origin from the ventricular system or choroidal plexus. The patient
showed clinical signs of von RECKLINGHAUSEN's neurofibromatosis. Case
2, a 16-year-old girl, had a large fronto-precentral meningioma of the
falx on the right side, which was associated with long-standing histiocytosis-x. Xanthogranuloma had to be ruled out in the differential
diagnosis. Total resection of the tumor was possible in either case
without any neurological deficits.

REFERENCES

1. BARCIA-GOYANES, J. J., CALVO-GARRA, W.: Meningiomas without arachnoid attachment. Acta Neurochir. 3, 241 - 247 (1953).

2. GROSZBERG, D., BLUMENTHAL, I. J.: Subcortical fibroblastoma of the
   brain. Amer. J. Path. 23, 741 - 753 (1947).

3. HEPPNER, F.: Das Vorkommen meningealer Tumoren bei Kindern. Öst.
   Z. Kinderheilk. 8, 38 - 56 (1953).

4. HUCKMAN, M. S., NEER, D., NORTON, Th.: Convexity Meningioma Presenting Angiographically as "Peudosubdural Hematoma". Neurochirurgia 17, 66 - 69 (1974).

5. JELLINGER, K.: Korrelationspathologische Aspekte kindlicher Hirngeschwülste. In: Pädiatrische Neurochirurgie, S. 57 - 72. (Hrsg.
   H. KRAUS, M. SUNDER-PLASSMANN). Wien: Wiener Med. Akademie 1970.

6. JELLINGER, K., SUNDER-PLASSMANN, M.: Connatal intracranial tumors.
   Neuropädiatrie 4, 46 - 63 (1973).

7. KOOS, W. Th., MILLER, M. H.: Intracranial Tumors of Infants and
   Children. Stuttgart: Georg Thieme 1971.

8. LANGHEIM, W., MESSERT, R.: Gehirnmeningeome, die Metastasen ent-
   halten. In: Fortschritte auf dem Gebiet der Neurochirurgie (Hrsg.
   K.-A. BUSHE), S. 283 - 290. Stuttgart: Hippokrates 1970.

9. MATSON, D. D.: Neurosurgery of Infancy and Childhood, p. 624.
   Springfield/Ill.: C. C. Thomas 1969.

10. NEWELL, G. B., STONE, O. J., MULLINS, J. F.: Juvenile xanthogranu-
    loma and neurofibromatosis. Arch. dermat. 107, 262 (1973).

11. PORRAS, C. L.: Meningioma in the foramen magnum in a boy aged 8
    years. J. Neurosurg. 20, 167 - 168 (1963).

12. SALCMAN, M., QUEST, D. O., MOUNT, L. A.: Histiocytosis-x of the
    spinal cord. J. Neurosurg. 41, 383 - 386 (1974).

13. SKULTETY, F. M.: Meningioma Simulating Ruptured Aneurysm. J.
    Neurosurg. 28, 380 - 382 (1968).

14. TENG, P., PAPATHEODOROU, Ch.: Suprachiasmal and Intraventricular
    Meningioma in a 4-Year-Old Child. J. Neurosurg. 20, 174-176 (1963).

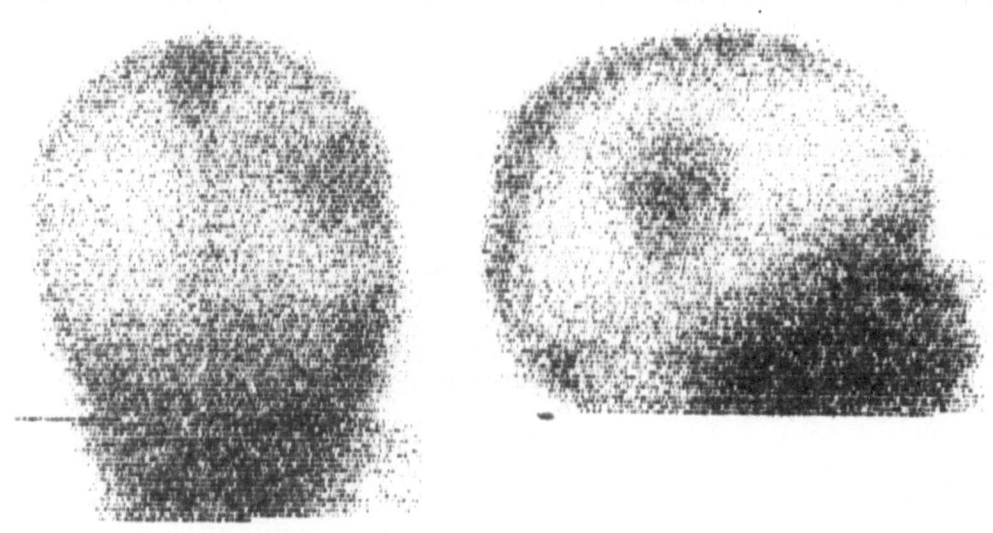

Fig. 1. Technetium brain scan in a 4-year-old boy with a history of von RECKLINGHAUSEN's disease. Isotope activity in the right parietal region is suggestive of meningioma

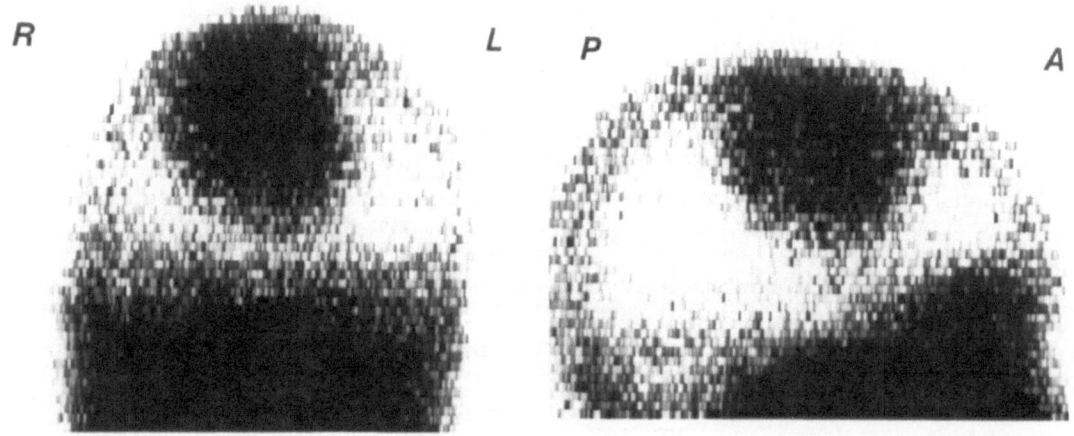

Fig. 2. Technetium brain scan of a 16-year-old girl with a history of histiocytosis-x. The pronounced activity in the right frontoparietal region near the midline is suggestive of meningioma rather than granuloma

Multiple Sclerosis
Misdiagnosis

Neuropathology of Multiple Sclerosis

J. PFEIFFER

Multiple sclerosis (MS) is a disease with no indication for neurosurgical intervention. If, nevertheless, it has become the subject of this Neurosurgical Congress as "misdiagnosis", this is probably because the differential diagnosis between MS and tumor always causes difficulties. NONNE (77) had already pointed out the problems of differential diagnosis between compression of the spinal cord and MS. The difficulties of MS diagnosis are also reflected in our own material.

In the last 10 years we diagnosed MS morphologically 22 times. These are about 0,5 % of our annual autopsy material. Among these 22 morphologically confirmed cases of MS a different clinical diagnosis had been made in 8, i. e. in more than one third of the cases. Clinically, a tumor was erroneously diagnosed twice, amyotrophic lateral sclerosis twice, and arachnitis optico-chiasmatica, cerebral venous thrombosis, LANDRY's paralysis and an endogenous psychosis once each. In 3 other cases MS had been considered, together with systemic degeneration, cerebrospinal syphilis and hysteria.

On the other hand, MS had been diagnosed clinically 4 times without morphological confirmation. We have never seen coincidence of MS and brain tumor. CURRIE and URICH (23), however, collected not less than 18 such cases.

The morphological diagnosis begins with the CSF cytogram. It reflects the intravital morphological processes in the CNS. For the morphologist the main interest is due to the immunologically relevant lymphoid and plasma cells (10, 11, 34, 95, 103, 73).

In 10.000 unselected CSF sediments we saw lymphoid cells (immunoblasts) in 14 %, plasma cells in 2 %. Among the 1426 cases with lymphoid cells (14 %) the clinical diagnosis of MS was the most frequent (15 %), followed by the diagnosis of abacterial meningitis (13 %). Among the 227 cases with plasma cells (2 %), MS was clinically diagnosed in 10 %. In 143 cases of "clinically certain" MS we saw a lymphocytic reaction in the CSF in 48,1 %, a monocytic reaction in 20,1 %, in a mixed lympho-monocytic reaction in 12,6 %, and furthermore lymphoid cells in 52,3 % and plasma cells in 4,2 %.

This combination of a lymphocytic reaction with numerous lymphoid cells is a characteristic criterium to facilitate the diagnosis of MS. According to those cytological criteria, the CSF cytogram of 601 cases of MS suspected was considered typical in 28 %, and suspicious of MS in further 32 %. In 7 % the cytogram revealed another diagnosis. Correlative examinations between light- and electronmicroscopic cell preparations confirmed our criteria for differentiating lymphoid and plasma cells by the light microscope (102). SCHLOTE and ROSS (102)

also found significant correlations between the left wave of the nor-
momastix reaction and the degree of lymphocyte transformation in our
material.

Morphologically the picture of MS is well defined and familiar to you.
There are multilocular foci with a definite tendency to affect the
ventricle walls, especially the tissue around the ventricle corners
(Fig. 1), and also the areas near to the surface of the brain stem
and spinal cord (Fig. 2), although here there occasionally is a fine
edge of preserved medullary sheaths below the pia mater. In view of
this distribution, the question has been raised again and again as
to whether some noxious agent enters the cerebral tissue by way of
the CNS. Convincing investigations (69), with the aid of consecutive
serial sections, show a close correlation between the foci and the
venous plexus which is, in fact, particularly well evidenced around
the ventricle corners or the lower cornua (Fig. 1). LUMSDEN (69) was
able to correlate the partly wedge-shaped foci near to the surface
with corresponding radiating veins. His investigations confirm earlier, similarly careful investigations by FOG (39, 40) and MACCHI
(70). The distribution of foci is therefore not quite hazardous but
related to certain angio-architectonical distribution patterns. This
is why sometimes a remarkable symmetry of foci can be observed.
PUTNAM's (85, 86) conception of the role of thrombosis, nevertheless,
could not be confirmed (70, 69).

Besides the discontinuity of the foci, it is the mode of distribution
and the pattern of damage that characterises MS morphologically. The
foci, sometimes visible only with a magnifying glass or microscope,
develop like a sleeve around thin-walled veins with a lumen of 0.5 -
0.1 mm around which such foci of demyelinization can also be arranged
like a string of pearls (69). Larger foci form by confluence. On their
margins the finger-like tongues of demyelinisation described by DAW-
SON can sometimes be seen following the veins. This linkage with vessels, however, is only one aspect of the distribution, while another
is distribution per continuitatem over neighbouring medullary segments.

It has long been known that cyto-architectonic boundaries do not affect the distribution of demyelination foci. At the first sight demyelination is undoubtedly the most impressive morphological finding,
especially in the old, "burned-out" foci in which no medullary sheath
substance is demonstrable any more, and where the focal borders may
be extremely sharply defined (Fig.3a). In more recent foci they are
indistinct. The regions show varicosities and bud-shaped loosening of
the medullary sheaths. According to the age of the focus, the lipho-
phages which have taken up the medullary sheath decomposition products
lie densly packed or more loosely and migrating towards the vessels
(Fig. 3 b). This is certainly the characteristic picture of the classical plaque but there are also medullary shadow foci (Fig. 4) in
which only a more or less distinct bleaching of the medullary sheath
covering is recognizable without there being a complete destruction
of the medullary sheath. Destruction of the medullary sheath, i. e.
damage of the oligodendroglia cells forming the medullary sheaths,
is one characteristic. The other is lively proliferation of astrocyte
fibers. This fiber gliosis gave rise to the denomination of the disease. For a long time the gliosis leading to sclerosis was considered
only a reaction to the medullary sheath damage. According to recent
electron-microscopic examinations it is probable that the astrocytic
fiber proliferation is essential in MS since - as pointed out by JACOB
(61) - especially in the medullary shadow foci the fiber gliosis may
greatly exceed the extent of the medullary sheath damage. Thus, it is

even possible to find preserved medullary sheaths sheated by astrocyte processes. PERIER and GREGOIRE (83) confirmed this astrocytic
reaction, with the electron-microscope mainly a wrapping up of the
axons, which remain largely preserved within the foci, as known for
a long time. The nerve cells, too, are preserved where a MS focus
extends into the gray matter (Fig. 5). However, neither the type of
demyelination nor excessive fiber gliosis, nor preservation of axons,
are specific, since similar pictures are found e. g. in parainfectious
encephalitis (60). Electron-microscopically, narrowing of medullary
sheaths and, occasionally, pictures which must probably be regarded
as signs of remyelination are also seen e. g. where an oligodendroglia
cell wraps up several naked axons (89). The assumption based on light-
microscopy that mesenchymal cells also take part in the regeneration
and formation of medullary sheaths (34) loses in weight in view of
the electron-microscopic findings (99, 51). On the other hand, McDONALD
(71) considers that the clinical remissions are also related to a reduction of edema in the focal regions. This edema may lead to distinct
focal swellings presenting the picture of tumor-like space-occupying
lesions and, therefore, is of differential diagnostic importance. In
my experience, however, the focal swelling is due to edema only in
the initial stage of acute episodes. HERRMANN and JACOB (57), and
JACOB (61) attributed the swelling, especially in the medullary shadow
foci, to glia cell proliferation. This agrees with LUMSDEN's (69)
electron-microscopic pictures, which show intracellular edema of the
astrocytic processes as being the source of the swelling. Only in
later stages signs of shrinking develop, restricted to the densely
gliotic foci, which may lead to dilatation of the ventricles. There
has been repeated discussion as to whether there are pathogenetic relations between the marked fiber gliosis and glioma formation in confirmed MS (91, 23). This idea is particularly appealing in the case
of astrocytomas or subependymal gliomas. In view of the great rarity
of their co-existence, however, this should be considered with reserve.

The role of astrocytes in demyelinating diseases, however, gains special importance from the immunological studies of WEINRAUDER and LACH
(113). These authors found an immunofluorescence of brain-specific
antigens only in astrocytes.

So far we have dealt with the foci which are, of course, the most
obvious manifestation to the morphologist. However, as regards the
question of whether MS is based on a generalized pathological process
of glial tissue, we are also interested in examinations of tissue outside the demyelination foci. Chemical studies have shown that here,
too, the chemical composition is not normal (20, 21, 22, 27, 32, 47 -
50). The total phospholipid content is reduced, even in apparently
normal regions, as is the content of highly unsaturated fatty acids.
The triglyceride and cholesterol ester content, on the other hand,
is raised (31). Nevertheless, LUMSDEN (69) warns against prematurely
concluding from these data that morphologically apparently intact regions are also affected, since serial sections have shown that small
foci are far more common than one is inclined to assume on the basis
of routine examinations (114).

The weakness of overall chemical analyses is overcome by enzyme histochemistry, with the aid of which it has been possible to demonstrate
changes in the marginal zone of the foci (9, 59, 46). Combined biochemical and electron-microscopic examinations of biopsy material
proved a significant increase in acid proteinases and a reduction of
cerebrosides outside the foci (89, 8, 90). According to BOWEN and
DAVISON (12) the monocytes and according to LAPRESLE (64) the lymphocytes (52) are the carriers of proteinases.

Electron-microscopic examinations have also shown that especially the thicker medullary sheaths not uncommonly present splitting up of lamellae and formation of buds (89). Often axons were only partially covered by thin medullary sheaths. Astrocyte processes showed increased and enlarged lysosomes. Signs of remyelination were also found. The nuclei contained tubular and microfilamentary material (87). Of special importance was the electron-microscopic demonstration of lysosome-rich mononuclear cells.

These studies of seemingly normal areas outside the foci demonstrable by light microscopy are of great importance for our understanding of the pathogenetic process. RINNE's (89) studies showed a considerable alteration of the astrocytes outside the foci. He discusses whether these astrocytes with increased hydrolases digest the bud formations of the myelin sheaths, and whether, in connection with this, it comes to an autoimmune processes, caused by an escape of encephalitogenic protein into the intercellular substance, since liberated encephalitogenic protein was demonstrated biochemically (2) in these regions.

The problem of neuroallergy or of a possible virus ethiology has a long tradition in German medical literature. I need only to mention PETTE (84), SCHALTENBRAND (100) and HALLERVORDEN (53 - 55). Morphological analogies of MS to complications of rabies inoculation (109, 110), to post-vaccinal reactions (29), or to the picture of demyelination encephalitis after repeated brain dry cell injections (62) may be mentioned as examples. The morphological similarities between acute disseminated encephalomyelitis and experimental allergic encephalomyelitis in animals have been familiar to us for a long time. Conclusions by analogy have been drawn from this, as done by HALLERVORDEN (53, 54), who compared the ring spot foci of tobacco mosaic virus disease with the peculiar lamination picture of demyelination observed in all transitional forms from the typical MS focus to the complete picture of concentric sclerosis (Fig. 6 a - c). Such concentric foci led ULE and KRAEMER (111) to establish the foci's rate of growth at 0.24 to 0.46 mm per day in a case with acute clinical course and, therefore, easily observable. With similar calculations LUMSDEN (69) arrived to rates of 1 cm per month to 2 - 4 mm per year. The range of variation is therefore considerable. Anyhow, it is interesting that the foci can progress very rapidly.

It is just in these recent foci that the inflammatory reaction - not yet discussed in detail - is especially impressive. Similar to the CSF sediment, we find, besides small lymphocytes, above all enlarged lymphoid cells and plasma cells, as already described 1908 by OPPENHEIM (82). The importance of these transformed lymphocytes and of the plasma cells for immune processes has meanwhile been confirmed many times. In the marginal focal zones most strongly infiltrated by mononuclear cells SIMPSON et al. (97, 98) found intensive local IgG formation with the aid of immunofluorescence methods. These findings confirmed investigations (42) of an enrichment of gamma-globulin in the foci with the aid of iodine 131-labelled gamma-globulin. It has been known for some time (62, 112) that CSF of MS patients contains relatively more gamma-globulin or IgG than the serum. The studies of TOURTELOTTE and PARKER's (107), which showed no increased passage of bromide or albumin, i. e. substances that pass the barrier easily, from the blood to the MS foci, but a local enrichment of IgG, support the fact that this is not a consequence of a disturbance of the blood-brain barrier. Studies with labelled gamma-globulin also indicate local immunoglobulin formation, in the damaged brain tissue (25, 26). TOURTELOTTE's investigations (108) suggest that the infiltrated mononuclear cells act as IgG formers. He assumes that an antigen sensitizes the lymphocytes

locally and induces them to form myelin-toxic antibodies. He sees
good correlations between the local IgG level and the degree of demyelination. A similar concept of continuous antigen stimulation with
proliferation of antibody-producing cell clones in MS was arrived at
by LINK (68).

HALPERN et al. (56) found a pronounced destructive tendency in the effect of such stimulated MS lymphocytes on cultures of embryonic rat
nerve cells when the lymphocytes were obtained from patients in an
acute episode. HAUW et al. (58) observed such an effect of MS-lympho-
cytes on human fetal cell cultures.

Similar toxic effects on oligodendroglia cell cultures were also found
with sera of MS patients (88), i. e. not only with the aid of a cell-
bound immunoactive substance. The myelinolysis in the tissue culture
was accompanied by growth stimulation of edematous, swollen astrocyte
processes as also occures in foci of MS. Knowing that transformed lymphocytes may become aggressive towards nerve tissue, we have to ask
what agent induces the transformation. The finding that serum and CSF
of MS patients have toxic effects on glia cells has a parallel in investigations of a transformation effect of serum and CSF of MS patients
on lymphocytes. FOWLER et al. (41) demonstrated a statistically significant lymphocyte transformation following the effect of CSF of MS patients. Similar results were obtained by FRICK and STICKL (43), who
attributed the cell-specific effect of the CSF of MS patients to im-
munoglobuline.

DAU and PETERSON (30) saw the same lymphocyte transformation due to
the effect of an encephalitogenic protein which plays an important
part in the development of experimental allergic encephalomyelitis.
The lymphocyte transformation due to the effect of this basic protein,
however, is only slightly more pronounced in MS patients as compared
with the effect on controls. As stressed by CASPARY and FIELD (16)
this is not a MS-specific effect.

This phenomenon of significant but not MS-specific immune reactions
is found in quite a number of other experiments, such as the RNA-
synthesis inhibition in normal lymphocytes by MS sera (78), in the
macrophage or leucocyte migration inhibition test (115), or in lymphocyte stimulation by phytohaemagglutinin. These experiments (45)
showed a clear correlation between the stimulation rate of MS lymphocytes by basic protein and the activity or severity of the disease.
However, they were not MS-specific. Nevertheless, these results indicate immunological processes originating in the destruction of medullary sheath tissue (45, 30). Remarkable is the cellular hypersensitivity to the synaptosome-like fraction (5). Although, admittedly,
any intravital damage of central nervous tissue leads to alterations
of the immunity situation with sensibilization of the lymphocytes, FIELD
and CASPARY (35) are probably right in asking why does not any cerebral trauma or any cerebral circulatory disorder leading to tissue
destruction, induce autoimmune processes such as are assumed to exist
in MS.

The just published analysis of 60 MS-cases by CURRIER et al. (24),
however, showed, indeed, more cases with trauma, perinatal hypoxia,
combustion, appendectomies and tonsillectomies in the anamnesis as
compared to controls. Possibly the activation of the autoimmune-pro-
cess, respectively the outbreak of a new MS-bout, depends on a serum
factor which hampers the sensibilization of lymphocates by antigens.

FIELD and CASPARY (35) demonstrated such a serum factor in a test assessing the mobility of the macrophages in an electrophoretic field under the influence of patient's serum. The serum factor inhibits the lymphocyte response to specific antigens. They postulate an imbalance between lymphocyte reactivity on the one hand and the degree of suppression activity of the lymphocyte-inhibiting factor in the serum on the other. This factor is more pronounced in MS patients, but also in patients with other brain lesions, as compared with controls. Thus again, we have a significant but unspecific effect in the immune system (see also OFFNER et al., 81).

Not only the lack of specificity but also the fact that the immune responses in the various suitable tests are by no means the same in all MS patients (92, 43), are reasons for reserve in the interpretation of the above findings in looking for a full explanation of the pathogenesis of MS. Still, the immunopathological findings correlate well with the neuropathological findings of focus infiltration by mononuclear cells. However, the fact that oligodendroglial damage, i.e. myelin sheath damage, and astrocyte proliferation, occur outside the foci in areas where no infiltrating cells can be found, obliges to look for additional pathogenic factors. It may be said that attempts to provide a therapy by antilymphocyte serum or immunosuppressants, or a combination of these agents intervening in the autoimmune process, did not stand critical examination (44, 76, 31, 72) as opposed to original expectations (28, 104).

Although numerous methodically unobjectionable findings support the importance of pathological, albeit non-specific immune reactions in MS, it is necessary to search for the antigen or another additional inducing factor. We must here cast a side glance at results of geographical medicine. The peculiar distribution of MS is well known. The comparison of MS-risk in immigrants from different civilized countries to Israel, South Africa and Hawaii gave important results (3, 33, 65). Immigrants from technologically advanced communities with good sanitary facilities, especially with a good water sanitation show the highest MS-risk. ALTER (3, 4) postulated that "MS is caused by an environmental factor, probably infectious and acquired from unsanitary drinking water. If it is acquired in early life before the CNS is well myelinated, protective antibodies develop and the individual is immune against MS. If the factor is acquired later in life, when the nervous system is better myelinated, demyelinating antibodies develop which can produce clinically apparent MS, perhaps in response to nonspecific events such as a febrile illness, emotional disturbance or trauma". The causative agent is unknown. Some points support the virus-hypothesis:

In view of the nonendemic occurence of MS, the non-monophasic course and the totally different pattern of morphological distribution, any ordinary virus infection could be excluded, as rightly pointed out by SCHRADER and STOCHDORPH (105). Quite definite, however, is the finding of antibodies against measles antigen in MS as well as in van BOGAERT's subacute sclerosing leucoencephalitis. ADAMS and IMAGAWA (1) were the first to report on measles virus antibodies in the CSF of about 75 % of MS patients. This was confirmed by many later investigators (19, 15, 14, 17, 18, 13, 93, 68, 79, 80). In contrast to subacute sclerosing leucoencephalitis, a progressive process without remissions and always starting before the age of 20, titre movements do not occur in MS (79). The measles virus antibody content in the CSF was distinctly higher than that in the serum, suggesting an origin within the nervous system (79). Difficulties in establishing a relation between MS and measles virus infection, however, resulted from the fact as much as about 1/4 of MS patients do not have an elevated measles antibody level (14). Healthy brothers and sisters of MS patients had equally high antibody titres (13). Another complication is the demonstration of raised titres against herpes zoster (66), herpes simplex (17) or mumps virus (96). CASPARY and FIELD (15) thought of the role of measles virus or other banal virus infections as auxiliary agents in the development of a slow virus infection and SALMI et al. (93) stressed the widespread infection of the population with measles which would explain the raised measles antibody titres, though measles virus could possibly induce a demyelination process as a carrier mechanism. Another possibility is that in an ethiologically quite different disease, with destruction of glia cells an escape of inactive measles virus components originating from a measles infection in childhood may occur as a secondary phenomenon.

One thing that could make the discussion easier has not yet succeeded, namely the demonstration of the virus itself. Virussuspicious particles (67), or the tubular substances in astrocytes (75), certainly arouse a certain suspicion of viral cell inclusions. However, the authors themselves are as reserved in the interpretation of their findings as are RAINE and FIELD (87) with regard to the inclusions in nerve cell nuclei observed by them. The only finding of virus, based on tissue cultures and inoculation, and supported by electronmicroscopy, was obtained by ter MEULEN et al. (74), and showed filament structures resembling the nucleocapsides of the paramyxo-virus.

Recently ARGYRAKIS et al. (6) reported a case with paramyxovirus-nucleocapsid-like structures in nuclei of monocytes and with papovavirus-like inclusions in axons. These findings require further confirmation.

We have seen that immune processes are of importance for MS and that a virus infection, presumably acquired in childhood, probably measles, is important for the pathogenesis of MS. Probably genetic factors must also be taken into account as a link in the pathogenetic chain. SIMPSON et al. (98) demonstrated a definitely increased incidence of MS in humans with blood group A, and ARNASON et al. (7), as well as FOG et al. (38), examining histocompatibility in MS, found an increase of the histocompatibility antigen HL-A = and, to a lesser degree, of A 7 and A 8. It is noteworthy that the incidence of MS tallies with that of HL-A 3, which is rare in Japan and relatively common in Northern Europe. ARNASON et al. (7) found a linkage between the incidence of HL-A 3 and raised measles antibody level, quite independent of MS affection. They therefore raise the question as to whether the raised measles antibody level may not be connected with the histocompatibility antigene rather than with MS.

On the basis of the available information one arrives to a hypothetical schema (Fig. 7) of a biphasic phenomenon with a virus contact at its start, possibly leading only to a slight disseminated oligodendroglial lesion if there is a genetic predisposition and if certain environmental conditions, e. g. the degree of civilization (3, 4, 65) prepare the way. In the second phase, possibly during an imbalance with the lymphocyte response depression factor (35, 36) and influenced by the linolic acid level (37), a transient or persistent flare-up of an autoimmune process takes place. Through the liberation of basic protein, i. e. the encephalitogenic factor, and through release of lysosomal hydrolases, this can have a deleterious effect on the myelin sheath-forming oligodendroglia and stimulate the proliferation of astrocytic fibres. It cannot be stated clearly enough that these thoughts are hypothetical speculations which, however, correlate with the clinical course (106) and, if confirmed, could have consequences for the therapy in the various phases.

To summarize, in MS we have a number of statistically clearly repeated but non-specific findings. The genetic factors have just been mentioned. Participation of a virus infection is suggested by raised measles antibody titres. An autoimmune process is suggested by the local IgG rise with antibodies against autogenous brain tissue. Morphologically there are the myelin sheath destruction processes with preservation of axons, the astrocyte fibre proliferation, the inflammatory reaction with lymphoid cells and plasma cells and, finally, corresponding enzyme reactions of glia and mononuclear cells associated with tissue destruction. The venous proximity of the foci is also characteristic.

In conjunction with the characteristic pattern of distribution, the morphology still provides the safest basis for the diagnosis of MS, with the interpretation of familiar findings adapted to recent knowledge. It also allows important insights into the pathogenetic process. However, it is not yet able to give an unequivocal answer to the essential question as to what provokes the onset of MS.

REFERENCES

1. ADAMS, J. M., IMAGAWA, D. T.: Measles antibodies in multiple sclerosis. Proc. Exp. Biol., N. Y. 111, 562 - 566 (1962).

2. ADAMS, C. W M., HALLPIKE, J. F., BAYLISS, O. B.: Histochemistry of myelin. XIII Digestion of basic protein outside acute plaques of multiple sclerosis. J. Neurochem. 18, 1479 - 1483 (1971).

3. ALTER, M.: The distribution of multiple sclerosis and environmental sanitation. In: Progress in multiple sclerosis (ed. U. LEIBOWITZ), p. 99. New York - London: Academic Press 1972.

4. ALTER, M., OKIHIRO, M.: When is multiple sclerosis acquired? Neurology 21, 1030 - 1036 (1971).

5. ALVORD, E. C., HSU, P. C., THRON, R.: Leukocyte sensitivity to brain fractions in neurological diseases. Arch. Neurol. 30, 296 - 299 (1974).

6. ARGYRAKIS, A.: Detection of nueclocapsid- and papova-like structures in brain sections of multiple sclerosis. Proc. VII. Internat. Congress Neuropath. Budapest 1974 (in preparation).

7. ARNASON, B. G. W., FULLER, T. C., LEHRICH, J. R., WRAY, S. H.: Histocompatibility types and measles antibodies in multiple sclerosis and optic neuritis. J. neurol. Sci. 22, 419 - 428 (1974).

8. ARSTILLA, A. U., RIEKKINEN, P. RINNE, U. K., LAITINEN, L.: Studies in the pathogenesis of multiple sclerosis. Europ. Neurol. 9, 1 - 20 (1973).

9. ASHBEL, R., ALEXANDER, L., RASKIN, N.: Histochemical studies of active carbonyl groups (proteolipids) in brains with multiple sclerosis. J. Neuropath. & Exp. Neurol. XII, 293 - 301 (1953).

10. BAMMER, H.: Über die Beziehungen der Plasmazellen im Liquor zur Aktivität der Multiplen Sklerose. Verh. dtsch. Ges. inn. Med. 72, 733 - 736 (1967).

11. BISCHOFF, A.: Das Vorkommen von Plasmazellen im Liquor cerebrospinalis bei der Multiplen Sklerose. Dtsch. Z. Nervenheilk. 185, 606 - 617 (1964).

12. BOWEN, D. M., DAVISON, A. N.: Macrophages and cathepsin A activity in multiple sclerosis brain. J. neurol. Sci. 21, 227 - 231 (1974).

13. BRODY, J. A., SEVER, J. L., EDGAR, A., McNEW, J.: Measles antibody titers of multiple sclerosis patients and their siblings. Neurology 22, 492 - 499 (1972).

14. BROWN, P., CATHALA, F., GAJDUSEK, D. C., GIBBS, C. J.: Measles antibodies in the cerebrospinal fluid of patients with multiple sclerosis. Proc. Soc. Exp. Biol. & Med. 137, 956 - 961 (1971).

15. CASPARY, E. A., CHAMBERS, M. E., FIELD, E. J.: Antibodies to measles antigen, control antigen, and monkey kidney antigen. Neurology 19, 1038 - 1042 (1969).

16. CASPARY, E. A., FIELD, E. J.: Sensitized lymphocytes in blood. A study of human neurological disease and experimental allergic encephalomyelitis. In: Progress in multiple sclerosis (ed. U. LEIBOWITZ), pp. 154 - 163. New York / London: Academic Press 1972.

17. CATALANO, L. W.: Herpesvirus hominis antibody in multiple sclerosis and amyotrophic lateral sclerosis. Neurology 22, 473 - 478 (1972).

18. CENDROWSKI, W., POLNA, I., NIEDZIELSKA, K.: Serum measles antibodies in multiple sclerosis. J. Neurol. Neurosurg. Psychiat. 36, 57 - 60 (1973).

19. CLARKE, J. K., DANE, D. S., DICK, G. W. A.: Viral antibody in the cerebrospinal fluid and serum of multiple sclerosis patients. Brain 88, 953 - 962 (1965).

20. CUMINGS, J. N.: The cerebral lipids in disseminated sclerosis and in amaurotic family idiocy. Brain 76, 551 (1953).

21. CUMINGS, J. N.: Lipid chemistry of the brain in demyelinating diseases. Brain 78, 554 (1955).

22. CUMINGS, J. N.: Abnormalities of lipid chemistry in cerebral lipidoses and demyelinating conditions. In: Modern Scientific Aspects of Neurology, p. 330. London: Arnold 1960.

23. CURRIE, S., URICH, H., Concurrence of multiple sclerosis and glioma. J. Neurol. Neurosurg. Psychiat. 37, 598 - 605 (1974).

24. CURRIER, R. D., MARTIN, E. A., WOOSLEY, P. C.: Prior events in multiple sclerosis. Neurology 24, 748 - 854 (1974).

25. CUTLER, R. W. P., WATTERS, G. V., HAMMERSTAD, J. P., MERLER, E.: Origin of cerebrospinal fluid gamma globulin in subacute sclerosing leukoencephalitis. Arch. Neurol. (Chic.) 17, 620 (1967).

26. CUTLER, R. W. P.: Diskussionsbemerkung. In: Neuropath. & Exp. Neurol. 27, 160 - 161 (1968).

27. CUZNER, M. L., DAVISON, A. N.: Changes in cerebral lysosomal enzyme activity and lipids in multiple sclerosis. J. neurol. Sci. 19, 29 - 36 (1973).

28. DANIELCZYK, W.: Immunosuppressiva bei der multiplen Sklerose. Wien. Med. Wschr. 118, 934 - 937 (1968).

29. DASTUR, D. K., SINGHAL, B. S.: Two unusual neuropathologically proven cases of multiple sclerosis from Bombay. J. Neurol. Sci. 20, 397 - 414 (1973).

30. DAU, P. C., PETERSON, R. D. A.: Transformation of lymphocytes from patients with multiple sclerosis. Arch. Neurol. 23, 32 - 40 (1970).

31. DAVIS, L. E., HERSH, E. M., CURTIS, J. E., LYNCH, R. E., ZIEGLER, D. K., NEUMANN, J. W., CHIN, T. D. Y.: Immune status of patients with multiple sclerosis. Neurology 22, 989 - 997 (1972).

32. DAVISON, A. N., WAJDA, M.: Cerebral lipids in multiple sclerosis. J. Neurochem. 9, 427 - 432 (1962).

33. DEAN, G.: Annual incidence, prevalence, and mortality of multiple sclerosis in white South-African-born and in white immigrants to South-Africa. Brit. Med. J. 2, 724 (1967).

34. FEIGIN, I., POPOFF, N.: Regeneration of myelin in multiple sclerosis. Neurology 16, 364 - 372 (1966).

35. FIELD, E. J., CASPARY, E. A.: Lymphocyte response depressive factor in multiple sclerosis. Brit. Med. J. 4, 529 - 532 (1971).

36. FIELD, E. J., CASPARY, E. A.: Lymphocyte sensitization to thymus and lymphe node antigen in multiple sclerosis and other neurological diseases. J. Neurol. Neurosurg. Psychiat. 36, 604 - 606 (1973).

37. FIELD, E. J., SHENTON, B. K., JOYCE, G.: Specific laboratory test for diagnosis of multiple sclerosis. Brit. Med. J. 1, 412 - 414 (1974).

38. FOG, T., JERSILD, C., PLATZ, B., SVEJGAARD, A., MIDHOLM, S.: Histocompatibility / HL-A antigens / and immuneresponses in multiple sclerosis. Proc. VII. Internat. Congress Neuropath. Budapest 1974 (in preparation).

39. FOG, T.: Rygmarvens patologiske anatomie ved disseminerat sclerose og disseminerat encephalomyelitis. Disputats. Copenhagen: Einar Munksgaard 1948.

40. FOG, T.: The topography of plaques in multiple sclerosis. Acta neurol. scand. 41 Suppl. 15, 1 - 162 (1965).

41. FOWLER, I., MORRIS, Ch. E., WHITLEY, Th.: Lymphocyte transformation in multiple sclerosis induced by cerebrospinal fluid. New Engl. J. Med. 275, 1041 - 1044 (1966).

42. FRICK, E., SCHEID-SEYDEL, L.: Untersuchungen mit J^{131}-markiertem gamma-globulin zur Frage der Abstammung der Liquoreiweißkörper. Klin. Wschr. 36, 66 und 857 (1958).

43. FRICK, E., STICKL, H.: Lymphocytentransformation bei Multipler Sklerose: Untersuchungen mit Liquor cerebrospinalis, Immunglobulinen und encephalitogenem Protein. Klin. Wschr. 46, 1066 - 1067 (1968).

44. FRICK, E., ANGSTWURM, H., SPÄTH, G.: Immunsuppressive Therapie der Multiplen Sklerose. Münch. med. Wschr. 112, 221 - 231 (1970).

45. FRICK, E., STICKL, H., ZINN, K.-H.: Lymphocytentransformation bei Multipler Sklerose. Nachweis einer Sensibilisierung gegen basisches Markscheidenprotein. Klin. Wschr. 52, 238 - 245 (1974).

46. FRIEDE, R. L., KNOLLER, M.: Quantitative enzyme profiles of plaques of multiple sclerosis. Experientia 20, 1 - 6 (1964).

47. GERSTL, B., KAHNKE, M. J., SMITH, J. K., TAVASTSTJERNA, M. G., HAYMAN, R. B.: Brain lipids in multiple sclerosis and other diseases. Brain 84, 310 - 319 (1961).

48. GERSTL, B., HAYMAN, R. B., TAVASTSTJERNA, M. G., SMITH, J. K.: Fatty acids of white matter of human brain. Experientia (Basel) 18, 131 - 133 (1962).

49. GERSTL, B., TAVASTSTJERNA, M. G., HAYMAN, R. B., SMITH, J. K., ENG, L. F.: Lipid studies of white matter and thalamus of human brains. J. Neurochem. 10, 889 - 902 (1963).

50. GERSTL, B., ENG, L. F., HAYMAN, R. B., TAVASTSTJERNA, M. G., BOND, P. R.: On the composition of human myelin. J. Neurochem. 14, 661 - 670 (1967).

51. GLEDHILL, R. F., HARRISON, B. M., McDONALD, W. I.: Pattern of re-myelination in the central nervous system. Nature (Lond.) 244, 443 - 444 (1973).

52. GOVINDARAJAN, K. R., OFFNER, H., CLAUSEN, J., FOG, T., HYLLESTED, K.: The lymphocytic cathepsins B-1 and D activities in multiple sclerosis. J. neurol. Sci. 23, 81 - 87 (1974).

53. HALLERVORDEN, J.: Die Multiple Sklerose als Viruskrankheit. Der Nervenarzt 23, 1 - 9 (1952).

54. HALLERVORDEN, J.: L'histopathologie de la sclérose multiple et de la sclérose diffuse chez l'homme et chez l'animal. Acta Neurol. et Psychiat. Belg. 8, 517 - 530 (1953).

55. HALLERVORDEN, J.: Anatomie und Pathogenese der Multiplen Sklerose. Münch. med. Wschr. 97, 509 - 516 (1955).

56. HALPERN, B., BAKOUCHE, P., MARTIAL-LASFARGUES, Chr.: Destruction des cellules nerveuses cultivées "in vitro" par les lymphocytes de malades atteints de sclérose en plaques. Presse Méd. 77, 2103 - 2106 (1969).

57. HERRMANN, E., JACOB, H.: Multiple Sklerose mit pseudotumoralem Verlauf. J. neurol. Sci. 7, 1 - 13 (1968).

58. HAUW, J. J., BERGER, B., ESCOUROLLE, R.: Etude de la cytotoxicité lymphocytaire sanguine en systeme homologue, au cours de la sclérose en plaques en poussée. Proc. VII. Internat. Congress Neuropath. Budapest 1974 (in preparation).

59. IBRAHIM, M. Z. M., ADAMS, C. W. M.: The Relationship between enzyme activity and neuroglia in plaques of multiple sclerosis. J. Neurosurg. Psychiat. 26, 101 - 110 (1963).

60. IIZUKA, R., JACOB, H., SOLCHER, H.: "Multiple-Sklerose" - Plaques nach Rubeolenerkrankung. J. neurol. Sci. 15, 327 - 338 (1972).

61. JACOB, H.: Tissue process in multiple sclerosis and parainfections and post-vaccinal encephalomyelitis. In: Pathogenesis and Etiology of Demyelinating Diseases. Add. ad. Int. Arch. Allergy 36, pp. 22-34. Basel - New York: Karger 1969.

62. JELLINGER, K., SEITELBERGER, F.: Akute tödliche Entmarkungs-Encephalitis nach wiederholten Hirntrockenzellen-Injektionen. Klin. Wschr. 36, 437 - 441 (1958).

63. KABAT, E. A., MOORE, D. H., LANDOW, H.: An electrophoretic study of the protein components in the cerebrospinal fluid and their relationship to serum proteins. J. Clin. Invest. 21, 571 (1942).

64. LAPRESLE, C.: Rabbit cathepsins D and E. In: Tissue proteinases (eds. A. J. BARRET, J. T. DINGLE) p. 135 - 155. Amsterdam: North Holland 1971.

65. LEIBOWITZ, U., ALTER, M.: Multiple sclerosis - clues to its cause. North Holland: American Elsevier 1973.

66. LENMAN, J. A. R., PETERS, T. J.: Herpes zoster and multiple sclerosis. Brit. med. J. 2, 218 (1969).

67. LHERMITTE, F., ESCOUROLLE, R., CATHALA, F., HAUW, J.-J., MARTEAU, R.: Etude neurophathologique d'un cas de sclérose en plaques. Rev. Neurol. (Paris) 129, 3 - 19 (1973).

68. LINK, H.: Immunoglobulin abnormalities in multiple sclerosis. Ann. Clin. Res. 5, 330 - 366 (1973).

69. LUMSDEN, C. E.: The neuropathology of multiple sclerosis. In: Handbook of Clinical, Neurology, Vol. 9: Multiple Sclerosis and other demyelinating Diseases (eds. P. J. VINKEN, G. W. BRUYN), pp. 217 - 319. Amsterdam: North-Holland-Publ. Comp. 1970.

70. MACCHI, G.: The Pathology of the blood vessels in multiple sclerosis. J. Neuropath. Exp. Neurol. 13, 378 - 384 (1954).

71. McDONALD, W. I.: Pathophysiology in multiple sclerosis. Brain 97, 179 - 196 (1974).

72. McFADYEN, D. J., REEVE, Ch. E., BRATTY, P. J. A., THOMAS, J. W.: Failure of antilymphocytic globulin therapy in chronic progressive multiple sclerosis. Neurology 23, 592 - 598 (1973).

73. MEYER-RIENECKER, H. J., OLISCHER, R. M.: Aspekte der diagnostischen Kriterien und Klassifikation der Multiplen Sklerose. Fortschr. Neurol. Psychiat. 42, 385 - 418 (1974).

74. Ter MEULEN, V., KOPROWSKI, H., IWASAKI, Y., KÄCKELL, Y. M., MÜLLER, D.: Fusion of cultured multiple sclerosis brain cells with indicator cells: Presence of nucleocapsids and virions and isolation of parainfluenza-type virus. Lancet 3, 1 - 5 (1972).

75. NARANG, H. K., FIELD, E. J.: An electron-microscopic study of multiple sclerosis biopsy material: some unusual inclusions. J. neurol. Sci. 18, 287 - 300 (1973).

76. NEUMANN, J. W., ZIEGLER, D. K.: Therapeutic trial of immuno-suppressive agents in multiple sclerosis. Neurology 22, 1268 - 1271 (1972).

77. NONNE, M.: Kasuistisches zur Differentialdiagnose zwischen multipler Sklerose und Rückenmarkskompression. Dtsch. med. Wschr. 37, 1 - 16 (1910).

78. NOORT, St. van den, STJERNHOLM, R. L.: Lymphotoxic activity in multiple sclerosis serum. Neurology 21, 783 - 793 (1971).

79. NORRBY, E., SALMI, A. A., LINK, H., VANDVIK, B., OLSSON, J.-E., PANELIS, M.: The measles virus antibody response in subacute sclerosing panencephalitis and multiple sclerosis. In: Slow Virus Disease (eds. W. ZEMAN, E. H. LENNETTE), pp. 72 - 85. Baltimore: The Williams & Wilkins Comp. 1974.

80. NORRBY, E., LINK, H., OLSSON, J.-E.: Measles virus antibodies in multiple sclerosis. Arch. Neurol. 30, 285 - 292 (1974).

81. OFFNER, H., AMMITZBOLL, T., CLAUSEN, J., FOG, T., HYYLESTED, K., EINSTEIN, E.: Immune response of lymphocytes from patients with multiple sclerosis to phytohemagglutinin, basic protein of myelin and measles antigens. Acta Neurol. Scandinav. 50, 373 - 381 (1974).

82. OPPENHEIM, G.: Zur pathologischen Anatomie der multiplen Sklerose mit besonderer Berücksichtigung der Hirnrindenherde. Neurol. Centralblatt 19, 1 - 13 (1908).

83. PERIER, O., GREGOIRE, A.: Electron microscopic features of multiple sclerosis lesions. Brain 88, 937 - 952 (1965).

84. PETTE, E., PETTE, H.: Zur Ätiopathogenese der Entmarkungsencephalomyelitis (einschließlich der akuten Multiplen Sklerose) und der Polyneuritis. Klin. Wschr. 34, 713 - 720 (1956).

85. PUTNAM, T. J.: Studies in multiple sclerosis: "encephalitis" and sclerotic plaques produced by venular obstruction. Arch. Neurol. Psychiat. (Chic.) 33, 929 - 940 (1933).

86. PUTNAM, T. J.: Evidence of vascular occlusion in multiple sclerosis and "encephalomyelitis". Arch. Neurol. Psychiat. (Chic.) 37, 1298 - 1321 (1937).

87. RAINE, C. S., FIELD, E. J.: Nuclear structures in nerve cells in multiple sclerosis. Brain Res. 10, 266 - 268 (1968).

88. RAINE, C. S., HUMMELGARD, A., SWANSON, E., BORNSTEIN, M. B.: Multiple sclerosis: Serum-induced demyelination in vitro. J. neurol. Sci. 20, 127 - 148 (1973).

89. RINNE, U. K., RIEKKINEN, P. J., ARSTILLA, A. U.: Biochemical and electron microscopic alterations in the white matter outside demyelinated plaques in multiple sclerosis. In: Progress in Multiple Sclerosis (ed. U. LEIBOWITZ), pp. 76 - 98. New York - London: Academic Press 1972.

90. RÖYTTÄ, M., FREY, H., RINNE, U. K., RIEKKINEN, P.: Mechanism of myelinbreakdown in MS and SSPE autopsy and biopsy samples. Proc. VII. Internat. Congress Neuropath. Budapest 1974 (in preparation).

91. RUSSELL, D. S., RUBINSTEIN, L. J.: Pathology of tumors of the nervous system. 3rd edition, p. 179. London: Arnold 1971.

92. SALMI, A., PANELIUS, M., VAINIONPÄÄ, R.: Antibodies against different viral antigens in cerebrospinal fluid of patients with multiple sclerosis and other neurological diseases. Acta Neurol. Scandinav. 50, 183 - 193 (1974).

93. SALMI, A. A., PANELIUS, M., HALONEN, P., RINNEN, U. K., PENTINNEN, K.: Measles virus antibody in cerebrospinal fluids from patients with multiple sclerosis. Brit. med. J. 19, 477 - 479 (1972).

94. SAYK, J.: Liquorsyndrome. Schweiz. Arch. Neurol. Neurochir. Psychiat. 93, 75 - 97 (1964).

95. SAYK, J., SCHMIDT, R. M.: Zur Liquordiagnostik bei der multiplen Sklerose. Ärztl. Wschr. 11, 788 - 793 (1956).

96. SEVER, J. L., KURTZKE, J. F.: Delayed dermal hypersensitivity to measles and mumps antigens among multiple sclerosis and control patients. Neurology 19, 113 - 115 (1969).

97. SIMPSON, Ch. A., VEJJAJIVA, A., CASPARY, E. A., MILLER, H.: ABO blood groups in multiple sclerosis. Lancet 1, 1366 (1965).

98. SIMPSON, J. F., TOURTELOTTE, W. W., KOMEN, E., PARKER, J. A., ITABASHI, H. H.: Fluorescent protein tracing in mulitple sclerosis brain tissue. Neurology 20, 373 - 377 (1969).

99. SUZUKI, K., ANDREWS, J. M., WALTZ, J. M, TERRY, R. D.: Ultrastructural studies of multiple sclerosis. Lab. Invest. 20, 444 - 454 (1969).

100. SCHALTENBRAND, G.: Die multiple Sklerose der Menschen. Leipzig: Georg Thieme 1943.

101. SCHALTENBRAND, G.: Multiple Sklerose. Mat. Med. Nordm. 24, 57 - 72 (1972).

102. SCHLOTE, W., ROSS, W.: Gibt es ein charakteristisches Liquorzellbild bei multipler Sklerose? Nervenarzt 45, 12 Seiten (1974).

103. SCHMIDT, R. M.: Der Liquor cerebrospinalis. Berlin: Volk und Gesundheit 1968.

104. SCHRADER, A.: Multiple Sklerose: Versuch mit Immunsuppression. Münch. med. Wschr. 110, 2842 (1968).

105. SCHRADER, A., STOCHDORPH, O.: Diagnostische und pathologische Aspekte der multiplen Sklerose. Klin. Wschr. 47, 501 - 507 (1969).

106. SCHULLER, E., DELASNERIE, N., DELOCHE, G., LORIDAN, M.: Multiple sclerosis: A two-phase disease? Acta neurol. Scandinav. 49, 453 - 460 (1973).

107. TOURTELOTTE, W. W., PARKER, J. A.: Postmortem evaluation of the blood-brain barrier in multiple sclerosis. J. Neuropath. Exp. Neurol. 27, 159 - 163 (1968).

108. TOURTELOTTE, W. W.: Interaction de l'immunité locale du système nerveux central et de l'immunité général au cours de la sclérose en plaques. Rev. Neurol. 127, 497 - 504 (1972).

109. UCHIMURA, Y., SHIRAKI, H., HARUHARA, Ch.: Zur Histopathologie und Pathogenese der Entmarkungsencephalomyelitiden mit besonderer Berücksichtigung der Entmarkungsprozesse infolge der Lyssaschutzimpfung. Psychiat. et Neurol. Jap. 56, 505 - 535 (1955).

110. UCHIMURA, Y., SHIRAKI, H.: A contribution to the classification and the pathogenesis of demyelinating encephalomyelitis. J. Neuropath. Exp. Neurol. 16, 139 - 203 (1957).

111. ULE, G., KRAEMER, R.: Konzentrische Sklerose der Brücke. Arch. Psychiat. Zschr. Neurol. 192, 613 - 619 (1954).

112. YAHR, M. D., GOLDENSOHN, E. S., KABAT, E. A.: Further studies on the gamma globulin content of cerebrospinal fluid in multiple sclerosis and other demyelinating disease. Ann. N. Y. Acad. Sci. 58, 613 (1954).

113. WEINRAUDER, H., LACH, B.: Immunfluorescence studies on the localization of the brain-specific antigen S in the central nervous system of the rat. Proc. VII. Internat. Congress Neuropath. Budapest 1974 (in preparation).

114. WENDER, M., FILIPEK-WENDER, H., STANISLAWSKA, B.: Cholesteryl esters in apparently normal white matter in multiple sclerosis. Europ. Neurol. 10, 340 - 348 (1973).

115. WROBLEWSKI, T.: L'inhibition de la migration de macrophages de cobaye au cours de E.A.E., avec différantes antigènes. Proc. VII. Internat. Congress Neuropath. Budapest 1974 (in preparation).

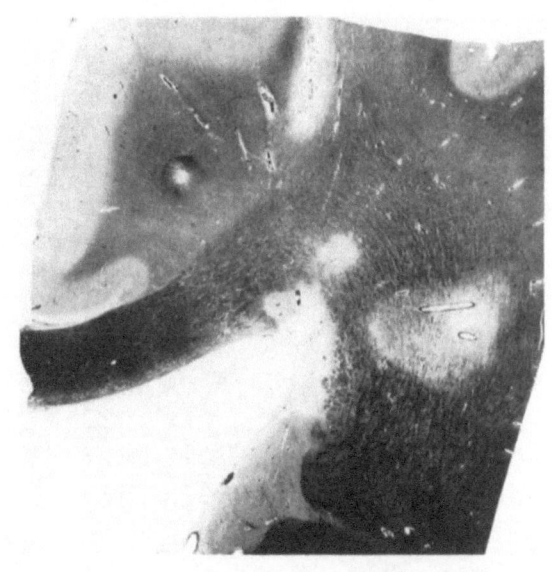

Fig. 1. Perivenous and periventricular demyelination in the white matter (van GIESON)

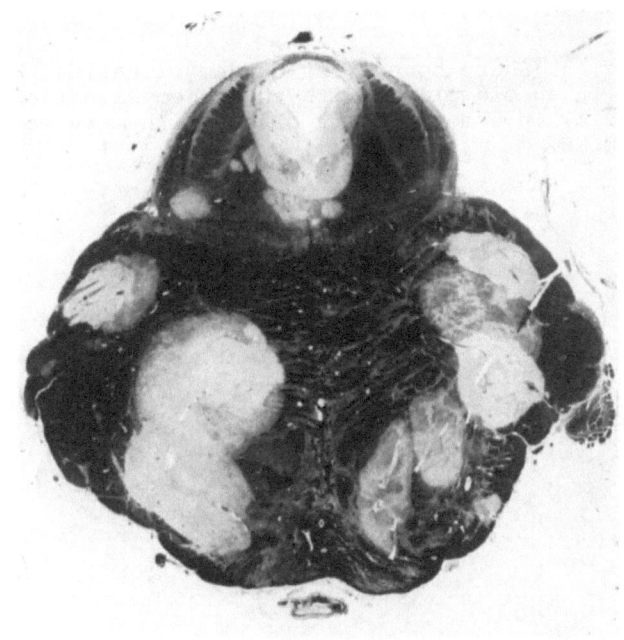

Fig. 2. Demyelination around the aqueduct. Disseminated plaques of different age in the pons, partly with typical correlation to the venous system (HEIDENHAIN-WOELKE)

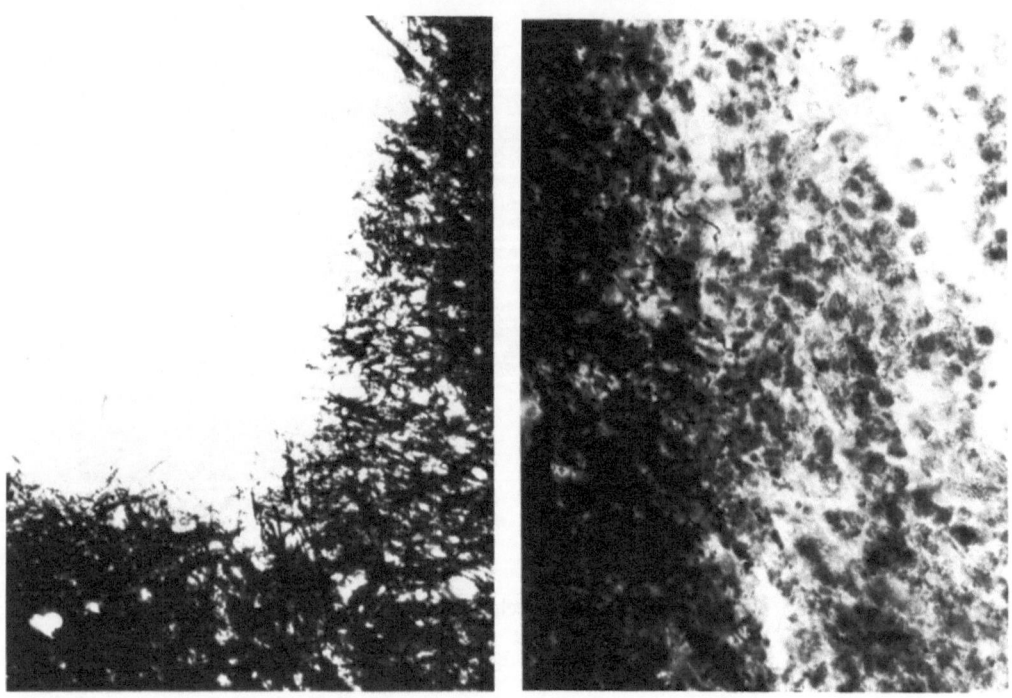

Fig. 3. Sharp boundaries of demyelination
a) in an old plaque with total demyelination without any macrophages,
and b) in a more recent plaque with many macrophagues (HEIDENHAIN-
WOELKE)

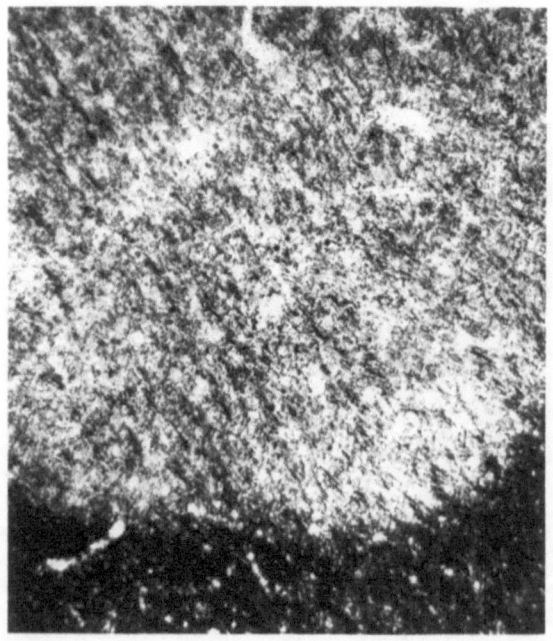

Fig. 4. Shadow plaque with a
rarefaction of myelin sheats

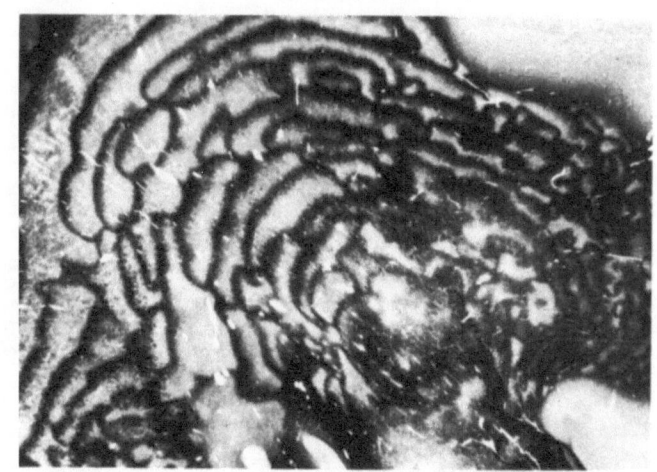

Fig. 5. Well preserved nerve cells between macrophages and proliferating astroglial cells in a fresh focus of demyelination. Small perivascular cuffs of lymphocytes (van GIESON)

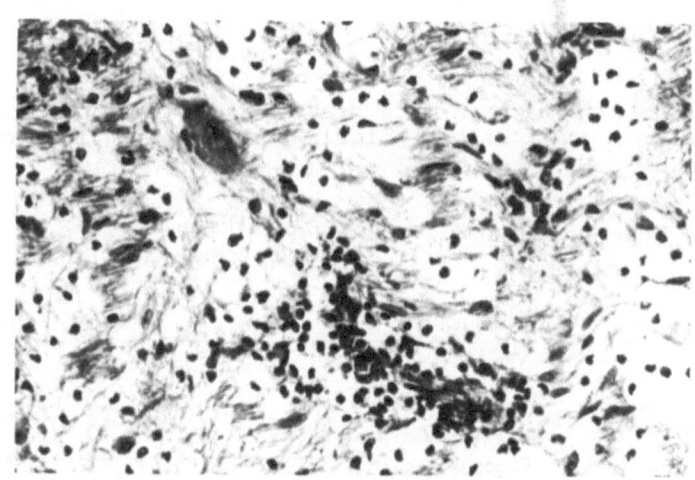

Fig. 6. Concentric sclerosis
a) concentric pattern of parallel rings of demyelination

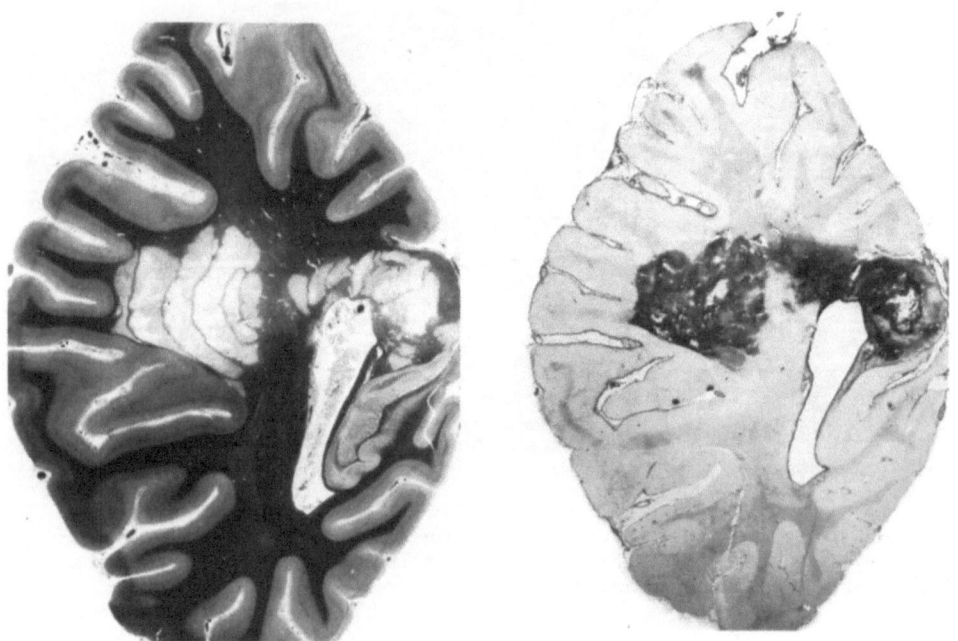

Fig. 6. (continued)
b) mosaic pattern in a transitional type (van GIESON)
c) astrocytic fibre gliosis corresponding to Fig. 5 b (HOLZER)

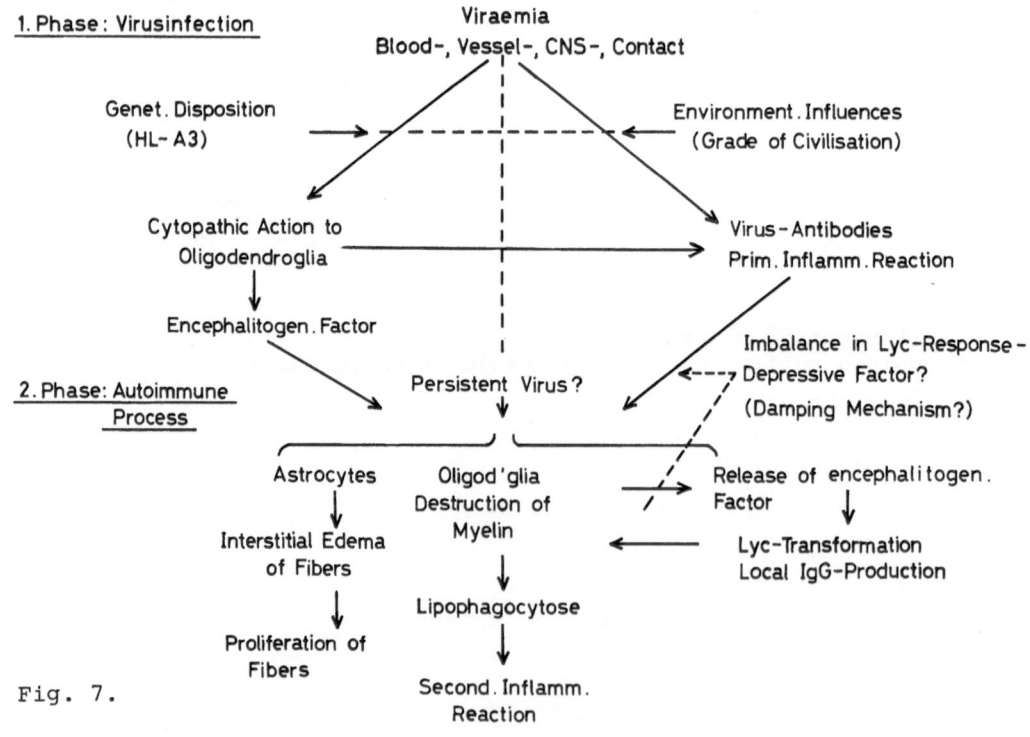

Fig. 7.

144

Neurological Aspects of False Diagnosis and Failure to Diagnose Multiple Sclerosis[*]

H. J. BAUER, H. ORTHNER, and S. POSER

Unquestionably, the consequence of a false diagnosis of multiple sclerosis (MS) are usually more serious than failure to diagnose this disease. Fear of provoking an exacerbation by lumbar puncture is unjustified, and MS is not an adequate reason for the omission of myelography, an arteriogram or an air study of the cerebrospinal fluid (csf) - spaces if an indication for such diagnostic measures exists. However, every neurologist has seen cases in which technical procedures appear to have prepared the way for rather sudden episodes of worsening, sometimes with irreversible results.

MS in a 16-year old male patient was characterized by a course of bouts and remissions, with brain stem symptomatology predominating and suggesting a brain stem tumor. Angiography of the vertebral artery was performed. The artery appeared somewhat stretched and displaced with respect to the clivus, this was taken as evidence for a space-occupying lesion. Operation revealed no tumor. In spite of this negative result, an intrapontine tumor was further suspected and a course of roentgen ray therapy was given. Relentless rapid deterioration ensued and the patient died 5 months after operation. Autopsy revealed extensive demyelination in the brain stem and other areas of the central nervous system.

This case may serve to exemplify the necessity of caution in the performance and evaluation of exacting diagnostic and therapeutic measures in MS. Where the clinical condition permits, meticulous history-taking and careful, repeated examination should not be bypassed because technical procedures promise quicker results.

In Table 1 a survey is given of the frequency of neurological symptoms in MS[1]. Spasticity, sensory disturbances, impairment of cranial nerve function, disturbances of bladder-, bowel- and sexual function lead the list. Fig. 1 shows the regional distribution of symptoms and indicates that symmetry is characteristic. Undeniably, lateralization is encountered frequently in the individual case. Analogous to the presence of a craniocaudal level in spinal lesions, however, the persistence of lateralization and the absence of contralateral disturbances demand a reconsideration of diagnosis.

---

[*]Supported by the Deutsche Forschungsgemeinschaft, Schwerpunkt "Ätiologie und Pathogenese der Multiplen Sklerose und verwandter Erkrankungen".

[1]The statistical data are derived from the documentation pool of the Multiple Sclerosis Research program of the DEUTSCHE FORSCHUNGSGEMEINSCHAFT.

Table 1. Frequency of neurological symptoms in MS

Type of Disturbance	Pool N = 812	R. Müller (1949) N = 582	J. K. Kurtzke (1961); N = 408 VA Bronx-Series
Pyramidal tract signs	757 (93 %)	a	93 %
Paresis of limbs	598 (74 %)	436 (75 %)	a
Impairment of coordination		a	87 %
"balance disturbance"	343 (42 %)	287 (49 %)	a
Impairment of sensory funtions	651 (80 %)	a	65 % (excl. subjective complaints)
"figure writing"		359 (81 %)	
Impairment of vegetative functions	413 (51 %)		53 %
micturition	399 (49 %)	290 (50 %)	a
defecation	158 (19 %)	145 (25 %)	a
Visual impairment	289 (36 %)	a	40 % (N = 93)
Impairment of cranial nerve/brain stem functions (excl. trigem. neuralgia)	562 (69 %)	a	81 %
Impairment of cerebral functions	451 (56 %)	a	20 % (N = 93)
euphoria	192 (24 %)	102 (18 %)	a
dementia	35 (4 %)	164 (28 %)	a

a   No comparable data

The diagnosis "spinal form of MS" in cases of spastic paraplegia is a dangerous diagnosis. In MARSHALL's series of 52 patients with spastic paraplegia the diagnosis remained unclear in 27, of the other 25 only 10 proved to be MS. PIA reports on a series of 93 cases of "spinal MS" in whom vascular malformations (angioma) were found; he points out that the risk of arteriography is warranted in view of the possibility of effective treatment.

Disturbances not encountered as often as those in Table 1, but play-ing an important role in the false diagnosis of MS, are listed in Table 2. *Pain*, usually described as rheumatic, not definitely local-ized and often accompanied by paraesthesias was registered in 30 % of our cases. In patients presenting pain in conjunction with spinal cord symptomatology diagnosed as "spinal MS", vascular malformations should always be considered as a diagnostic possibility. In a series of 60 cases of this type, AMINOFF and LOGUE observed pain as an initial symptom in 42 %, later in 100 % of their patients.

Vascular malformations of the spinal cord may have a recurrent course simulating the bouts and remissions of MS. Important differentiating signs are a craniocaudal boundary of sensory disturbances, high cere-brospinal fluid protein values without the IgG increase characterizing MS, and lesions in the peripheral neuron.

Table 2. Symptoms less often found in MS

	pool n	n = 812 %	lit.
Pain, all forms	241	30	10 - 27 %
headache	89	11	
trigeminal pain	41	5	1 - 2 % (only neuralgia)
vertigo	85	10	5 - 31 %
seizures	9	1	0,5 - 3 %
disturbances of consciousness	8	1	1 - 4 %
aphasia	2	<1	< 1 %

The course of vascular myelopathies due to disturbances of venous circulation may be characterized by bouts and remissions leading to the false diagnosis of MS.

A 50-year old female patient died after 4 bouts of "spinal MS". Even the histopathology on first glance appeared strongly suggestive of MS: a myelin stain, showing the cross section of the spinal cord at the level of C 6, revealed large areas of demyelination bilaterally in the posterior bundles and an additional plaque in the lateral tracts of the left side. An area of preserved myelin fibers in the marginal areas was unusual for MS, however and much more typical for venous lesions as described by JELLINGER and STOCHDORPH. A cresyl violet stain showed an area of total necrosis invaded by granular cells and sharply deliminated at the edge of the anterior horn.

Headache was encountered in 10 - 26 % of MS cases in the literature and in 11 % of our own cases (Table 2). Retrobulbar neuritis and acute brain stem lesions with meningeal reactions may be the cause of transient headache in MS. Tension- (migraine-like) headache, usually experienced long before the clinical manifestations of MS, hypertension and cervical spondylosis in older patients (which we encountered in 12 % of a series of 150 patients) are common causes of persisting headache.

Transient *trigeminal nerve pain* was experienced by 5 % of the patients in our series of 812 MS cases at some time in the course of their disease, without adequate differentiation of tic douloureux from pain of a more continuous type, however. In the literature, typical tic douloureux is described in approximately 1 % of MS cases.

Epileptic seizures are a rare symptom of MS. Our own figure of 1 % in the series of 812 patients correlates well with the figures reported by other authors. Occasionally, symptomatic epilepsy, due to perinatal or early childhood lesions or due to a space-occupying intracranial lesion, may concur with MS. In this connection, the concurrence of glioma and MS appears noteworthy. CURRIE and URICH listed 12 cases from the literature and 3 cases observed by them. These authors discuss the possibility that gliomas may develop from MS plaques.

Vertigo as an isolated symptom is transient, but a fairly frequent complaint of MS patients. The brain stem symptomatology often encountered in MS makes vertigo a symptom difficult to evaluate if other symptoms strongly suggestive of disseminated symptomatology are not present.

In this connection, *retrobulbar neuritis* is of particular value. However, the presence of this sign may also be misleading. Particular caution is required in evaluating residual signs of retrobulbar neuritis such as temporal pallor of the optic disks. This sign should never be accepted as evidence of prior retrobulbar neuritis if ophthalmological examination reveals no visual defects (scotomas).

Visual defects were registered in only 36 % of the 812 cases of our documentation pool. By the measurement of evoked potentials using the pattern stimulation method, HALLIDAY et al. found a retarded cortical response indicating a lesion of the optic pathways in 90 % of their patients. Pallor of the optic disks may be seen in severe malnutrition, anemia, exogenous intoxications (SMON), nicotine addiction (tobacco amblyopia), systemic lupus erythematosis. A list of conditions, in which transient disturbances of vision may occur, is given in Table 3.

Table 3. Transient impairment of vision in various disorders of the central nervous system may occur in:

Stenosis of carotid artery
Ischemia of basilar artery
Aneurysms at base of brain
Space-occupying process in region of optic chiasma
Diabetes
Temporal arteriitis
Neurosyphilis
Migraine accompagné
Cerebral seizures
Spinocerebellar heredodegenerative disease
Hormonal contraceptive drugs

It is generally accepted that *dissemination in place and time* is an essential feature justifying the clinical diagnosis of MS. It should not be forgotten, however, that a number of other conditions may present a disseminated symptomatology and a course suggestive of bouts and remissions. As shown in Table 4, cerebrospinal fluid findings may provide important criteria for differentiating such conditions.

Table 4. Diseases of the central nervous system characterized by disseminated symptoms and a course of bouts and remissions

	Disseminated symptoms	Course in bouts and remissions	MS-type csf alterations
MS	+	+	+
Monocyclic encephalomyelitis	+	−	+
M. Boeck	+	+	(+)
Neurosyphilis	+	(+)	+
Panarteriitis	+	+	−
Arteriosclerosis	+	(+)	−
Embolism	+	+	−
Dysglobulinemias	+	(+)	(+)
Multilocular tumors	+	+	−

Parasitosis may produce disturbances suggestive of MS.

A chronic-progressive disorder of the central nervous system in a 30-year old man characterized by tetraspasticity, and subeuphorea was interpreted as the classical, full-blown picture of MS. Cerebrospinal fluid findings also seemed to be suggestive of MS, total protein, with persisting concentrations of about 80 mg %, appeared rather high, however. This and the unusual occupational history of the patient - he repaired manure bins - made a reconsideration of the established diagnosis of MS advisable. A broad spectrum of serological studies finally revealed an infection with cysticerosis. The therapy with cyclophosphamide resulted in a gradual disappearance of the serological reactions, which initially were strongly positive. The neurological condition remained chronic-progressive, however.

Unquestionably, failure to diagnose a space-occupying lesion of the central nervous system is the greatest hazard in the differential diagnosis of MS. There is hardly a tumor, vascular malformation or spinal compression due to skeletal anomalies and degenerative alterations that has not erroneously and prematurely been tagged as MS, with the result, that vitally important neurosurgical measures were not taken.

On the other hand, the failure to diagnose MS may also have serious consequences. In 40 autopsies in which MS was histopathologically confirmed, there were 6 patients in whom a psychotic condition led to permanent confinement in a mental hospital; 5 of these were marked as schizophrenia. Fortunately cases of this kind are rare. Far more frequent consequences of the failure to diagnose MS are misguidance in the choice of profession and in family planning. In this connection, inadequate information of the patient with respect to the diagnosis may have grave consequences.

In spite of all technical progress, false diagnosis of MS and the failure to diagnose this disease will remain a serious problem confronting neurologists and neurosurgeons. Continuous reexamination and reassessment of the diagnosis of MS are obligatory; in practice these are dependent on an efficient organization of follow-up care for the patient.

Note: Neurological departments cooperating in the formation of an MS-documentation pool (MS-Research program of Deutsche Forschungsgemeinschaft.

Neurologische Univ.-Klinik Göttingen, Taunusklinik Falkenstein, Kamillus-Klinik Asbach, Med. Akademie Lübeck, Medizinische Hochschule Hannover, Neurologische Univ.-Klinik Würzburg, MS-Centrum Melsbroek, Kommunehospitalet Kopenhagen, Karl-Bonhoeffer-Nervenklinik Berlin, Allgem. Krankenhaus St. Georg Hamburg, Neurologische Univ.-Klinik Hamburg, Neurologische Klinik Essen, Schloßparkklinik Berlin, Klinikum Steglitz Berlin, Rudolf-Virchow-Krankenhaus Berlin, Neurologische Klinik Darmstadt, Department of Neurology Fukuoka, Klinik Dr. Evers Langscheid, Univ.-Nervenklinik Bonn, Nervenklinik der Universität München.

Summary

A survey of the diagnostic features of multiple sclerosis is given and problems encountered in the differential diagnosis are discussed. False diagnosis of MS is a hazard in a wide variety of diseases of the central nervous system. One of the most tragic consequences is failure to recognize space-occupying processes amenable to neurosurgical therapy. On the other hand, failure to diagnose MS may also lead to serious disadvantages for the patient. A number of cases is described to exemplify this.

Key words: Multiple sclerosis cysticercosis, epileptic seizures, pain syndromes, psychosis, retrobulbar neuritis, spinal angioma, vascular myopathy.

REFERENCES

AMINOFF, M. J., LOGUE, V.: Clinical features of spinal vascular malformations. Brain 97, 197 - 210 (1974).

BAUER, H., FIRNHABER, W.: Zur Leistungsprognose Multiple-Sklerose-Kranker. Dtsch. Med. Wschr. 88, 1357 - 1364 (1963).

BUSHART, W.: Fehldiagnose MS bei spinalen Prozessen. Internist 7, 157 - 166 (1966).

CURRIE, S., URICH, H.: Concurrence of multiple sclerosis and glioma. J. Neurol., Neurosurg. Psychiat. 37, 598 - 605 (1974).

FARAGO, I., DUX, A. M.: Atypische klinische Aspekte der Multiplen Sklerose. Schweiz. Arch. Neurol., Neurochir., Psychiat. 109, 217 - 227 (1974).

FULFORD, K. W. M., CATTERALL, R. D., DETHANTY, J. J., DONIACH, D., KREMER, M.: A collagen disorder of the nervous system presenting as multiple sclerosis. Brain 95, 373 - 386 (1972).

HACKETT, E. R., MARTINEZ, R. D., LARSON, P. F., PADDISON, R. M.: Optic neuritis in systemic lupus erythematodes. Arch. Neurol. 31, 9 - 11 (1974).

HOWE, J. R., TAREN, J. A.: Foramen magnum tumors-pitfalls in diagnosis. Jama 225, 1061 - 1066 (1973).

JANZEN, R.: Differentialdiagnostische Schwierigkeiten bei Multipler Sklerose. Dtsch. Med. Wschr. 92, 764 - 765 (1967).

JANZEN, R.: Entstehung von Fehldiagnosen. Stuttgart: Georg Thieme 1970.

JELLINGER, K.: Vascularization of the spinal cord. Acta Neurochirurgica 26, 327 - 338 (1972).

KREINDLER, A., MACOVEI-PATRICHI, M.: Recurrent cranial nerve palsies of dysglobulinemic orgin. J. Neurol. Sci (Amst.) 6, 117 - 123 (1968).

KURTZKE, J. F.: Clinical Manifestations of multiple sclerosis. In: Handbuch der klinischen Neurologie (Hrsg. P. J. VINKEN, G. W. BRUYN), Bd. 9, S. 161 - 216. Berlin - Heidelberg - New York: Springer 1970.

McALPINE, D., LUMSDEN, Ch., ACHESON, E. D.: Multiple Sclerosis - A reappraisal. Livingstone: Churchill 1972.

NEUMAYER, E.: Die vasculäre Myelopathie. Wien - New York: Springer 1967.

RINTELEN, F.: Zum Wesen und zur Differentialdiagnose der "Retrobulbärneuritis" bei Multipler Sklerose. Ophthalmologica 167, 100-113 (1973).

SCHRADER, A.: Multiple Sklerose. In: Differentialdiagnose neurologischer Krankheitsbilder (Hrsg. G. BODECHTEL), S. 342 - 367. Stuttgart: Georg Thieme 1974.

STOCHDORPH, O.: Vascular pathology of the spinal cord. Acta Neurochir. 26, 330 (1972).

STRÖTKER, H.: Quantitative morphologisch-klinische Studien an 25 Fällen von chronischer Multipler Sklerose. Dissertation, Göttingen 1968.

VERON, J. P., ESCOUROLLE, R., BUGE, A., CASTAIGNE, P.: Acute necrotic myelopathy. Europ. Neurol. II, 83 - 96 (1974).

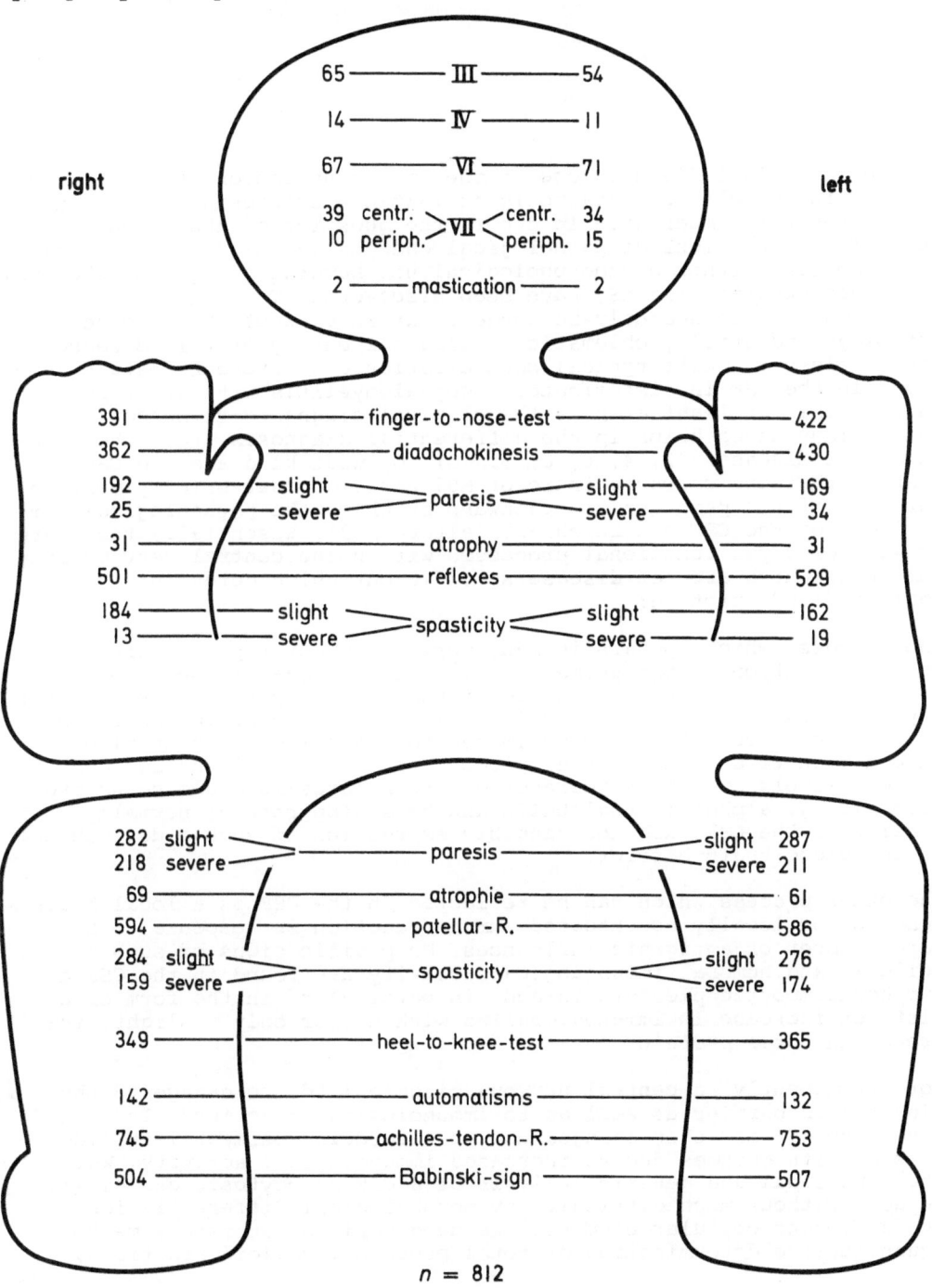

Fig. 1. Regional distribution of symptoms in MS

Cerebrospinal Fluid in Multiple Sclerosis and Its Clinical Diagnostic Value

H. W. DELANK

The cerebrospinal fluid is one of the important components to be considered in the clinical diagnosis of multiple sclerosis (MS). Main
reason for this importance is due to the question of the value and
specific informations of pathological changes in the CSF in this disease. So far neither cytomorphological nor humoral changes of the CSF,
which are specific for MS, have been discovered. This inadequacy of
CSF diagnosis can scarcely be wondered at in view of the obscure
aetiology and still problematic nosological entity of this disease.
Nevertheless, a quite typical constellation of different features are
found in the CSF in disseminated encephalomyelitis with great regularity. This at least enables the clinical diagnosis to be confirmed
and in many cases helps in the differential diagnosis from other neurological diseases (2, 4, 6, 8, 9, 10). Of what kind are the CSF
changes that are characteristic of MS? First we must briefly mention
our idea of the pathogenetic pathways by which the physiological composition of the CSF can be chiefly altered (3). Essentially there are
two pathological functional processes within the central nervous system (CNS) which are not disease specific but which determine the pathological CSF picture:

One process, which appears in many very different types of disease,
is an alteration in the permeability of the blood-brain barrier. As
a result, that is, in consequence of the greater permeability of this
physiological barrier, the CSF loses its typical profile due to the
barrier and increasingly approximates to the composition of blood.
In addition to a haematogenous pleocytosis, greatly increased CSF
protein levels and the appearance of other large-molecule serum proteins (e. g. alpha$_2$-macroglobulin and beta lipoprotein) normally
foreign to the CSF, are the tangible expression of such a disturbance
in the blood-brain barrier.

The other process which can be reflected in the CSF is a local brain
reaction or locally accentuated immune reaction in response to a
large number of antigenic influences. Unspecific signs of such a
cellular and humoral immunological activity are found in the CSF as
lymphoplasmocytic pleocytosis and, in particular, in the form of a
distinct increase in immunoglobulins with no, or only a slight, increase in total protein.

Not infrequently, a central nervous disease leads to damage to the
blood-brain barrier as well as to immunological reactions. In these
cases the CSF may show changes due to disordered permeability side
by side with changes due to increased immunological activity. While
the functional and genetic analysis of a CSF pleocytosis can usually
be done without much difficulty by morphological differentiation of
the different cellular elements, we need various laboratory methods
(quantitative determination of total proteins, colloid reactions,

electrophoresis, immunoelectrophoreses and MANCINI's immunodiffusion method) for the detection of changes in the CSF protein pattern, i. e. a CSF dysproteinosis (2). Now, in MS, the CSF changes typical of the disease are produced by immunological processes and not, or hardly ever by a disturbance of the blood-brain barrier function (the "immunoreactive CSF syndrome") (Table 1).

Table 1. Frequency of the abnormalities in the immunoactive CSF syndrome in multiple sclerosis (compiled from the literature and own observations)

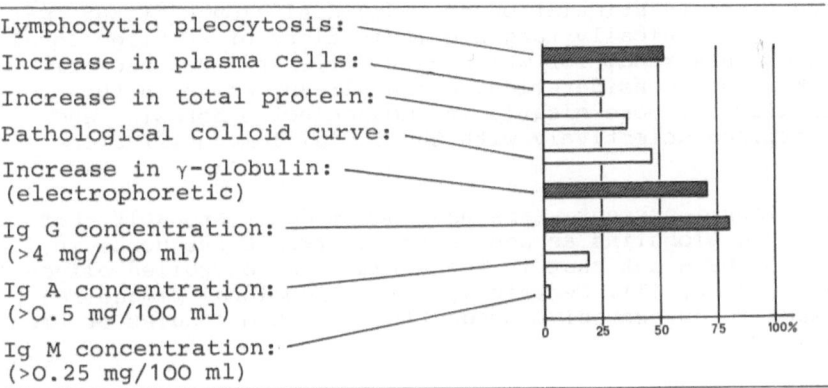

Lymphocytic pleocytosis:
Increase in plasma cells:
Increase in total protein:
Pathological colloid curve:
Increase in γ-globulin: (electrophoretic)
Ig G concentration: (>4 mg/100 ml)
Ig A concentration: (>0.5 mg/100 ml)
Ig M concentration: (>0.25 mg/100 ml)

If one enquires into the frequency of the individual findings in this immunoreactive CSF syndrome in MS, it is seen that, without taking into consideration the various types and courses of the disease, in more than half of the cases there is a moderate lymphoplastocytic pleocytosis (scarcely more than 100/3 cells) and in about 70 %, the gammaglobulin values detectable by electrophoresis are increased. This increase in gammaglobulins is caused very largely by an increase in the IgG content, contrary to many other inflammatory disorders, in which other Ig types may be considerably involved in the increase of Ig, depending on the stage of the disease.

As characteristic for the CSF pattern typical of MS can be considered: the moderate lymphoplasmccytic pleocytosis and the marked increase in immunoglobulins of the IgG type accompanied by only an insignificant rise in total protein. It is also worthy of note that these changes in the CSF are largely independent of the activity, duration and nature of the clinical picture, and are seen as a permanent finding. In MS we speak, therefore, of a "persistent immunoactive CSF syndrome" (4).

The question as to whether, and with what significance, immunoactivity is characterized by disorders or conspicuous features of protein synthesis in this disease has long been discussed as a question of basic research in MS (1, 7, 9). In other words whether the immunoglobulins found in particular in the CSF are characterized by definite structural peculiarities. The question seems the more justified since atypical globulin fractions have long been observed in the protein spectrum, particularly in agar electrophorectic separation of the CSF proteins in MS patients (1, 7).

But in order to indicate the clinical importance of the present state of our knowledge, the basic structure of an immunoglobulin must first be recalled briefly. Immunoglobulin molecules are made up of two kinds of polypeptide chains, the heavy H-chains and the light L-chains. The H-chains define the Ig class (i. e. the IgA, IgG, IgM type etc.) and the L-chains the type of immunoglobulin. The L-chain of an immunoglobulin is either of the kappa or the lambda type. Normal human serum and also the CSF contain immunoglobulins of the kappa and lambda types in definite proportions. Today it can be assumed that molecules of an Ig class which are very heterogenous in the amino acid sequence in the variable parts of the molecule and, probably associated with this, in their electrical charge, are formed by different cell clones. If it is found that in a certain Ig class there is increase of a particular type of Ig, e. g. the kappa or lambda type, then it can be inferred that there is an elective stimulation of individual clones of the immunocompetent cells. Clinically tangible indications of an oligoclonal immune reaction of this kind, for which very different possible origins must be taken into consideration, often already arise in the electrophoretic diagram, more clearly in immunoelectrophoresis, and they can be determined selectively with the radial immunodiffusion method.

Clinical observations in recent years have now made it probable that the production of Ig globulins as seen with remarkable frequency in the CSF in cases of MS - not that in the serum - is controlled oligoclonally (1, 4, 6, 7, 8, 11). Certainly, this oligoclonal immune reaction in MS leads to an excessive production of IgG molecules of the kappa type (Table 2).

Table 2.

Electrophoretic Agar and PA electrophoresis	Immunoelectrophoretic	Radial immunodiffusion Mancini-method

Findings:
"γ zoning"
  γ c globulin
  γ E globulin
"unusual" IgG
	Findings:
	Doubling of IgG precipitate
	
	Extra (cathodic)-precipitate
	
	IgG "splitting"
		Findings:
		Increase of K/λ-relation (>1,8)
		
		Double ring of the K-precipitate?

Indications for oligoclonal immunoreactions in the CSF in multiple sclerosis

As already mentioned, we first succeeded in demonstrating homogenous oligoclonal immunoglobulins in the CSF by protein electrophoresis, especially by agar and polyacrylamide electrophoresis. The findings obtainable by this method show an accentuated prominence of some subfractions in the range of moderately slowly migrating globulins. These gammaglobulins, the striking increase of which is almost characteristic in the CSF of MS patients, have been variously described and named.

Immunoelectrophoretically, there are indications of an oligoclonal immunoactivity in MS in the form of various abnormalities of the IgG line of precipitation.

Ever since antisera have become available for the determination of free and combined kappa and lambda chains, it is also possible, with the MANCINI method, to investigate the proportion of the different light chains in the CSF immunoglobulins in MS quantitatively. This showed in a very striking manner that, in a large percentage of MS patients, there was at times an extreme predominance of kappa chains, i. e. a considerable increase in the physiological kappa-lambda relationship (5, 7,). It has also very recently been shown that the kappa precipitates obtained by this method frequently have a unique double ring (5) which is caused by free kappa chains, i. e. chains no longer attached to the rest of the molecule. We, too, saw several double rings of this type in the kappa precipitate in the CSF of MS patients. But, strikingly, the IgM content was also always raised in an unusual manner, so that, in our opinion, it is conceivable that with these double rings the kappa chains of the IgG and those of the IgM molecules are being represented side by side.

From the clinical diagnostic point of view, the question of where and how and oligoclonal immune reaction can be demonstrated in the CSF, not only in MS, but also in other neurological diseases, must now be of interest (Table 3).

Table 3. Demonstration of oligoclonal. Ig production in CSF

	in MS	in other inflammatory diseases	in non-inflammatory diseases
Agar electrophoretic: (R. Bader et al.)	47 % (H. Link: 94 %)	35 %	8 %
Immunoelectrophoretic: (H. Link et al.)	44 %	21 %	15 %
K/λ-Relation (>1.8): (H. Link et al.)	53 % (55 %)	0 % (0 %)[a]	3 % (14 %)

() own observations,
[a]without polyneuropathies

This review shows, firstly, that agar and immunoelectrophoresis also give an indication of an abnormal CSF immunoglobulin synthesis in other inflammatory and noninflammatory diseases of the CNS, even though with a markedly lower frequency. These cannot, therefore, be findings in the CSF specific for MS, even though some authors have observed abnormalities of the kind mentioned in agar electrophoresis in over 90 % of all MS cases (7). In contrast, the increased kappa-lambda relationship appears to be a striking feature of CSF protein which, although it does not appear in all MS patients, is only rearly seen in other neurological diseases and not all in other inflammatory processes. In our own investigations, surprisingly high kappa-lambda ratios were found in the CSF of cases of polyneuropathy and occasionally of cases of tumors of the CNS. The number of these cases observed is still too small to attempt to make any comment, but the hoped-for differential diagnostic value of a raised kappa-lambda ratio in MS seems, unfortunately, to be restricted by it.

If finally, we ask what is the diagnostic and, consequently, the differential diagnostic value of CSF investigations in MS, then we can state, in summary that a persisting immunoreactive CSF syndrome is characteristic of the regular, case of MS. This CSF syndrome, typical of MS, is largely independent of the duration and activity of the disease and comprises a moderate lymphoplasmocytic pleocytoses and a marked increase in immunoglobulins of the IgG class, usually with only a insignificant rise in total protein. Furthermore, if an indication of abnormal immunoglobulin synthesis can be obtained by agar, polyacrylamide or immunoelectrophoresis, or if an increased kappa-lambda ratio can be found by frequency analysis of the light chains in the Ig molecules as an expression of an oligoclonal immune reaction, then the clinical suspicion of MS can be confirmed with great probability. But it must be emphasized that, conversely, the absence of many or even all of the changes in the CSF which have been mentioned does not exclude MS with absolute certainty. But, in any case, it may have become clear, how a differentiated diagnosis in the CSF, without finally specific findings, can make an important contribution to the clinical diagnosis of MS.

Summary

Changes in the CSF, typical but not specific for MS, appear in the form of a "persistent immunoactive CSF syndrome" with moderate lymphoplasmocytosis and a marked increase in immunoglobulins of the IgG class. For the diagnostic differentiation from other inflammatory disorders agar electrophoretic or immunoelectrophoretic indication for the presence of abnormal immunoglobulin synthesis can be useful. Such synthesis is believed to be an oligoclonally controlled immune reaction which is characterized by excessive production of IgG molecules of the kappa type.

REFERENCES

1. BADER, R., RIEDER, H. P., KAESER, H. E.: Die Bedeutung der diskontinuierlichen Zonierung des Immunglobulinbereiches für die Diagnose neurologischer Erkrankungen. Z. Neurol. 206, 25 - 38 (1973).

2. DELANK, H. W.: Das Eiweißbild des Liquor cerebrospinalis. Darmstadt: Dr. D. Steinkopff 1965.

3. DELANK, H. W.: Klinische Liquordiagnostik. Nervenarzt 43, 57 - 68 (1972).

4. DELANK, H. W.: Liquorbefunde bei der multiplen Sklerose. Fortschr. Neurol. Psychiatr. 40, 440 - 453 (1972).

5. IWASHITA, H., GRUNWALD, F., BAUER, H.: Double Ring Formation in Single Radiol. Immunodiffusion for Kappa Chains in Multiple Sclerosis Cerebrospinal Fluid. J. Neurol. 207, 45 - 52 (1974).

6. KOLAR, O. J., ROSS, A. T., HERMAN, J. T.: Serum and cerebrospinal fluid immunoglobulins in multiple sclerosis. Neurology 20, 1052 - 1061 (1970).

7. LINK, H., MÜLLER, R.: Immunoglobulins in Multiple Sclerosis and Infections of the Nervous System. Arch. Neurol. Vol. 25, 326-344 (1971).

8. MEYER-RIENECKER, H. J.: Immunologisch bedeutsame Zell- und Eiweiß-
befunde im Liquor bei neuroallergischen Erkrankungen. Psychiat.
Neurol. med. Psychol. 24, 256 - 264 (1972).

9. MEYER-RIENECKER, H. J., HITZSCHKE, B.: Ätiopathogenetische Probleme der Multiplen Sklerose. Nervenarzt 45, 133 - 141 (1974).

10. SCHMIDT, R. M.: Der Liquor cerebrospinalis. Berlin: VEB-Verlag
Volk und Gesundheit 1968.

11. WALLER, M., HOFFMANN, P. F.: Observation on the Double Gamma
Globulin Lines Seen on Gel Diffusion. Am. J. clin. Path. 656,
645 - 652 (1971).

Neurophysiological Examination (SEP) for the Objective Diagnosis of Spinal Lesions*

T. FUKUSHIMA and Y. MAYANAGI

For the diagnosis of spinal lesions, various neurophysiological procedures can be applied. EMG and Nerve Conduction Velocity are not always sufficient to make a differential diagnosis. Cerebral somatosensory evoked potential (SEP), which was first reported by DAWSON (3), have been subjected to many studies in both normal pathological cases (1, 4, 5, 6, 7, 9). This method has been employed in our clinic to verify clinical findings in cases with various neurological disorders. The present report deals with a proposal of criteria for defining abnormal SEP and results of SEP-recordings in patients with spinal and radicular lesions.

Material and Methods

The individuals examined were 50 normal volunteers, 30 male and 20 female, ranging between 18 to 67 years, with an average of 43 years, and 66 patients with various spinal and radicular lesions. These included 18 MS cases (we want to thank Prof. SCHLIACK and the neurological department for their help), 7 vascular disorders, 7 space-occupying lesions, 4 spinal traumas, 8 cervical spondyloses, 16 lumbar root compression syndromes and 6 other spinal processes.

Recording electrodes were placed on the scalp above the sensory area corresponding to the stimulation site. The responses were amplified through a conventional EEG apparatus, stored in a magnetic tape and fed to a digital computer (NICOLET 1072). A summation was taken over a sequence of 128 responses with an analysis time of 100 msec. Electrical stimuli, consisting of 0.1 msec rectangular pulses were applied 1 c/sec with a pair of disc electrodes. Stimulus intensity was adjusted just above the motor threshold for the nerve stimulation and 5 times above the sensory threshold for the skin stimulation.

Results

1. Criteria for Determining Abnormal SEP

The SEPs in normal subjects were extremely consistent. Examples of normal SEP are illustrated in Fig. 1, which shows a proportional increase in latency according to the distance between the head and the stimulation site. Normal SEP had usually a reversed W-shape irrespective of the site of stimulation. The components of SEP were designated according to LARSSON (8) as shown in Fig. 1. Out of 132 recordings in 50 normal subjects, the mean value, standard deviation and range of peak latencies of these components were calculated (Table 1). The peak

* Supported by a grant of the Deutsche Forschungsgemeinschaft.

Table 1. Statistical analysis of normal SEP values to the stimulation of upper and lower extremities.
A) Average, standard deviation and range of peak latencies of each component are illustrated. Amplitudes represent the general magnitude between the peak of IN and that of Pmax (P1 or P2). The values of normal limit are indicated in frame
B) Side differences between right and left are shown based on 36 bilateral recordings in 20 normal volunteers. The normal limits are also indicated in frame

Site of stimulation	IN	P 1	ND	P 2	Amplitude IN-Pmax	No.
N. med. (Hand)	19.6 ± 0.9 (18.0 - 21.5)	28.2 ± 1.9 (24.1 - 32.0)	35.5 ± 3.5 (29.8 - 46.0)	45.8 ± 5.3 (39.6 - 60.2)	6.5 ± 2.5 (2.5 - 12.0)	53
Middle finger	23.2 ± 1.5 (21.0 - 25.0)	32.5 ± 2.3 (27.1 - 36.0)	40.2 ± 4.3 (32.1 - 52.0)	51.2 ± 4.4 (42.0 - 59.1)	3.4 ± 1.2 (1.2 - 5.6)	25
N. pern. (knee)	30.5 ± 2.9 (25.0 - 36.3)	39.1 ± 4.2 (30.0 - 50.0)	49.5 ± 4.6 (43.0 - 63.0)	59.8 ± 6.6 (48.9 - 76.1)	1.6 ± 0.8 (0.8 - 4.5)	31
Toes (I, II, V)	42.1 ± 1.8 (39.2 - 45.0)	50.6 ± 2.8 (45.0 - 56.6)	60.5 ± 3.4 (54.1 - 67.3)	69.6 ± 5.4 (60.0 - 84.8)	1.6 ± 0.7 (0.8 - 4.0)	23

(B)

Latency difference (msec)				Amplitude difference (uV)
IN	P 1	ND	P 2	
0.5 (0 - 2.0)	1.8 (0 - 10.0)	2.6 (0 - 13.8)	3.1 (0 - 17.0)	26 % (0 - 49)

159

latencies of IN and Pl were considerably constant, however, those of
ND and P2 were more variable. The amplitudes of SEP, measured from IN
to the maximal positive deflection, showed a wide range of distribution. Comparing both sides, the latencies and wave forms were bilaterally almost the same, whereas the amplitudes were fairly different.
The values circumscribed in frames (Table 1) indicate the normal limits of the latencies and amplitudes. On the basis of these data, the
following criteria may be proposed to determine the abnormality of
SEP. 1. Delay of IN over the normal limit, 2. Delay of Pl over the
normal limit, particularly significant in absence of IN, 3. Decrease
of amplitude below the normal limit, 4. Side differences in latency
and amplitude, 5. Deformity of waveform. The SEP abnormality was classified in three grades, mainly depending upon the latency delay:
1. mild change (+)-- delay up to 5 msec, 2. moderate change (++)--
delay from 5 to 10 msec, 3. severe change (+++)--delay more than 10
msec. The decrease of amplitude, deformity and side difference were
additionally taken into account to determine the grade of abnormality.

2. SEP Changes in Spinal Lesions

Totally 244 SEPs were recorded from 66 patients with various spinal
lesions. Four representative cases will be described in detail.

Case 1: C. L., a 61 year old woman with a meningioma at the level of
Th 7 (Fig. 2). Neurologically spastic paraplegia and distally dominant
sensory disturbances below Th 9 were noted. Stimulation to the area
of moderate sensory loss produced normal responses, whereas the responses evoked by the right foot stimulation where the sensory loss
was severe, were almost absent.

Case 2: W. J., a 43 year old woman who had tetraparesis and moderate
sensory disturbances below Th 10 caused by a vascular lesion (Fig. 3).
In this case, the SEPs after the leg stimulation showed only minimal
latency delay in spite of moderate sensory deficit. The SEP to the
median nerve stimulation was normal.

Case 3: R. H., a 59 year old man, with a history of MS for 15 years
(Fig. 4). Neurological examination revealed spastic paraparesis, loss
of vibration sense as illustrated in the figure and right optic atrophy. The SEP to the median nerve stimulation were bilaterally abnormal. In spite of relatively mild sensory deficit, a marked delay of
latencies was noted. The amplitudes were well preserved. In the responses evoked by stimulation of the lower extremities, the latency
delay was also prominent.

Case 4: W. G., a 42 year old man, with a history of multiple sclerosis
since 8 years. Neurological findings were internuclear ophthalmoplegia
on the right side, nystagmus, spastic paraparesis and mild impairment
of vibration sense on both legs as illustrated in Fig. 5. It is interesting to note that the SEPs produced by stimulation of the intact
upper extremities showed significant latency delay (5 msec delay of
IN) with preserved amplitudes and waveforms. The SEPs to stimulation
of the lower extremities with sensory impairment showed relatively
stronger changes, also characterized by latency delay.

The results of 244 SEP recordings are summarized in Fig. 6 to show
the correlation between the severity of sensory disturbances and the
grade of SEP abnormality. These both did not always run parallel. As
to the MS cases, 15 out of 49 SEPs produced by stimulation of the area
with sensory deficit showed stronger alterations than those expected
from the severity of the sensory impairment. The alterations of the

other 34 SEPs corresponded with the sensory loss. The other feature to be stressed is that 22 out of 63 recordings (35 %) after stimulation of sensory unaffected areas presented abnormal responses, characterized by a delay of latencies. On the contrary, the SEP changes in other spinal lesions such as vascular, traumatic, radicular or space-occupying were generally rather mild, in so far as the sensation was not severely impaired.

Findings in 13 patients with dissociated sensory loss are listed in Table 2. In 4 cases exclusively with pain and temperature disturbances, the SEPs were all normal. In contrast, the SEPs obtained from the patients with vibration and position sense impairment showed considerable abnormality.

Discussion

The standardization of normal SEP was worked out in order to have objective criteria for abnormal SEP. The results as to the upper extremity seem to correspond with previous observations (1, 4, 8, 9). Concerning the lower extremity, however, the latency values in this study are somewhat different from the results of other reports (2, 11). The fact that the SEP changes are related to the impairment of vibration and position sense suggests the important role of the posterior fascicle of the spinal cord for the manifestation of SEP. This has been also confirmed by HALLIDAY (6) and GIBLIN (4).

Although it may be difficult so far to make a precise differential diagnosis of spinal lesions by means of SEP, the present study reveals some differences in SEP alterations between MS and other spinal processes. In accordance to NAMEROW (10), it is noteworthy to point out that in MS patients about 30 % of SEPs to stimulation of the extremities even without sensory loss were abnormal. In addition, latency delay without amplitude decrease and disproportionally altered SEP appear to be the features of MS. This relatively severe SEP changes in MS cases may be due to the block of myelinated fast conducting fibers in disseminated lesions.

Conclusion

1. Criteria for diagnosis of abnormal SEP are proposed.
2. SEP seems to be formed by impulses mediated through the posterior fascicle.
3. The following features suggest the existence of MS:
   abnormal SEP to stimulation even of unaffected extremity, latency delay without amplitude decrease, and relatively severe SEP change disproportional to sensory impairment.

Table 2. A list of 13 cases with dissociated sensory loss. Severity of sensory loss is classified into 4: intact (O), mild (+), moderate (++) and severe (+++), for pain and temperature disturbance (the third column from the last) and for vibration and position sense disturbance (the next column) respectively. SEP change is classified also into 4 grades: normal (N), minimal change (+), moderate (++) and severe (+++). Note the good correlation of SEP change only with vibration and position sense disturbance, but not with pain and temperature disturbance

No.	Patient	Sex	Age	Diagnosis	Limb stimulated	Pain-temperature	Vibration-position	SEP change
1	M. J.	F	68	Anterior spinal artery syndrom	L. leg	+++	O	N
2	J. M.	M	49	MS	L. leg	++	O	N
3	D. A.	M	64	Vascular lesion	R. leg	+++	O	N
4	H. J.	M	49	Cervical injury	L. arm	+	O	N
					L. leg	+++	+	N
5	T. S.	M	52	Spinal multiple myeloma	R. leg	+++	+	N
					L. leg	+++	++	+
6	U. J.	F	34	Vascular lesion	L. leg	+++	++	+
7	W. G.	M	33	MS	R. & l. legs	+	++	+++
8	J. M.	M	57	Vascular lesion	L. leg	+++	+	+
					R. leg	O	+	+
9	O. D.	F	74	Paraneoplastic myelopathy	R. leg	O	+++	+++
					L. leg	O	+	+
10	O. Z.	M	61	Vascular lesion	L. leg	O	++	+++
11	M. L.	M	21	Friedreich's ataxia	R. & l. arms	O	+	+++
					R. & l. legs	O	++	+++
12	K. L.	M	70	Tabes dorsalis	R. & l. legs	O	++	+++
13	B. W.	M	72	Unknown spinal lesion	R. & l. legs	O	++	++

REFERENCES

1. ALLISON, T.: Recovery functions of somatosensory evoked responses in man. Electroenceph. clin. Neurophysiol. 14, 331 - 343 (1962).

2. BAUST, W., ILSEN, H. W., JÖRG, J., WAMBACH, G.: Höhenlokalisation von Rückenmarksquerschnittssyndromen mittels corticaler Reizantwortpotentiale. Nervenarzt. 43, 292 - 304 (1972).

3. DAWSON, G. D.: A summation technique for the detection of small evoked potentials. Electroenceph. clin. Neurophysiol. 6, 65 - 84 (1954).

4. GIBLIN, D. R.: Somatosensory evoked potentials in healthy subjects and in patients with lesions of the nervous system. Ann. N. Y. Acad. Sci. 112, 93 - 142 (1964).

5. GOFF, W. R., ROSNER, B. S., ALLISON, T.: Distribution of cerebral somatosensory evoked responses in normal man. Electroenceph. clin. Neurophysiol. 14, 697 - 713 (1962).

6. HALLIDAY, A. M.: Changes in the form of cerebral evoked responses in man associated with various lesions of the nervous system. Electroenceph. clin. Neurophysiol. Suppl. 25, 178 - 192 (1967).

7. LARSON, S. J., SANCES, Jr., A., CHRISTENSON, P. C.: Evoked somatosensory potentials in man. Arch. Neurol. 15, 88 - 93 (1966).

8. LARSSON, L. E., PREVEC, T. S.: Somato-sensory response to mechanical stimulation as recorded in the human EEG. Electroenceph. clin. Neurophysiol. 28, 162 - 172 (1970).

9. NAKANISHI, T., SHIMADA, Y., TOYOKURA, Y.: Somatosensory evoked responses to mechanical stimulation in normal subjects and in patients with neurological disorders. J. Neurol. Sci. 21, 289 - 298 (1974).

10. NAMEROW, N. S.: Somatosensory evoked responses in multiple sclerosis patients with varying sensory loss. Neurology (Minneap.) 18, 1197 - 1204 (1968).

11. TSUMOTO, T., HIROSE, N., NONAKA, S., TAKAHASHI, M.: Analysis of somatosensory evoked potentials to lateral popliteal nerve stimulation in man. Electroenceph. clin. Neurophysiol. 33, 379 - 388 (1972).

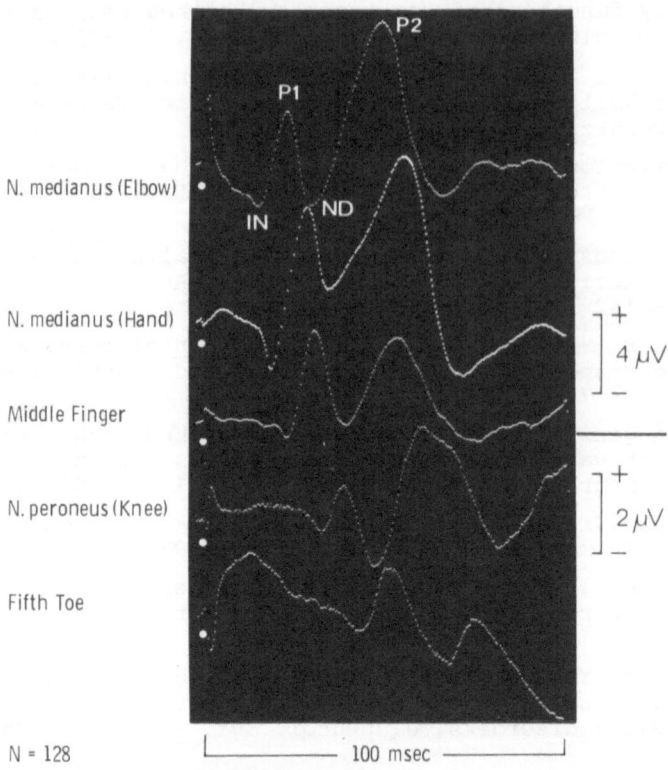

N. medianus (Elbow)

N. medianus (Hand)

Middle Finger

N. peroneus (Knee)

Fifth Toe

N = 128

100 msec

Fig. 1. Examples of normal SEPs produced by stimulation at various locations in one volunteer. Note proportional increase in latency from the top to the bottom according to the distance between the brain and the stimulation sites. IN: initial negative deflection, P1: first positive deflection, ND: second negative deflection, P2: second positive deflection, according to LARSSON's nomenclature. Vertical scales indicate 4 microvolts for the upper 3 SEPs and 2 microvolts for the lower two

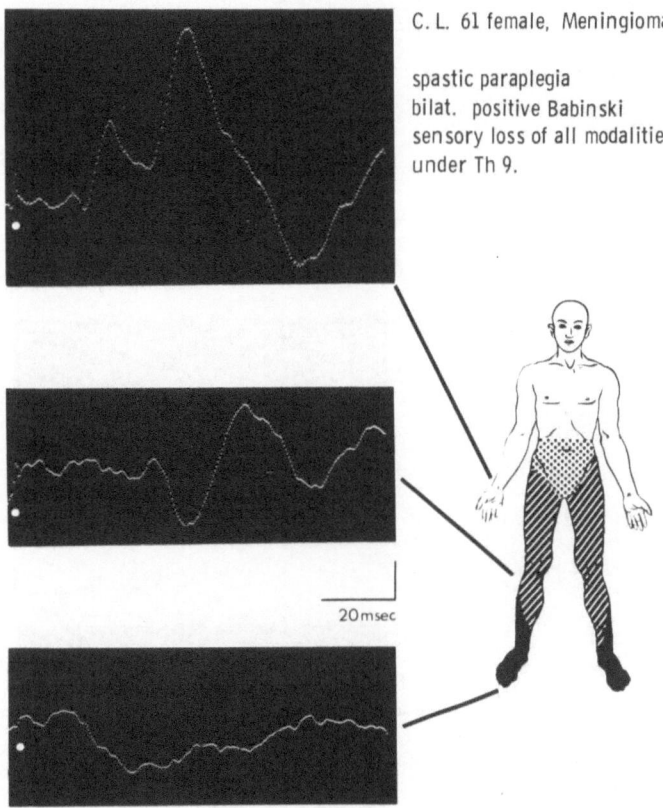

C. L. 61 female, Meningioma

spastic paraplegia
bilat. positive Babinski
sensory loss of all modalities
under Th 9.

20 msec

Fig. 2. Case 1. 61 year old woman, with a meningioma at the level of Th 7. Sensory map in this and following figures shows the degree of vibration and position sense disturbance: slight (dotted), moderate (hatched) and severe impairment (black area). Indication lines show that the uppermost SEP is caused by stimulation of the median nerve, the middle one by that of the peroneal nerve and the lowest one by that of the big toe. The vertical line at the right border indicates 2 microvolts for the uppermost SEP and microvolt for the other. N=128

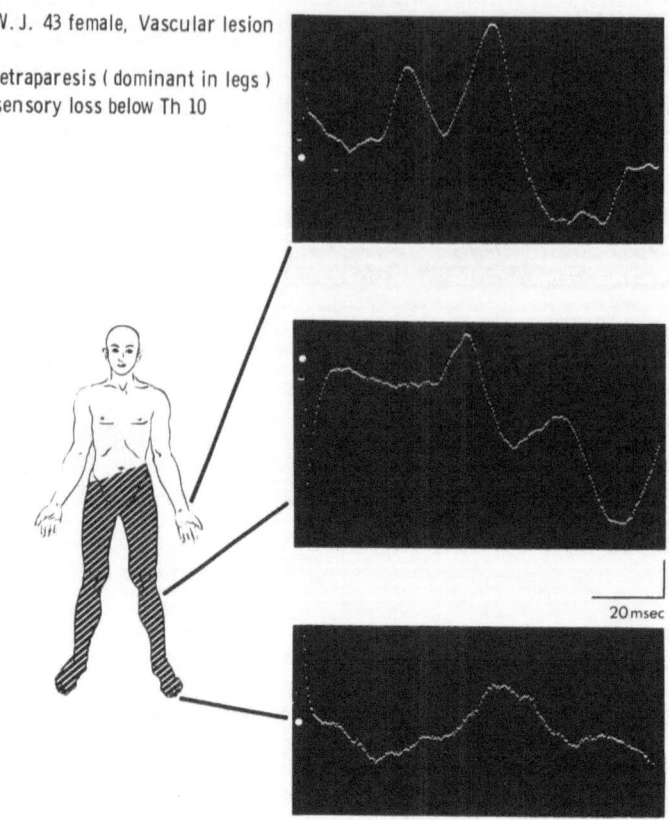

W. J. 43 female, Vascular lesion

tetraparesis (dominant in legs)
sensory loss below Th 10

20 msec

Fig. 3. Case 2. 43 year old woman with a vascular lesion of the lower cervical spinal cord. Note the minimal SEP changes with moderate sensory deficit at the stimulation sites (hatched)

Fig. 5. Case 4. 42 year old man with a history of MS for 8 years. Neurological findings are written in the Figure. Note the relatively strong SEP changes with no or minimal sensory loss, particularly the significant delay of latency in the SEPs produced by stimulations of the sensory intact upper extremities

▷

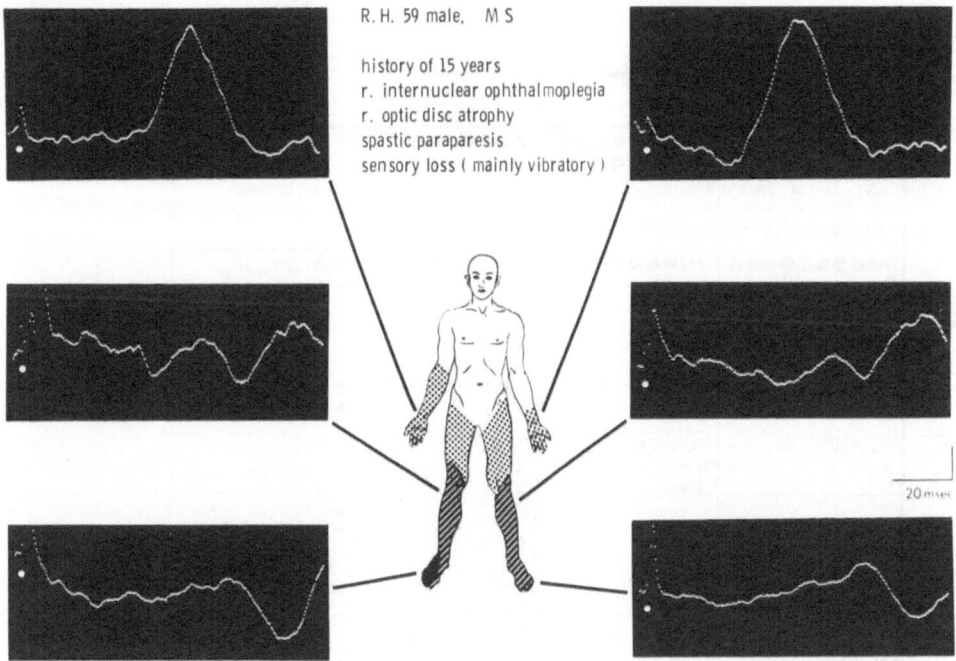

Fig. 4. Case 3. 59 year old man with a history of MS for 15 years. Neurological findings are written in the Figure. In spite of the minimal sensory deficit, the SEPs to the median nerve stimulation showed the marked latency delay (IN: right 18 msec, left 9 msec delay). The wave form altered into a reversed V-shape, but the amplitudes were well preserved. The SEPs to the leg stimulation were also markedly delayed

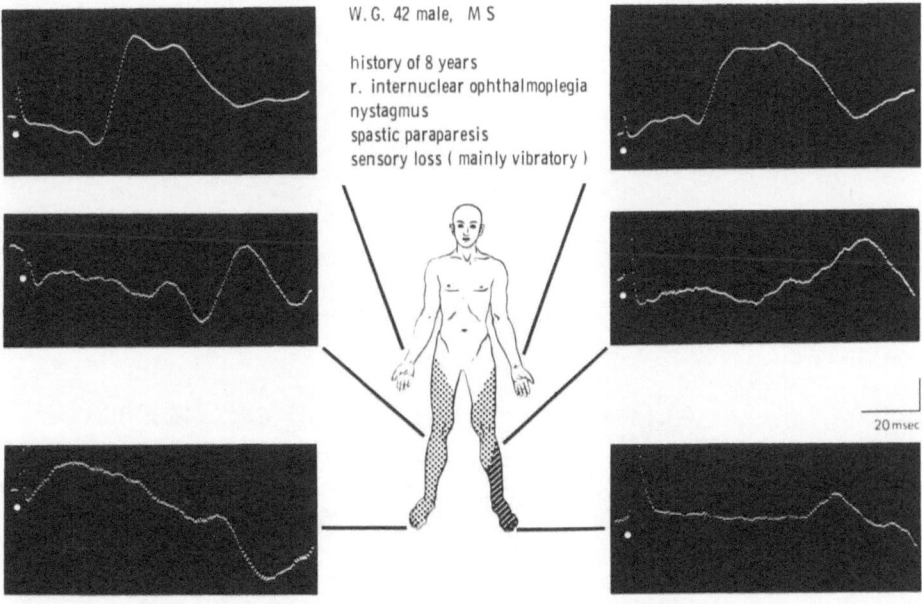

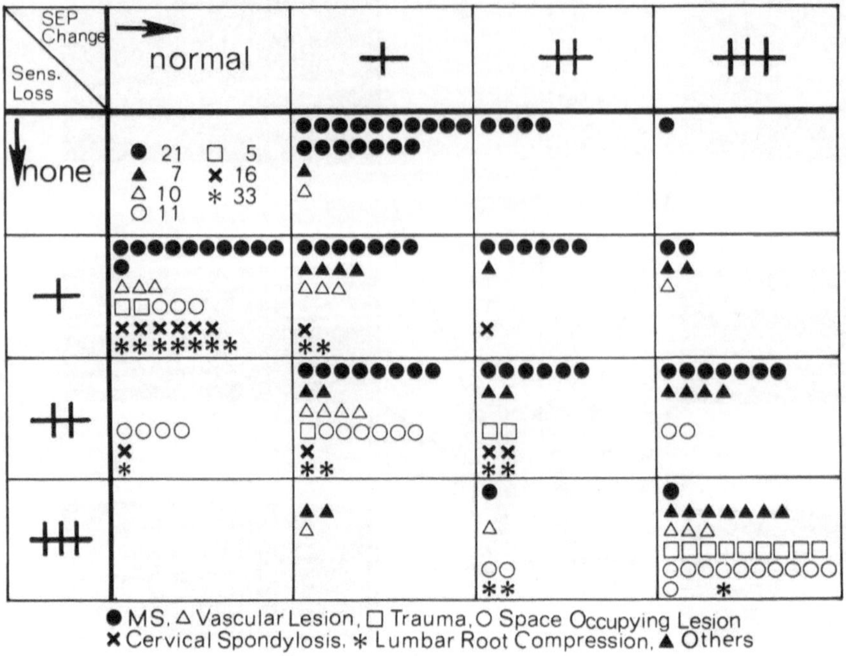
SEP Change
Sens. Loss
normal
none
● 21 □ 5
▲ 7 × 16
△ 10 ✱ 33
○ 11
● MS, △ Vascular Lesion, □ Trauma, ○ Space Occupying Lesion
× Cervical Spondylosis, ✱ Lumbar Root Compression, ▲ Others

Fig. 6. A diagram to show the correlation between the severity of sensory disturbances and SEP abnormality, for 244 recordings from 66 patients. Each marker represents one SEP recording and is placed in one of the frames to show the grade of its abnormality (horizontally) and the severity of sensory loss at the stimulation site (vertically). Seven different kinds of spinal lesions are indicated as shown by the symbols at the bottom

Misdiagnosis – Cerebral Form of Multiple Sclerosis

G. Lausberg, E. Farhoumand, H. Collmann, N. Nicola, H. Waldbaur,
P. Dragoun, K. v. Wild, J. Zierski, J. Wickbold, G. Simon, A. Kühner,
H. Palleske, K. P. Wisplinghoff, P. Oldenkott, M. Gaab, and T. Demirel

Multiple sclerosis was first described by CRUVEILHIER in 1835 (5) and
the anatomicophathological picture was first given by CARSWELL in
1838 (4). It was FRERICHS (7), who diagnosed multiple sclerosis clinically for the first time in 1849 and CHARCOT published an extensive
clinical review in 1868. In the second half of the 19th century the
disease aroused such an interest that E. MÜLLER (19) was able to col-
lect over 1000 literature references in his monograph, which appeared
in 1904.

The possibility of erroneous diagnosis of brain tumor in patients
with multiple sclerosis and, on the other hand, of multiple sclerosis
in patients with brain tumor was known since the beginning of our
century. The first type of this misdiagnosis was described by GUSSEN-
BAUER in 1902 (10), who reported on a patient in whom intracranial
exploration of the left parietal region was performed because of
Jacksonian fits followed by paresis. The patient died and the post-
mortem examination revealed typical multiple sclerosis. Further cases
of similar misdiagnosis were reported by EISELSBERG and RANZI in 1913
(6) and OPPENHEIM in 1905 (22). In both cases posterior fossa tumors
were suspected. MARBURG (17) critizised in his review this act of
misinterpretation of neurological findings upon which the operative
indications were based and added another case of multiple sclerosis
in which exploration of the posterior fossa was performed.

Introduction and development of contrast medium investigations and
scintigraphy reduced drastically this type of misdiagnosis and surgical explorations in patients with multiple sclerosis have become
extremely rare nowadays. In contrast to this type of misdiagnosis,
erroneous diagnosis of multiple sclerosis in patients harbouring a
brain tumor is not so infrequent and has not lost its critical importance, as we will demonstrate further on. Review of the literature
revealed a case with multiple CNS-sarcomas diagnosed as multiple sclerosis, reported by v. HIPPEL in 1892 (12). MARBURG (17) described a
tumor in the ventral part of the posterior fossa misdiagnosed as
multiple sclerosis in 1921. Similar misinterpretations were reported
by SUNDER-PLASSMANN (29) in a case of right parasagittal tumor,
OESTERREICH (21) in four cases of intracranial tumors and WIECK in
1964 (31) in a case of an acoustic neurinoma. In 1951 de GISPERT (9)
pointed out misdiagnosing multiple sclerosis in cases of cerebello-
pontine angle tumors. ARATJUNOV (1), RENNERT (24) and SCHRADER (26)
described misdiagnosis of multiple sclerosis in patients with tumors
of the caudal brain stem.

Our report comprises 120 cases collected from 15 neurosurgical departments in Germany (Table 1). 21000 patients with brain tumors were
treated in these departments in the period analysed, so that the incidence of misdiagnosed multiple sclerosis corresponds to 0.57 %. The

Table 1. Misdiagnosis: cerebral form of "MS". Review of 120 cases, localization and histology

Supratentorial		Brain stem and infratentorial	
Frontobasal tumors	22	Brain stem tumors	13
Craniopharyngiomas	7	Caudal brain stem	7
Pituitary adenomas	7	Thalamus	1
Tub. sellae meningiomas	6	IIIrd ventricle	1
Olfactory groove meningiomas	2	Cerebello-pontine angle tumors	17
Parietal tumors	15	Acoustic neurinomas	7
Meningiomas	7	Epidermoids	4
Angiomas	4	Meningiomas	4
Glioblastomas	2	Other tumors	2
Astrocytomas	2	Cerebellar tumors	16
Other hemispheric localizations	23	Spongioblastomas	7
Meningiomas	6	Haemangioblastomas	5
Glioblastomas	5	Medulloblastomas	3
Astrocytomas	3	Other tumors	1
Angiomas	2	Other processes of the posterior fossa	11
Metastases	2	Tentorium meningiomas	4
Other gliomas	2	Arachnoiditis	2
Other tumors	3	Basilar impressions	2
Other supratentorial processes	3	Other tumors	3
Hydrocephalus	2		
A. c. a. aneurysm	1		
Supratentorial processes	63	Brain stem and infratentorial processes	57

difficulties of such retrospective analysis are well known but, in spite of incomplete information in some cases, a general review was possible. As seen from Fig. 1 the first cases date back to 1933. This was possible thanks to the report of WISPLINGHOFF in 1968 (32), who published the statistics of patients who were under the care of Prof. TÖNNIS and traced the first patients back to 1933. An increase of correctly diagnosed cases since the middle fifties is most probably due to the increase of number of contrast medium investigations performed.

Analysis of histological findings in 63 supratentorial and 57 brain stem and infratentorial tumors (Table 2) shows that the majority of neoplasms erroneously diagnosed as multiple sclerosis were slowly growing tumors. Among supratentorial tumors there were 21 meningiomas (i. e. 18 %), 7 craniopharyngiomas, pituitary adenomas and glioblastomas respectively, 6 angiomas, 5 astrocytomas, 2 other gliomas and 2 metastases. Other misdiagnosed processes include 1 case of sarcoma, 2 not differentiated tumors, 2 cases of hydrocephalus and 1 case of complex aneurysm of the anterior communicating artery with recurrent vascular spasm.

Table 2. Misdiagnosis: cerebral form of "MS". Histological classification of the 120 misdiagnosed cases

Supratentorial		Brainstem and infratentorial	
Meningiomas	21	Meningiomas	8
Craniopharyngiomas	7	Spongioblastomas	7
Pituitary adenomas	7	Acoustic neurinomas	7
Glioblastomas	7	Angioblastomas	5
Angiomas	6	Cholesteatomas	4
Astrocytomas	5	Medulloblastomas	3
Other gliomas	2	Other tumors	7
Metastases	2	Brain stem tumors	11
Other tumors	3	Other processes	5
Other processes	3		
Total	63	Total	57

Among the infratentorial lesions there were 8 meningiomas, 7 spongioblastomas and acoustic neurinomas respectively, 5 hemangioblastomas, 4 epidermoids and 3 medulloblastomas. In 7 cases of other tumors and in 11 cases of brain stem tumors no histology was available. Other lesions include 2 cases of arachnoiditis of the posterior fossa, 2 cases of basilar impression and 1 case of basilar artery aneurysm.

Fig. 2 shows the localization of 60 from 63 supratentorial tumors. The largest group is constituted by 22 cases of frontobasal tumors and includes 7 craniopharyngiomas, 7 pituitary adenomas, 6 sellar meningiomas and 2 olfactory groove meningiomas. The second largest group is formed by 15 purely parietal lesions and comprises 7 meningiomas, 4 angiomas and 4 gliomas. The remaining 11 tumors were located in the frontal, frontotemporal and temporal region. This group includes 5 meningiomas, 4 more occipitally localized processes and 2 cases of diffuse lesions - glioblastomatosis and carcinomatosis.

57 brain stem and infratentorial lesions (Fig. 3) comprise 13 histologically not verified brain stem tumors and include 1 case of a tumor of the 3rd ventricle. Among 17 cerebellopontine angle tumors there were 7 acoustic neurinomas, 4 epidermoids and meningiomas re-

spectively, 1 metastasis and 1 unclassified tumor. Among 16 tumors
localized exclusively in the cerebellum there were 7 spongioblastomas,
5 hemangioblastomas, 3 medulloblastomas and 1 unclassified tumor. The
other lesions of the posterior fossa had different localization and
comprised 6 tumors including 4 tentorial meningiomas, 1 hypoglossal
nerve neurinoma, 1 tumor of the fourth ventricle and already mentioned
cases of arachnoiditis, basilar impression and aneurysm of the basilar
artery.

As far as the age of patients at the time of the misdiagnosis is concerned - 27 % were in the forties and fifties (Fig. 4). Only 51 % of
patients showed symptoms of the disease between the second and fourth
decade of age, i. e. in the preference age for multiple sclerosis.
51 patients were men and 69 women. Average length of anamnesis from
the onset of the disease until the erroneous diagnosis of multiple
sclerosis was made was 2 years and so was the time for which diagnosis
was delayed.

The symptoms in each individual patient correlated well with the localization of the tumor, and were of little value for our analysis.
Therefore, we will only analyse the symptoms which are typical for
mulitple sclerosis. What makes the early diagnosis difficult is the
fact already noticed by KÄPPELI and coll. (14) among 200 patients
with mulitple sclerosis, that 35 % of patients show symptoms of a
single focal lesion at the onset of the disease. SCHRADER and STOCH-
DORPH (27) reported 500 cases of multiple sclerosis and noticed pyramidal signs in 88 % of cases, ataxia in 61 %, lack of abdominal reflexes in 97 %, nystagmus in 56 % and ocular signs in 41 % of cases.

In our series 47 % of patients had pyramidal signs and motor symptoms,
58 % ataxia, 14 % abolished abdominal reflexes, 15 % nystagmus and
16 % ocular symptoms at the time when the misdiagnosis of multiple
sclerosis was made. In 4 further cases papilledema was present. However, in one of them it was mistaken for neuritis. Occurence of papilledema in multiple sclerosis is extremely rare but was already
reported in a single case in 1900 by KAMPRAD (15). Cerebrospinal
fluid abnormalities were found in 18 patients. In 3 of them CSF protein was normal, but the fluid contained 20 - 100/3 cells. In 10
cases CSF protein was raised over 70 mg % with no excess of cells,
and in additional 5 cases there was an excess of cells apart from
protein raise. We would like to remind here the opinion of SCHRADER
and WEISE (28) as well as that of MEYER (18), who think that protein
content above 60 to 75 mg % speaks against multiple sclerosis.

Plain skull X-rays, considered by WÜTHRICH and coll. (33) as necessary
in every case of suspected multiple sclerosis, were performed only in
43 patients (36 %) of our series, in 3 cases the findings were described as abnormal. Investigations with contrast medium were performed
in only 18 cases at the time of the misdiagnosis of multiple sclerosis.
In 3 of them radiological signs pointing to the presence of space-
occupying lesions were found but the diagnosis of tumor was dropped
because of type of neurological symptoms.

Multiple sclerosis was diagnosed on the basis of neurological symptoms
in 70 cases (58 %). Additional or isolated ocular signs were the basis
for diagnosis in 22 cases (19 %). Remission of symptoms directed the
diagnosis towards multiple sclerosis in 21 cases, in 4 cases the diagnosis was based only on CSF-abnormalities. The course of the disease
was considered as progressive in 92 cases whereas remissions were observed in 26 cases.

The correction of misdiagnosis was due mostly (in 77 cases) to symptoms of deterioration. In other cases diagnosis was corrected by another team of physicians and in 7 cases it was established at postmortem examination.

Correct diagnosis was based on contrast medium investigations in 88 cases (73 %). In 15 cases further neurological, ophthalmologic and otologic examinations helped to diagnose the tumor. In further 10 cases EEG and scintigraphy established the diagnosis. In 102 correctly diagnosed cases a tumor was operated on. However, very often at a very late stage, as reflected by 33 postoperative deaths. 60 patients were cured or improved by operation, 9 patients remained unimproved or became worse. In 56 cases it was felt that the postoperative course could have been better had diagnosis been established earlier. In 44 cases the surgeon concerned thought that the late diagnosis had no particular influence on the postoperative course.

We have separated 5 groups according to localization of the lesion, and we have compared the length of history, first symptoms, main neurological signs and time and reasons for misdiagnosis. The groups compared are:

1. Frontobasal tumors (22 cases)
2. Parietal tumors (15 cases)
3. Brain stem tumors (13 cases)
4. Cerebello-pontine angle tumors (17 cases)
5. Cerebellar tumors (16 cases).

MUMENTHALER (20) and FRICK and coll. (8) pointed out possible misinterpretation of neurological and ocular signs of frontobasal tumors. In this group of patients, visual signs were the first signs of the disease in 17 cases (Table 3). Age distribution in this group does not differ from that of the whole series. There were twice as much women as men in this group. Mean duration of the clinical history up to the time at which multiple sclerosis was misdiagnosed was 36,8 months, approximately 1 year longer than for the whole series. The course of the disease was progressive in 20 cases, undulating in 2 cases. Main neurological signs at the time of misdiagnosis were visual and visual field disturbances (19 patients). Motor weakness, muscle tone disturbances and pathological reflexes were absent. Abdominal reflexes were absent in 1 case, sensory disturbances were found in 2 cases. None of the patients had coordination disturbances. Pathological findings in the eyeground were found in 73 % of patients during the first examination. Pallor of the temporal field of the disc was found in 3 patients, optic atrophy in 8 patients and optic neuritis in 5 patients. In 2 cases CSF protein content was over 50 mg % and CSF cell-count showed values around 50/3. X-ray examination of the skull was performed in 8 cases. In 7 of these the findings were normal. Contrast medium investigations, performed in 4 cases were considered to be normal. In 20 cases the diagnosis of multiple sclerosis was based on the interpretation of visual findings. The mean time during which the patient retained the diagnosis of multiple sclerosis was 14,5 months, and was below the average for the whole series. At the time of correct tumor diagnosis isolated or combined visual and visual field disturbances were present in all 22 cases. Except for 2 cases, one of them diagnosed post-mortem, the correct diagnosis was made by contrast medium investigations. Twenty patients were operated on, 2 dying postoperatively. In 16 cases the surgeons considered that an earlier correct diagnosis would have improved the postoperative course.

Table 3. Misdiagnosis: cerebral form of MS in frontobasal tumors (n = 22)

Duration of history until MS diagnosed	36,8 mths.	
Course of the disease until MS diagnosed	progressive	
First symptoms	visual	
First signs		
Cranial nerves	visual and visual field	
Extremities		Ø
Sensibility		(+)
Coordination		Ø
Eyeground	+++	
CSF		(+)
EEG		Ø
Skull X-rays		Ø
Contrast medium investigations		Ø
Reason for misdiagnosis	Ocular findings	
Misdiagnosed for		14,5 m.
Correct diagnosis through	Contrast medium investigations	
Operation	20	
Postoperative death		4
Unfavourable course because of delayed diagnosis	75 %	

As concerns parietal and, particularly, parasagittal tumors, MUMEN-THALER (20) as well as SUNDER-PLASMANN (29) pointed out that these tumors can be the cause of possible misinterpretation of neurological findings. In our 15 cases age and sex distribution revealed nothing particular (Table 4). Motor weakness of one lower extremity was the first symptom in 7 cases, while sensory disturbances affecting one side of the body were noticed in 3 cases. Seizure-like attacks were the first symptom in only 3 cases. The average length of the clinical history before multiple sclerosis was diagnosed was 9,1 months. The course was progressive in 2/3 of cases. At the time of misdiagnosis only 6 patients had disturbances of the cranial nerves, mostly of the facial and hypoglossal nerve. However, in 14 out of 15 cases of this group monoparesis or hemiparesis of central types was present. Abdominal reflexes were unilaterally or bilaterally diminished in 5 cases, sensory disturbances in one extremity or in one half of the body were found in 8 cases. Disturbances of coordination were present only in the extremity affected by weakness. In 7 cases neurological findings were attributed to a spinal lesion, and in only 3 cases there was pallor of the temporal part of the optic disc. In only one case the cerebrospinal fluid was abnormal, EEG showing general disturbances and focal changes in 2 cases. Skull X-rays, performed in 7 patients, wer normal. Contrast medium investigations were performed in 3 cases and were considered to be normal.

Misdiagnosis of multiple sclerosis was based on neurological findings in 11 cases. In the remaining patients the diagnosis was based on the course of the disease and eyeground changes, as well as on negative

Table 4. Misdiagnosis: cerebral form of MS in parietal tumors (n =15)

Duration of history until MS diagnosed		9,1 mths.
Course of the disease until MS diagnosed	Progressive	
First symptoms	Paresis	(Seizures)
First findings		
Cranial nerves		++
Extremities	Paresis	
Sensibility		++
Coordination		Ø
Eyeground		(+)
CSF		(+)
EEG		+
Skull X-rays		Ø
Contrast medium investigations		Ø
Reason for misdiagnosis	Neurol. findings	
Misdiagnosed for		24,8 m.
Correct diagnosis through	Contrast medium investigation	
Operation	15	
Postoperative death		1
Unfavourable course because of delayed diagnosis	40 %	

contrast medium investigations. In this group multiple sclerosis remained as diagnosis for 24,8 months in average, which corresponds to
the mean time of misdiagnosis for the whole series. In all 15 patients
correct diagnosis was established by contrast medium investigations.
All patients were operated on with one single operative mortality
(7 %). The question of whether earlier diagnosis could have improved
the postoperative course received a negative answer in 9 cases.

Space-occupying lesions localized in the brain stem are frequently
the cause of the misdiagnosis of multiple sclerosis, because of their
variety of symptoms and frequently intermittent clinical course. The
difficulties of differential diagnosis between multiple sclerosis and
brain stem tumors were already mentioned by PETTE in 1932 (23). This
subject was further discussed, among others, by BARNETT in 1952 (3),
WHITE 1963 (30), BAMMER 1968 (2), SARKARI and coll. 1969 (25). HIERONS
(11) and LESELL and coll. (16) discussed the diagnostic difficulties
with arteriovenous angiomas of the brain stem.

In our series the group of misdiagnosed brain stem tumors is the
smallest and comprises 13 cases. Both sexes were equally affected but
66 % of patients were aged under forty (Table 5). The mean length of
the clinical history until the erroneous diagnosis of multiple sclerosis was established was 30,6 months. The course of the disease was
progressive in 9 cases. The initial symptoms of the disease were very
variable in contrast to the previous groups. Headaches, visual disturbances, double vision and motor weakness of the extremities were
found with almost equal incidence. At the time when "multiple sclero-

Table 5. Misdiagnosis: cerebral form of MS in brain stem tumors (n = 13)

Duration of history until MS diagnosed	30,6 mths.		
Course of the disease until MS diagnosed	Progressive		
First symptoms		Diffuse	
First findings			
Cranial nerves			+
Extremities	Paresis		
Sensibility			+
Coordination		++	
Eyeground			(+)
CSF			(+)
EEG			Ø
Skull X-rays			Ø
Contrast medium investigations			
Reason for misdiagnosis	Neurol. findings and course		
Misdiagnosed for:			14 m.
Correct diagnosis through		Contrast med. investig.	
Operation	2		
Postoperative death			O
Unfavourable course because of delayed diagnosis	75 %		

sis" was diagnosed 2/3 of patients had paresis of one extremity or hemiparesis, 58 % of patients had coordination disturbances and only in 2 cases eyeground and CSF abnormalities were found. Skull X-rays and contrast medium investigations were performed in 3 cases, respectively, and were considered to be normal.

The diagnosis of "multiple sclerosis" was based on neurological findings in 6 cases and on the course of the disease with remissions in further 5 cases. Correct diagnosis was made after an average time of 14 months and was due to contrast medium investigations in 9 cases. Progression of neurological signs and symptoms was the indications for renewed investigation. Obviously, in 12 patients of this group the timing of correct diagnosis did not have any influence on the further course of the disease due to the impossibility of radical surgical cure.

Lesions located in the cerebello-pontine angle are also a frequent cause of misdiagnosis, as we already mentioned in the review of the literature. In this group there were three times more women than men, and the mean length of the clinical history previous to the diagnosis of "multiple sclerosis" was 42 months, being the longest of all groups of patients (Table 6). In 56 % of cases the course of the disease was progressive. Hearing and balance disturbances were the first symptoms in 8 cases and visual disturbances in further 4 cases. At the time of the first examination, abnormal signs of the cerebello-pontine angle nerves were found in 13 patients. Involvement of long tracts

Table 6. Misdiagnosis: cerebral form of MS in cerebello-pontine angle tumors (n = 17)

Duration of history until MS diagnosed	42 mths.		
Course of the disease until MS diagnosed	Progressive		
First symptoms	Auditory and balance		
First signs			
Cranial nerves	Cerebello-pontine angle		
Extremities		++	
Sensibility			Ø
Coordination	+++		
Eyeground			+
CSF		++	
EEG			Ø
Skull X-rays			Ø
Contrast medium investigations			Ø
Reason for misdiagnosis	Neurol. findings		
Misdiagnosed for	33 m.		
Correct diagnosis through		Contrast medium investigation	
Operation	15		
Postoperative death			8
Unfavourable course because of delayed diagnosis	76 %		

was found in 7 cases. Disturbances of abdominal reflexes and sensory loss, apart from trigeminal, were not found. Disturbances of coordination were present in 59 % of the cases. In 3 cases optic fundi changes were revealed. CSF was abnormal in 5 out of 10 cases in which it was examined. In 3 of these there was an isolated protein content increase and in 2 cases an isolated cell increase. EEG, performed in 7 cases, and skull X-rays, performed in 8 cases, were all normal. Contrast medium investigations were performed, at that time, in only 1 case, and revealed no abnormalities. The time for which the tumor was misdiagnosed as multiple sclerosis was 33 months on average and was longer than the average for the whole series. Correct diagnosis was made at further examinations in 82 % of the cases because of progression of the neurological syndrome. In 12 cases contrast medium investigations established the final diagnosis. Fifteen patients were operated on, with an operative mortality of 54 %. The treating surgeons felt that earlier correct diagnosis could have improved the postoperative course in 13 cases (76 %).

The last group comprises 16 cases of cerebellar lesions. Both sexes are equally represented. As far as age distribution is concerned, there were 7 patients aged under thirty, which indicates an earlier onset of symptoms in comparison to other groups (Table 7). The mean length of the clinical history was 15 months. The course of the disease was progressive in 75 % of the cases. In the remaining patients

Table 7. Misdiagnosis: cerebral form of MS in cerebellar tumors (n = 16)

Duration of history until MS diagnosed		15 mths.
Course of the disease until MS diagnosed	Progressive	
First symptoms	Disturbances of equilibrium	
First signs		
Cranial nerves	Nystagmus	
Extremities	++	
Sensibility		(+)
Coordination	+++	
Eyeground		+
CSF		(+)
EEG		+
Skull X-rays		(+)
Contrast medium investigations		ø
Reason for misdiagnosis	Neurol. findings	
Misdiagnosed for		20 m.
Correct diagnosis through	Contrast medium investigations	
Operation	13	
Postoperative death		3
Unfavourable course because of delayed diagnosis	55 %	

the course of the disease was undulating. In half of the cases disturbances of body balance were the first symptom. Nystagmus was present in 50 % of patients. Unexpectedly almost half of the number of patients showed signs of involvement of long tracts, whereas sensory disturbances were very infrequent. Seventy-five percent of the patients showed disturbances of coordination, their intensity and type depending on the localization of the localization of the tumor already at the first examination. Fundoscopic changes were described twice as temporal pallor and once misinterpreted as neuritis. Among the CSF abnormalities, isolated increase in protein content, isolated pleocytosis and general abnormalities were found in 3 cases, respectively. Six patients had an EEG examination in the early stage of their disease. In 3 of them focal changes or dysrhythmia were found. Skull X-rays were performed in 7 patients and showed no abnormalities. Contrast medium investigations were performed in 2 patients and were found normal. Misinterpretation of the findings as "multiple sclerosis" was based on the neurological syndrome in 15 cases. The average time for which a tumor was misdiagnosed as multiple sclerosis was 20 months. Correct diagnosis was made by contrast medium investigations in 13 patients. The same number of patients was readmitted because of progression of their neurological symptoms. Thirteen patients were operated on. Three (23 %) died. The late diagnosis was considered to have had unfavourable influence on the further course in 7 patients.

We do not expect the conclusions from this review to be the means of avoiding misdiagnosis of multiple sclerosis in patients with brain tumor. We have tried to isolate 5 groups from the total number of 83 cases, and analysed them according to uniform criteria. We feel that these considerations on localization and symptomatology should be taken into account in the differential diagnosis, in order "to accomplish a constant revision of the diagnosis of MS in probable as well as in doubtless cases, particular when one is faced with odd symptoms" as stated by JANZEN (13).

REFERENCES

1. ARATJUNOV, A. J.: Quoted by OESTERREICH 1962.

2. BAMMER, H. G.: Multiple Sklerose. Pathologie - Ätiologie - Epidemiologie. Fortschr. d. Med. 86, 713 - 715 (1968).

3. BARNETT, H. J., HYLAND, H. H.: Tumors involving the brain-stem. A study of 90 cases arising in the brain-stem, fourth ventricle and pineal tissue. Quart. I. Med. 21, 265 - 284 (1952).

4. CARSWELL, R.: Illustrations of the elementary forms of disease (Atrophy). London: Longman 1838.

5. CRUVEILHIER, L. J. B.: Atlas d'anatomie pathologique. Paris: J. B. Baillière 1842.

6. EISELSBERG, A. v., RANZI, E.: Quoted by MARBURG 1921.

7. FRERICHS: Über Hirnsklerose (MARBURG 1921).

8. FRICK, E., ANGSTWURM, H.: Diagnose Multiple Sklerose. Münch. Med. Wschr. 115, 1075 - 1081 (1973).

9. De GISPERT, J.: Quoted by OESTERREICH 1962.

10. GUSSENBAUER, K.: Quoted by MARBURG 1921.

11. HIERONS, R.: Brain-Stem Angioma Confirmed by Ateriography. Relapsing Symptoms and Signs Strongly Suggestive of Disseminated Sklerosis. Proc. Royal Soc. Med. 46, 195 - 196 (1953).

12. HIPPEL, E. v.: Ein Fall von multiplen Sarkomen des gesamten Nervensystems und seiner Hüllen verlaufend unter dem Bilde der multiplen Sklerose. Dtsch. Z. Nervenheilkde. 2, 388 - 413 (1892).

13. JANZEN, R.: Differentialdiagnostische Schwierigkeiten bei multipler Sklerose. Dtsch. Med. Wschr. 92, 764 - 765 (1967).

14. KÄPPELI, F., WÜTHRICH, R.: Untersuchungen über den Erstschub bei multipler Sklerose und dessen Bedeutung für die Diagnosestellung. Schweiz. Rdsch. Med. (Praxis) 61, 1226 - 1231 (1972).

15. KAMPRAD: Inauguraldissertation, Leipzig 1900 (quoted by MARBURG 1921).

16. LESSELL, S., FERRIS, E. I., FELDMAN, R. G., HOYT, W. F.: Brain Stem Arteriovenous Malformations. Arch. Ophthalmol. 86, 255 - 259 (1971).

17. MARBURG, O.: Hirntumoren und multiple Sklerose. Ein Beitrag zur Kenntnis der lokalisierten Form der multiplen Sklerose im Gehirn. Dtsch. Z. Nervenheilkde. 68, 27 - 39 (1921).

18. MEYER, G.: Die Encephalomyelitis disseminata (auch multiple Sklerose genannt). Fortschr. Med. 91, 611 - 615 (1973).

19. MÜLLER, E.: Die multiple Sklerose des Gehirns und Rückenmarks. Jena: G. Fischer 1904.

20. MUMENTHALER, M.: Die Multiple Sklerose, Diagnose und Differentialdiagnose. Praxis 15, 514 - 517 (1967).

21. OESTERREICH, K.: Zur Differentialdiagnose zwischen Multipler Sklerose und Rückenmarks- bzw. Hirntumor. Med. Welt 21, 1675 - 1693 (1963).

22. OPPENHEIM, H.: Der Formenreichtum der multiplen Sklerose. Dtsch. Z. Nervenheilkde. 52, 169 - 239 (1905).

23. PETTE, H.: Sklerose (Multiple Sklerose). Neue Deutsche Klinik 9, 761 - 798 (1932).

24. RENNERT, H.: Quoted by OESTERREICH 1962.

25. SARKARI, N. B. S., BICKERSTAFF, E. R.: Relapses and Remissions in Brain Stem Tumors. Brit. Medic. J. 2, 21 - 23 (1969).

26. SCHRADER, A.: Die multiple Sklerose. In: Handbuch der Inneren Medizin, Bd. V/2 (Hrsg. G. v. BERGMANN, W. FREY, H. SCHWIEGK), S. 649 - 740. Berlin - Göttingen - Heidelberg: Springer 1953.

27. SCHRADER, A., STOCHDORPH, O.: Diagnostische und pathologische Aspekte der multiplen Sklerose. Klin. Wschr. 47, 501 - 507 (1969).

28. SCHRADER, A., WEISE, H.: Kasuistischer Beitrag zur Differentialdiagnose zwischen spinaler Erscheinungsform der multiplen Sklerose und Rückenmarkstumor. Nervenarzt 22, 447 - 451 (1951). (Quoted by SCHRADER'1953).

29. SUNDER-PLASSMANN, P.: Neurochirurgischer Beitrag zur "multiplen Sklerose". Bruns Beitr. z. Klin. Chir. 181, 337 - 346 (1951).

30. WHITE, H. H.: Brain stem tumors occuring in adults. Neurology 13, 292 - 300 (1963).

31. WIECK, H. H.: Ein als Encephalomyelitis disseminata verkannter Hirntumor. Med. Welt 2, 975 - 976 (1964).

32. WISPLINGHOFF, K. P.: "Multiple Sklerose" als Fehldiagnose bei intracraniellen raumbeengenden Prozessen. Inaugural-Dissertation Köln 1968.

33. WÜTHRICH, R., KÄPPELI, F.: Diagnose und diagnostische Irrtümer bei der multiplen Sklerose. Schw. med. Wschr. 99, 1460 - 1464 (1969).

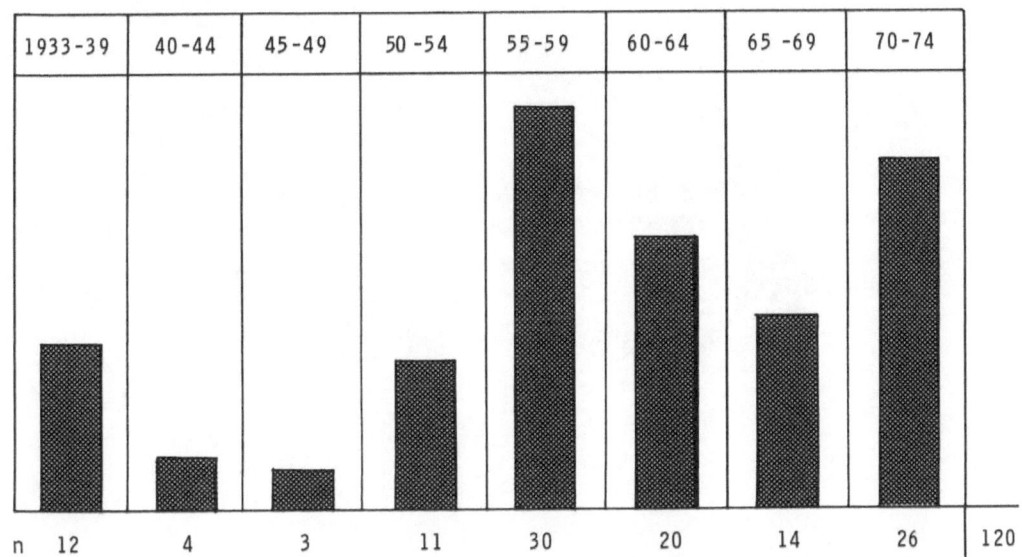

1933-39	40-44	45-49	50-54	55-59	60-64	65-69	70-74	
n 12	4	3	11	30	20	14	26	120

Fig. 1. Misdiagnosis - cerebral form of MS. Year of correct diagnosis after previous misdiagnosis MS

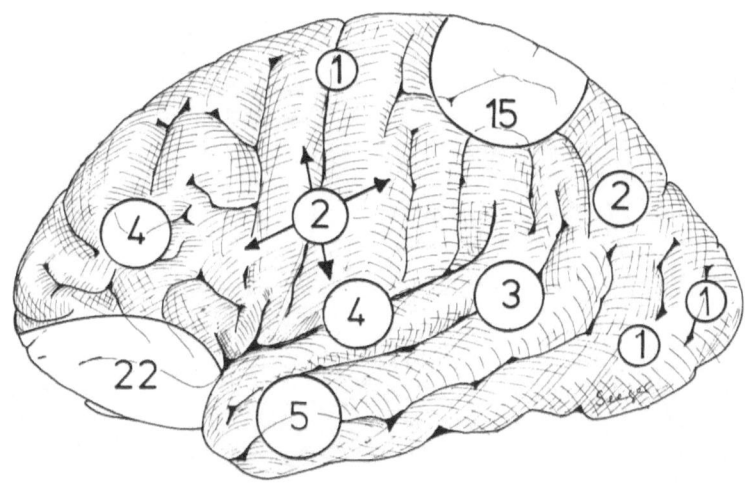

Fig. 2. Misdiagnosis - cerebral form of MS. Localization of supratentorial tumors (n = 60)

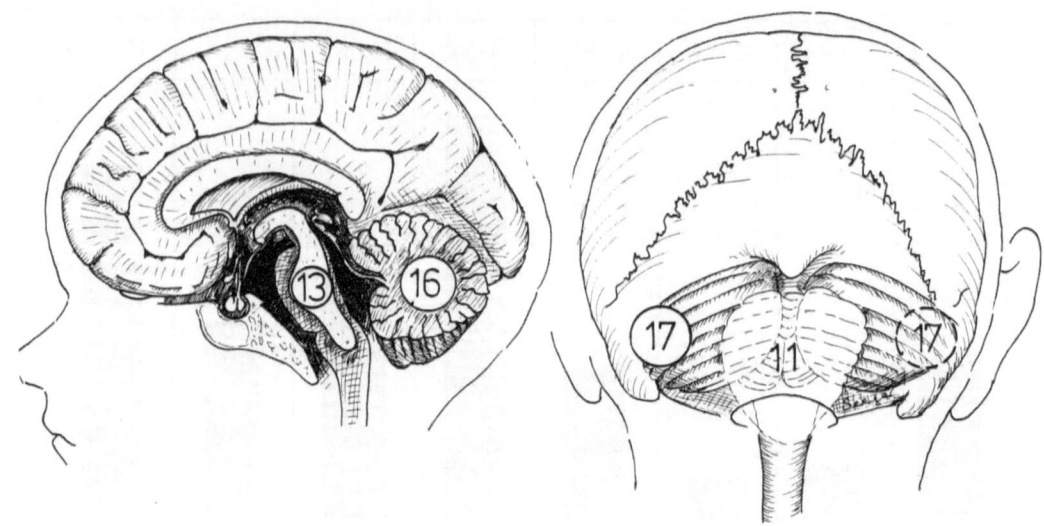

Fig. 3. Misdiagnosis - cerebral form of MS. Localization of infratentorial and brain stem processes (n = 57)

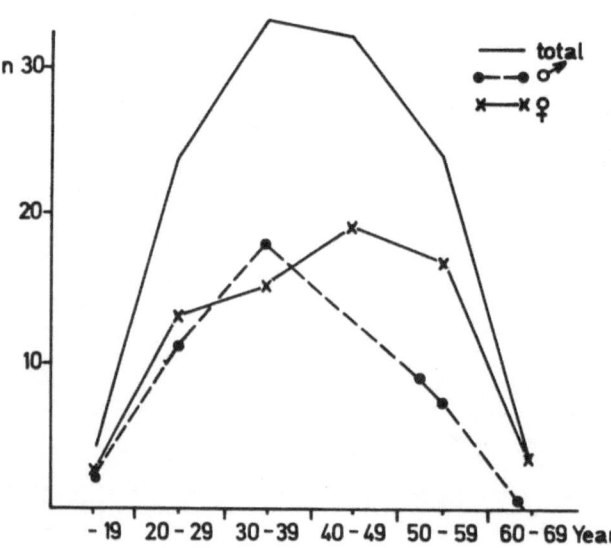

Fig. 4. Misdiagnosis - cerebral form of "MS". Age and sex distribution at the time of misdiagnosis

Multiple Sclerosis and Other Misdiagnoses in Spinal Processes

H. Kuhlendahl and W. Ischebeck with collaboration of K. Hartmann,
I. Iizuka, I. Kuske, H. Waldbaur, J. Brkic, H. v. Wild, H. Effinowicz,
Brendel, Friedrich, Th. Schaake, H. Palleske, K. Nittner, E. Hamel,
R.-I. Kahl, and W. Braun

We all make diagnostic mistakes at times! The fact that we here,
among neurosurgeons, are discussing false diagnoses which have in
most cases been made by our colleagues, must not be considered pre-
sumptuous. It is an effort to attract attention to the resulting
problems - of which, and there is no doubt about this, there are many.
We should always have in mind that, conversely, there are patients
with a definite clinical picture of multiple sclerosis who have undergone myelographies and sometimes even laminectomies without clear
indications! Here, we mainly want to investigate the reasons for the
relatively numerous wrong diagnoses.

The collected and revised material covers 2637 cases from 12 clinics.
In 24 %, that is one quarter of these cases, wrong diagnoses could
be found in the medical records. There is no doubt, however, that,
in fact, the percentage of wrong diagnoses, also among these 2637
cases, has been far layer, but the available sources and medical records could provide no proof of this. It is a common experience that
early diagnosis of a space occupying spinal process is rare. In this
sphere we have to take into account a fairly wide and 'grey' diagnostic margin. Thus, the statistical data given here cannot be completely flawless. They must, at least, represent the lowest limit of
reality.

This collection is restricted to 5 groups of spinal processes: meningiomas, neurinomas, angiomas and the cervical myelopathy. Table 1
shows the distribution of the total of 2637 cases according to these
5 diseases. (Because cervical myelopathy has only recently been recognized as a clinical entity and has not been accessible to surgical
treatment for long, the number of such cases in the various clinics
differs greatly).

Table 1. Distribution of 2637 cases

Meningiomas	Neurinomas	Intramedullary tumors	Cervical myelopath.	Angiomas
799 = <u>30 %</u>	713 = <u>27 %</u>	566 = <u>21 %</u>	389 = <u>15 %</u>	174 = <u>7 %</u>
Misdiagnosed cases:				
220 = <u>44 %</u>	141 = <u>28 %</u>	70 = <u>14 %</u>	36 = <u>7 %</u>	31 = <u>6 %</u>

700 of the total of 2637 cases had records documenting the wrong diagnosis. For various reasons we could only make use of 498 of these 700 in the following statistical report. The list on Table 2 gives a survey of the distribution of wrong diagnoses compiled from the cases we are dealing with here. "Multiple sclerosis" is by far the most frequent. When considering and evaluating this fact, one should have in mind that this diagnosis is almost exclusively made by specialists and probably almost always in special departments. This is certainly not true of the other wrong diagnoses, at least not to such an extent. It remains to be mentioned that the latter are mostly diagnosed as "circulatory disturbances", "rheumatism" and "neuralgia" without positive i. e. specific symptoms and signs.

Table 2. 498 cases with misdiagnoses

"Multiple sclerosis"	144	=	29 %
"Ischialgia"	84	=	17 %
"Circulatory disturbances"	58	=	12 %
"Rheumatism"	47	=	9 %
"Neuralgia"	47	=	9 %
"Spondylopathy"	39		
"Hip-joint disease"	17		
"Intraabdominal involvement"	16		
"Funicular myelosis"	15		
"Spinal paralysis"	12		
"Amytrophic lateral sclerosis"	7		
"Syringomyelia"	5		
"Intracranial process"	4		
"Arachnoiditis"	4		

The relatively frequent misdiagnosis of "multiple sclerosis" for space occupying spinal processes now becomes a point of interest. It is surprising that in the total material the diagnosis "multiple sclerosis" was made almost equally often for each of the 5 diseases (Table 3). However, when considering only the 498 cases of wrong diagnoses, the different significance of the "m. s." diagnosis for the various space occupying processes comes to light (Fig. 1).

The wrong diagnosis "m. s." is most frequent for cervical myelopathy (almost two thirds) and is made more often for spinal angiomas (one third) and intramedullary tumors (almost one third) than for neurinomas (26 %) and meningiomas (24 %). This corresponds to what general clinical experience has lead one to expect. *The localization* of the space occupying processes including angiomas (but excluding cervical myelopathy) which have had a wrong diagnosis corresponds to the general frequency-distribution in the localization of spinal tumors.

In our opinion, the essential aim of this investigation can only be to ascertain the causes of the diagnostic mistakes. We have to find out which symptoms or signs are misinterpreted. On the other hand, it is important to realize the extent and significance of the sequelae of the diagnostic errors.

Table 3. Misdiagnosis "multiple sclerosis" among

795	Meningiomas	52	=	6,5 %
713	Neurinomas	37	=	5,2 %
566	Intramed. tumors	22	=	4,0 %
389	Cerv. myelopathy	23	=	6,0 %
174	Angiomas	10	=	5,8 %
2637		144	=	5,5 %

When analyzing the clinical symptomatology of the wrongly diagnosed cases, the early symptoms and signs are obviously of primary importance, as the direction of diagnostic considerations and procedures is mainly dependent on them.

As expected, we see that paresthesias consitute 39 % of the symptoms in the cases of false "m. s." (Table 4).

Table 4. First sign in misdiagnosed cases

	Paresthesia	Paresis	Pain	Hypesthesia
"Multiple sclerosis"	39 %	31 %	17 %	13 %
"Circulat. disturb."	24 %	43 %	25 %	8 %

Pareses were present in almost one third of the cases. What is remarkable is that in 17 % of the cases pain was given as first symptom, which cannot really be regarded as very revealing for the diagnosis of multiple sclerosis!

In contrast, the first signs in the cases with false diagnosis of "circulatory disturbances" had been motor pareses in almost the half of these cases - a really most surprising discovery. They are followed, which is not as surprising, by pain and paresthesias.

With regard to the wrong diagnosis "multiple sclerosis" one can, thus, deduct that a diagnostic malassessment of paresthesias had taken place. But, in fact, these are the typical signs which, as primary signs, play such an important part in the slow-growing, extramedullary, non-malignant spinal tumors. Paradoxically and unfortunately they have led or often lead to a wrong diagnosis!

The result of the investigations of the neurological symptomatology ascertained at the time the wrong diagnosis "m. s." was made, is fairly surprising too. (Again we would like to point out the difficulties and the margin of error of these investigations based on medical records). It is alarming that of the 144 cases, 27 already had paraparesis and further 5 patients were already unable to walk. This was at the time the wrong diagnosis "multiple sclerosis" was made! (Table 5).

One third of the patients had already had micturition difficulties, which should also not have favoured the diagnosis of multiple sclerosis.

To return to the problem of the more or less serious consequences of the wrong diagnoses, it is impressive that of these 144 patients 70,

Table 5. 144 cases with the misdiagnosis MS

At the time of misdiagnosis:			At the time of definite diagnosis:
Paraparesis	low grade	6161	 15
	moderate	2424	.... 47 ┐
	severe	9 9	.... 74 ┘ = 89 %
Walking	little handi-cap	72	 18
	severe handi-cap	27	.... 53 ┐
	unable	5	.... 70 ┘ = 87 %
Micturition Disturb.		46	

i. e. one half, were not able to walk any more at the time the diagnosis was corrected, which was, in most cases, 6 to 18 months later! Two thirds of the patients had more or less severe micturition difficulties by then.

This means that the development of the clinical picture of severe paraplegia could have been avoided in 75 % of these cases, had the proper diagnosis not been missed before. In view of the fact that, in the majority of cases, we are dealing with non-malignant processes, this is of utmost importance. The difficulties of reascertaining a given diagnosis are illustrated in Fig. 2. It shows that, in many cases a considerable period of time, even a number of years, elapsed before the wrong diagnosis was corrected and the tumor was diagnosed.

The age of the patients is also an important factor concerning differential diagnosis. Multiple sclerosis begins at a fairly early age, as is well known: in the majority of cases between 20 and 40 years. (The age distribution curve for multiple sclerosis in Fig. 3 is based on data from the "Handbook of Clinical Neurology" and SCHALTENBRAND's statistics of 1956).

Thus, it is remarkable that the majority of patients with wrong diagnoses were much older. The essential difference is illustrated in Fig. 2. Although we have recorded the age at the time of the definitive diagnosis, we may shift the age distribution curve of our cases 2 to 3 years to the left without introducing any real difference, since 75 % of the wrong diagnoses had not been made more than 3 years before. The fact remains that the age of the patient at the time the wrong diagnosis "m. s." should have given rise to doubt in most cases.

A diagnostic procedure usually follows a first diagnostic concept based on the case history. A rigid concept can be misleading, as everyone knows, and lead to the finding of false or problematic signs. A "problematic symptom" is, for instance, the temporal pallor of the discs which was indeed (surely wrong) recorded in some findings. In 7 cases other cranial nerve signs were described (probably most of them had been "central pareses of the facial nerve"). Once the diagnosis "m. s." has been made, even a CSF protein content of more than 100 mg % can sometimes not dislodge it.

In this context, CSF diagnostic is certainly an especially important source of error. As well known, the CSF protein content plays an essential part in the diagnosis of space occupying spinal processes. However, what does not seem to be equally well-known or sufficiently taken into consideration, is that a lower CSF protein content does not exclude a space occupying lesion. It is surprising that the great significance of this fact with regard to diagnostic errors has not been adequately emphasized in the handbooks and in the literature at all. Thus, it seems to be necessary to stress the basic facts here again: especially in cases of spinal meningiomas a considerable number of patients had a normal or, at most, a slightly elevated CSF protein content. In the "Handbuch der Neurochirurgie" we find that 24 % of the cases of spinal meningiomas of the Cologne Clinic had a protein content below 50 mg %. In a thesis from the Duesseldorf Clinic a protein content below 50 mg % was recorded in even 30 % of 88 cases of spinal meningiomas.

The available material presented here provides the CSF findings of 188 meningiomas. One third of these cases had a protein content below 50 mg %. Almost in every 4th, or even 3rd, spinal meningioma a normal CSF protein content or only a slight and uncharacteristic increase of it is to be expected. Evidently, neither the localization nor the size of the tumor can be considered decisive (Table 6).

Table 6. CSF protein content

	30	50	60	200	100	mg %
188 Meningiomas	27	30	27	27	77	
	31 %			55 %		
122 Neurinomas	12	13	13	12	72	
	19 %			69 %		
38 False diagnosis "MS"	14	13	4	5	2	
	71 %			18 %		

Again, in the "Handbuch der Neurochirurgie" NITTNER quotes 50 mg % of protein in the CSF for 9 % of the *neurinomas*. This was the same in the Duesseldorf cases. In the present material low protein content was even recorded in 19 % of spinal neurinomas.

A normal or, at most, slightly increased protein content must be taken into account even more in connection with *intramedullary tumors* and spinal *angiomas*.

Considering these facts, we would like to conclude that the concept of "CSF blockade" should finally be given up, because there is no doubt that in the majority of cases without increased protein content the subarachnoid space had, nevertheless, been moderately or even totally obstructed. Factors other than the mechanics of CSF circulation must play an important role for the increase in protein content. The protein content in cases of neurinoma, which is often extremely high, proves that here an active transsudative process is the decisive factor.

In 70 % of the cases of space occupying lesions compiled here with the previous misdiagnosis of "m. s." a protein content below 50 mg % was recorded. Because this is so, we must conclude that in the cases the diagnosis of a space occupying process had been dropped mainly because an increase in the protein content in the CSF had been lacking!

It is even more surprising that, on the other hand, no further diagnostic measures were undertaken, since in 19 % - that is almost one fifth of the cases - a considerable increase of the protein content to above 100 mg % was found! According to the most recent report in the "Handbook of Clinical Neurology", a normal CSF protein content is found in 77 % of cases with multiple sclerosis, and, although extremely rare, 108 mg % is considered to be the upper limit.

In our opinion one of the especially important, although not new, conclusions to be reached on the basis of this statistical analysis is that there is an ignorance of the fact that a relatively large number of cases of spinal tumors are accompanied by a normal or only slightly increased CSF protein content. This is why, even in the course of clinical examinations, a space occupying lesion is far too frequently excluded on the basis of the CSF findings. -

The conclusions drawn from the evidence presented here confirm that, as regards the wrong diagnosis of "multiple sclerosis", there are four avoidable main sources of error:

1. the age of the patient at the onset of the illness is disregarded,
2. an omission of thorough analysis of the case history,
3. the diagnostic misinterpretation of early specific neurological symptoms and signs, especially paresthesias in the lower extremities, but also parapareses,
4. the malassessment of the CSF findings.

In short, it can be said that, if there is a patient older than 40 with paresthesia, hypoesthesia and/or with spastic symptoms, or perhaps paraparesis, one must concentrate on a tentative diagnosis of a space occupying lesion until there is counter-evidence enough based on perfect and, if necessary, repeated myelography to make this diagnosis most unlikely (to avoid the word "exclude"). We should also remember that BRAIN and WILKINSON (1957) have described 17 cases of association of cervical spondylosis (cervical myelopathy) with disseminated sclerosis (12 "beyond doubt" and 2 verified by post mortem examination). -

We have refrained from giving a casuistic report because it seemed more important, if possible, to establish generally valid facts for differential diagnosis and which may aid in avoiding wrong diagnoses followed by serious consequences. Our main task was the analysis of the reasons why at least every fourth patient with a spinal space occupying lesion is initially given a wrong diagnosis, especially multiple sclerosis.

We can learn from our own mistakes or from those of others if we analyze them thoroughly enough.

REFERENCES

ABB, L., SCHALTENBRAND, G.: Statistische Untersuchungen zum Problem der Multiplen Sklerose. Dtsch. Z. Nervenhk. 174, 199 - 218 (1955/ 1956).

BLINZINGER, K. H.: Querschnittsbilder bei der multiplen Sklerose. Zugleich ein Beitrag zur Differentialdiagnose zwischen Sclerosis multiplex und Tumor medullae spinalis. München: Thesis 1960.

BUSHART, W.: Fehldiagnose multiple Sklerose bei spinalen Prozessen. Internist 7, 157 - 166 (1966).

HIRSCHBIEGEL, H.: Remittierende Verläufe bei Spinaltumoren. Dtsch. Z. Nervenheilk. 190, 74 - 82 (1967).

KURTZKE, J. F.: Diagnosis and differential diagnosis of multiple sclerosis. Acta Neurol. Scand. 46, 484 - 492 (1970).

KURTZKE, J. F.: Clinical manifestations of multiple sclerosis. Hdb. Clinical Neurol. 9, 161 - 216 (1970).

NITTNER, K.: Raumbeengende Prozesse im Spinalkanal (einschließlich Angiome und Parasiten). In: Handbuch der Neurochirurgie, Bd. VII/2, S. 1 - 606 (1972).

OPPENHOFF, I.: Liquoreiweißgehalt bei Spinaltumoren. Düsseldorf: Thesis 1965.

RENNERT, H.: Zur Differentialdiagnose Spinaltumor - Multiple Sklerose. Psychiat. Neurol. Med. Psychol. (Leizpig) 2, 353 - 363 (1950).

RENNERT, H.: Weiteres zur Differentialdiagnose Spinaltumor - Multiple Sklerose (unter besonderer Berücksichtigung des Auftretens von Remissionen und supraläsionellen Störungen bei Spinaltumoren). Psychiat. Neurol. Med. Psychol. (Leipzig) 5, 414 - 422 (1953).

SCHRADER, A.: Differentialdiagnose der multiplen Sklerose. In: Differentialdiagnose neurologischer Krankheitsbilder, 3. Aufl. (Hrsg. G. BODECHTEL). Stuttgart: Georg Thieme 1974.

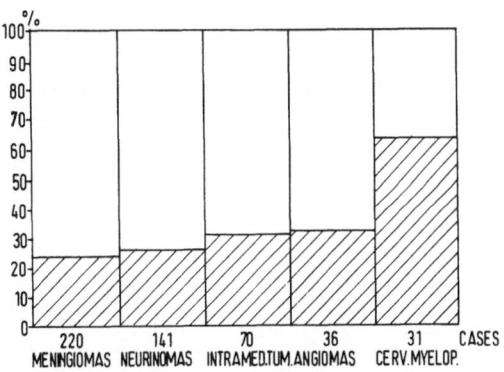

Fig. 1. Misdiagnosis "MS" in relation to the total number of wrong diagnoses in the 5 groups

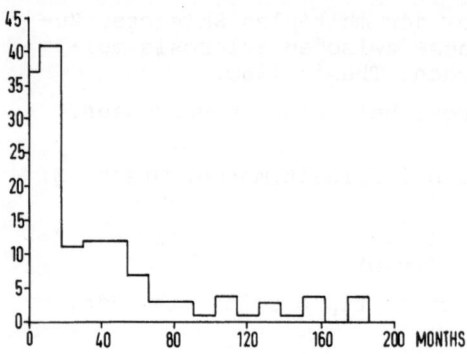

Fig. 2. Span of time between the misdiagnosis MS and subsequent operation (144 cases)

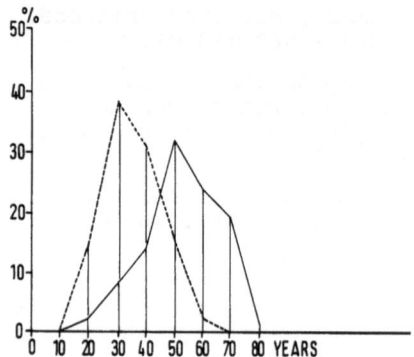

Fig. 3.
Age distribution ——————— multiple sclerosis
5000 cases
Age distribution ················ wrong diagnosis
multiple sclerosis
144 cases

Reasons for the Non-Recognition of Tumors of the Spinal Cord

K. NITTNER

Non-recognition of a tumor of the spinal cord in cases of narrowing in the spinal canal is, at least for a part of the cases, due to insufficient knowledge with respect to diagnostic findings: either they are not known well enough or they are not being attributed enough importance. This concerns particularly anamnestie findings, radiological findings with changes that are typical of a tumor or even specific with respect to the tumor species, as well as changes of composition and dynamics of CSF. In cases of spinal cord compression radiological changes are often underestimated as to their diagnostic importance, whereas the importance of pathological CSF is often overestimated.

Anamnesis

Generally, a slowly advancing progress is to be observed with tumors of the cord. Nevertheless, we also know of *intermittent* or *remittent* cases of e. g. gliomas (2, 5) or neurinomas and meningiomas (1, 3).

It is only in about 6 % of all cases of spinal cord tumors that diagnosis is possible based on one single symptom and in only about 11 % when there are 2 symptoms; thus, only every 6th patient is sure to receive surgical treatment at this stage of suffering from spinal cord compression (Fig. 1). On hospitalisation, more than one third of the cases showed 3 main symptoms of compression of the spinal cord and about half of the cases showed four symptoms, such as pain, pareses or plegia, perception disorders, rectovesical and sexual disturbances. On hospitalisation, up to two thirds of the cases exhibit a complete transverse syndrome. -

Pain is the leading early symptom of a compression of the spinal cord. It can, however, be missing, both at this stage and during the whole course of the disease. This was the case in 16 % of our patients [with meningiomas in 32,5 %, with gliomas in 17,6 % and in neurinomas in 14,6 % (Table 1)].

Table 1. Diagnosis in cases of tumors of the cord: normal

		Total number %	Gliomas + ependymom.	Neurinomas	Meningiomas
No pains		16 %	17,6 %	14,6 %	32,5 %
X-ray:	normal	60 %	90 %	60 %	86 %
CSF:	normal	15 %	21 %	9 %	24 %
Queckenstedt test:	normal	15 %	22 %	10 %	4 %
CSF + Qu. test	normal	5 %	16,3 %	1,8 %	1,6 %

Diagnosis

Spastic pareses or plegia, mostly para- or tetraspasticity, are the neurological disturbances that are to be expected. But there are also hypotonic pareses (23 % of the cases). If paresis develops quickly, a malignoma must be suspected in most of the cases. In our material malignomas amounted to 33 % (49 % of the cases with hyptonic pareses). Bleeding from tumor or angioma must be excluded in cases of acute hypotonic transverse lesions of the spinal cord with paraplegia. Such tumors were primarily localized at the D 3 - 6 level with a maximum at D 5 - i. e. in a region of inadequate spinal circulation - as well as at C 3 - 6 and D 12. In the hypotonic group, paraparesis was caused by gliomas in 30 %, by meningiomas in 18 % and by neurinomas in 15 %.

Evaluating 565 cases of spinal cord compression, observed over a 37-years period (6), the following criteria appeared to be of importance with respect to the diagnosis of tumors of the spinal cord:

Motor disturbances of any kind were rare at the early stage; it was in only 15 % of the cases that they were the first symptom. They were missing in 9 % of all tumors of the spinal cord during the whole course of the disease.

This is similarly true for *perception disorders*, as these were missing in 22 % of the cases.

Rectovesical disturbances appear, in most cases, in the final stage of a compression syndrome of the spinal cord, i. e. after the transverse lesion of the spinal cord has become complete. However, in 29 % of the cases rectovesical disorders were missing during the whole course of the disease.

The following criteria may help to *prevent false diagnoses*:

Radiological changes are present in about one third of all extra-modullary spinal cord tumors, and in about 10 % of intramedullary tumors. Localized changes in 1 - 2 segments of the vertebral arches and excavations on the vertebral body generally indicate a benign lesion, usually a neurinoma. If changes are limited to one segment and, then, mostly to the base of arch on one side, presence of a meningioma may be suspected. Massive changes on both sides of the arches, with excavations extending over several segments, indicate presence either of an ependymoma or an epidermoid. Generally, a more accurate radiological definition is not possible. Changes on larger parts of the spinal column, though not even very marked, may be found in cases of extradural sarcomas and intrademullary gliomas (about 10 % with intramedullary gliomas). Radiological changes in the shape of direct or indirect tumor symptoms are missing in 60 % of the cases, in 90 % of all gliomas, in 86 % of all meningiomas and in 60 % of all neurinomas.

Changes in the *protein content* of CSF are found in 85 % of all patients suffering from spinal cord compression; thus, 15 % (cf. Table 1) cannot be verified by this method. However, protein values between 40 mg % and 50 mg %, considered within the whole of the pathological findings, should not be underestimated with respect to their diagnostic significance (Table 2). 24 % of all meningiomas, 21 % of all gliomas and 9 % of all neurinomas (Table 3) cannot be verified by CSF studies. A minor pleocytosis of the CSF - not over 30/3 cells - is also found in 38 % of cases of spinal cord tumors, particularly gliomas.

Table 2. CSF total protein and Queckenstedt test

mg/%	No. of cases		Total	Part.	Normal	
> 100	134	60 %	91	34	9 =	7 %
50 - 100	38	17 %	21	11	6 =	16 %
40 - 50	16	7,5 %	3	9	4 =	25 %
< 40	34	15,5 %	14	8	12 =	35 %
	222	100 %	129 58 %	62 28 %	31	14 %

Table 3. Kind of tumor according to protein findings in CSF [from K. NITTNER, p. 162 (4)]

Kind of tumor		Protein normal		40 - 50 mg %	Patholog. increase
Gliomas	35	5	21 %	2	28
Ependymomas	17	3		1	13
Sarcomata	28	3		4	21
Plasmocytomas	6	-		-	6
Meningiomas	74	12	24 %	6	56
Neurinomas	64	5	9 %	1	58
Cysts	3	1		1	1
Angiomas	22	5	36 %	3	14
Carcinomata	23	4		1	18
Lipomas	5	3		-	2
Dermoids	6	1		2	3

As CSF dynamics show disturbances in 85 % of the cases, 15 % cannot be verified by dynamic studies [22 % of the gliomas and ependymomas, 10 % of the neurinomas, 4 % of the meningiomas (cf. Table 1)] .

It is only 5 % of the cases, about 16 % of the gliomas and ependymomas and nearly 2 % of the neurinomas and meningiomas respectively that cannot be verified by examination of b o t h *CSF changes* and *CSF dynamics*.

According to protein content in lumbar CSF and to the results obtained from the Queckenstedt Test, a compension of these two methods is possible as shown in Table 2.

Myelography is always clearly pathological and, thus, is indispensable only in case of doubt.

Summary

Reasons that may lead to non-recognition of tumors of the spinal cord are discussed on the basis of findings in 565 patients suffering from spinal cord compressive lesions. The importance of careful anamnesis, neurological and radiological examination as well as studies of the composition and dynamics of CSF are emphasized.

REFERENCES

1. ANTONI, N. R. E.: Über Rückenmarkstumoren und Neurofibrome; Studien zur pathologischen Anatomie und Embryogenese; mit einem klinischen Anhang. München - Wiesbaden: J. F. Bergmann 1920.

2. CASTEN, H. R.: Rückenmarkstumor. Berl. klin. Wschr. 48, 45 (1911).

3. MÜLLER, A.: Ein Fall von Rückenmarkstumor im oberen Cervicalbereich. Dtsch. Z. Nervenheilk. 71, 183 - 186 (1921).

4. NITTNER, K.: Raumbeengende Prozesse im Spinalkanal (einschließlich Angiome und Parasiten). In: Handbuch der Neurochirurgie, Bd. VII/2, S. 1 - 606. (Hrsg. W. KRENKEL, H. OLIVECRONA, W. TÖNNIS), Berlin - Göttingen - Heidelberg: Springer 1972.

5. SCHLAPP, M. G.: A neuroepithelioma developing from a central gliosis, after an operation on the spinal cord. J. nerv. ment. Dis. 38, 129 - 151 (1911).

6. TÖNNIS, W.: Clinical Reports on 565 patients: Chirurgische Universitätsklinik Würzburg 1932 - 1937, Neurochirurgische Universitätsklinik Berlin 1937 - 1945, Neurochirurgische Abteilung Knappschaftskrankenhaus Bochum - Langendreer 1945 - 1951, Neurochirurgische Universitätsklinik Köln 1951 - 1968.

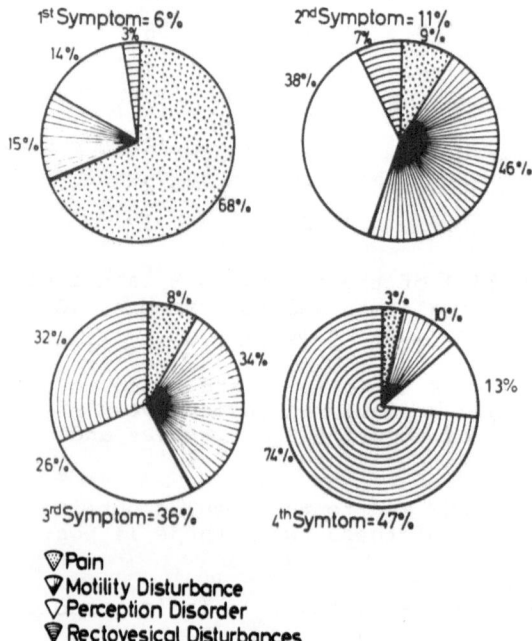

▽ Pain
▼ Motility Disturbance
▽ Perception Disorder
▼ Rectovesical Disturbances

Fig. 1. Sequence of disturbances [from: K. NITTNER, p. 138 (4)]

194

Unfavorable Effects of Lumbar Puncture and Other Diagnostic Procedures on the Course of Multiple Sclerosis?

B. WEISNER

Multiple sclerosis (MS) frequently is a wrong diagnosis. Differential diagnostic considerations often make necessary lumbar puncture (LP) as well as other operative diagnostic means.

It has been emphasized (2, 3) that MS may get worse by a single lumbar puncture. SCHAPIRA (4) and TOURTELOTTE (5), on the other hand, were unable to see any detremental effect by lumbar puncture on the course of MS.

We studied the development of neurological symptoms in patients suffering from MS over seven weeks following LP, pneumencephalography (PEG) and cerebral angiography. From 1965 up to 1973, 262 patients were studied using the scale of FOG (1). In the same way, the course of MS before and after PEG was evaluated in a long term study of 50 cases from 1 up to 18 years.

No acute deterioration of neurologic symptoms was observed following LP, PEG and angiography. In 93 patients there were no neurological changes, while in 45 cases there was some improvement. In 7 patients neurological signs appeared more severe, however deterioration had already started before LP. In a number of cases new symptoms developed, but they could not be correlated with the diagnostic procedure. Some patients showed the tendency of accusing LP as being responsible for deteriorioration.

In 9 cases (total 94) gait and spasticity deteriorated following PEG, however in all these 9 cases there had already been signs of deterioration of neurologic symptoms previous to PEG. In no case did PEG appear to have accelerated deterioration. In no case an increase of neurological symptoms was observed following cerebral angiography.

In our long-term observation of 50 patients with MS who had had PEG, there were two cases with acute deterioration. PEG did not, however, influence the overall course of MS.

Isolated observation of the period immediately following PEG might be indicative for deterioration. On the long run of the case, however, this does no longer appear to having been so (Fig. 1). Similarly, improvement is possible immediately following PEG (9 cases), again without influence on the long-run course (Fig. 2).

Summary

Diagnostic procedures such as lumbar puncture, pneumencephalography and angiography do not appear to have any unfavourable effect with respect to the course of multiple sclerosis. While it seems advisable to withhold temporarily such diagnostic procedures during an acute phase of the disease, their use is justified to insure that signs and symptoms are definitely of multilocular and not of locally restricted origin, the process being inflammatory in nature.

REFERENCES

1. FOG, T.: A scoring System For Neurologic Impairment in Multiple Sclerosis. Acta Neurologica Scandinavica 41 suppl. 13, 551 – 555 (1965).

2. HENNER, K.: Neurological Congress Brussels 1957, cited by SCHAPIRA, K.: Is Lumbar Puncture Harmful in Multiple Sclerosis? J. Neurol. Neurosurg. Psychiat. 22, 238 (1959).

3. PAYK, Th. R.: Iatrogene Schäden in der Neurologie. Fortschr. Neurol. Psychiat. 42, 97 – 111 (1974).

4. SCHAPIRA, K.: Is Lumbar Puncture Harmful in Multiple Sclerosis? J. Neurol. Neurosurg. Psychiat. 22, 238 (1959).

5. TOURTELOTTE, W. W.: Cerebrospinal Fluid in Multiple Sclerosis. In: Handbook of Clinical Neurology (eds. P. J. VINKEN, G. W. BRUYN), pp. 224 – 325. Amsterdam: North Holland Publ. Comp. 19 .

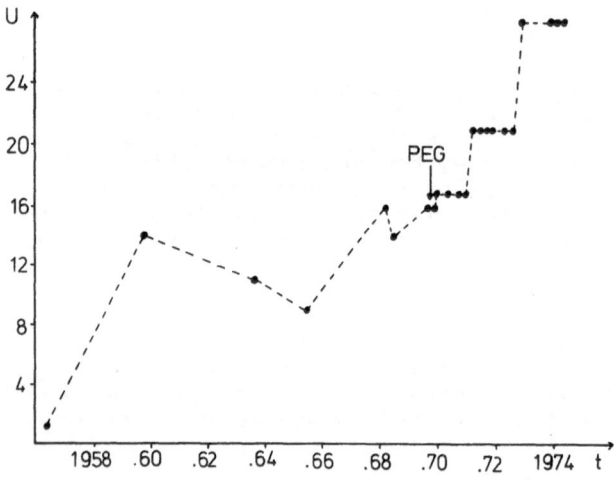

Fig. 1. H. G. 51 years old woman. Long-term observation over 18 years. Rating scale (U) of signs and symptoms as used by FOG (1). Signs of deterioration appeared already prior to PEG. The long-term development of the disease is not influenced

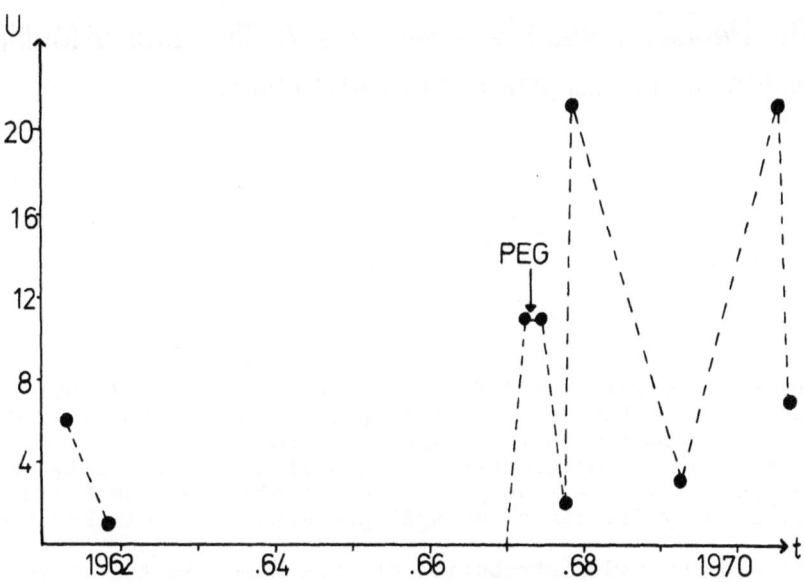

Fig. 2. K. J. 24 years old woman. Long-term observation. Rating scale (U) of signs and symptoms as used by FOG (1). Signs of improvement following PEG. The episodic course of the disease continues at unchanged rate

The Periadventitial Brain Sarcoma: A Simulator of Multiple Sclerosis

W. Entzian, F. Gullotta, and H. Vahar-Matiar

The parvicellular periadventitial brain sarcoma (PPBS) is actually subjected to the "malignant lymphomas" of the CNS (1). Generally, the tumor is located in the brain stem and in the periventricular regions. Because of its multicentric origin it grows diffusely and almost symmetrically with a wide spread infiltration of the brain tissue (Fig. 1). In very few cases the PPBS presents as a solitary tumor (3, 4).

The wide-spread distribution of this tumor is the cause for complex neurological deficits, that may simulate a multiple sclerosis. Therefore a case report is given to draw attention to this diagnostic problem.

Case Report

A 61 year old female patient was hospitalized because of slowly increasing headache, vertigo and nausea. She showed motoric aphasia, paresis and hypoflexia of the left extretimites, no cutaneous abdominal reflexes and severe ataxia. - Later on bilateral facial nerve paresis, intention tremor and transient dysphagia were observed. Papilledema did not develop.

Pneumencephalogram and right sided carotid and vertebral angiograms were normal. EEG showed paroxysms of deltawaves slightly accentuated on the left side.

CSF: 64/3 leucocytes and lymphocytes, total protein content 58 mg %; CSF-electrophoresis showed a mixed pherogram due to severely disturbed barriers, V- and T-fraction were missing, gamma-globulins were increased.

Death occurred six months after onset of symptoms without a definite clinical diagnosis being established. At authopsy multiple tumors with perivascular infiltrations were found in the cerebrum and in the cerebellum (Fig. 2).

Discussion

The great variety of neurological symptoms is impressive in this case as well as in some other personal cases and in the cases described in literature: mental changes, disorders of the pyramidal tracts, of the cranial nerves and of coordination may occur and may be combined in such a way, that the origin of the disease cannot be pinned down on one single supra- or infratentorial area. The clinical course in patients with PPBS may be a subacute or chronic one and may even be enhanced by remissions.

Due to the pathomorphologic distribution of the PPBS, neuroradiologic, isotope and EEG studies generally do not reveal a circumscript space occupying lesion.

A laboratory diagnosis appears to be possible by CSF-cell collecting methods in those cases with the tumor bordering CSF-pathways. Recently KOLAR (2) pointed out, that immunologic studies of serum and CSF should be done.

The prognosis of the disease is considered to be desolate, as irradiation or surgical treatment of the PPBS may prolonge the patients live only under the rare prerequisite, that the tumor has developed unifocally.

Finally the authors want to point out, that in the early phases of the disease, that is as long as signs of intracranial hypertension are missing, the neurological multifocal symptoms may simulate multiple sclerosis.

It is concluded therefore, that under the above mentioned conditions differential diagnosis should be extended to the PPBS.

Summary

The parvicellular periadventitial brain sarcoma is characterized by multicentric perivascular origin with preferrably localized in the brain stem and in the periventricular regions. Therefore, the neurological symptoms may simulate multiple sclerosis unless intracranial hypertension develops in the late course of the disease. Generally, intracranial contrast studies will not detect a solitary tumor; prognosis is poor.

REFERENCES

1. JELLINGER, K., RADASKIEWICZ, Th., SLOWIK, F.: Primary malignant lymphomas of the central nervous system in man (ed. K. JELLINGER), Malignant lymphomas of the nervous system, p. 23. International symposium, Aug. 29 - 31, 1974. Vienna: Facultas 1974.

2. KOLAR, O. J.: Differential diagnostic aspects in malignant lymphomas involving the central nervous system (ed. K. JELLINGER). Malignant lymphomas of the nervous system, p. 24. International symposium, Aug. 29 - 31, 1974. Vienna: Facultas 1974.

3. MEYER-LINDENBERG, J., GULLOTTA, F.: Das "Mikrogliom" als ortsspezifische mesenchymale Hirngeschwulst. Arch. Psychiat. Nervenkr. 213, 66 - 77 (1970).

4. MEYER-LINDENBERG, J., VLIEGEN, J.: Klinische, diagnostische und therapeutische Überlegungen bei Mikrogliomen. Der Nervenarzt 42, 370 - 376 (1971).

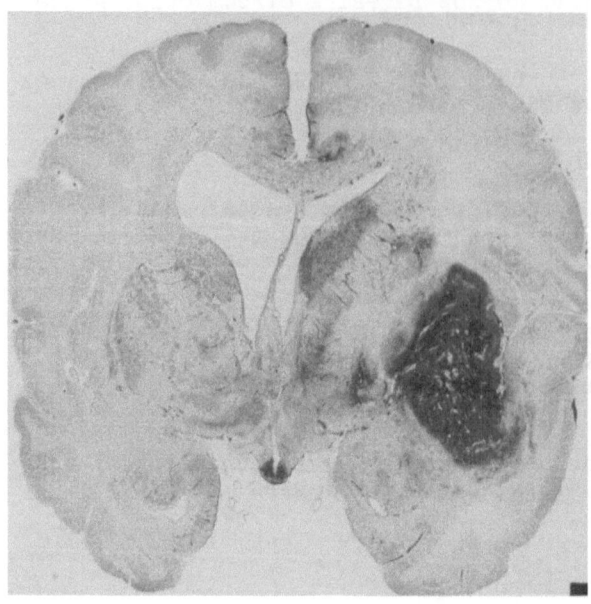

Fig. 1. Parvicellular periadventitial brain sarcoma (PPBS). Wide-spread neoplastic infiltration of the central and periventricular brain structures, tumor masses in the right insular cortex and infundibulum

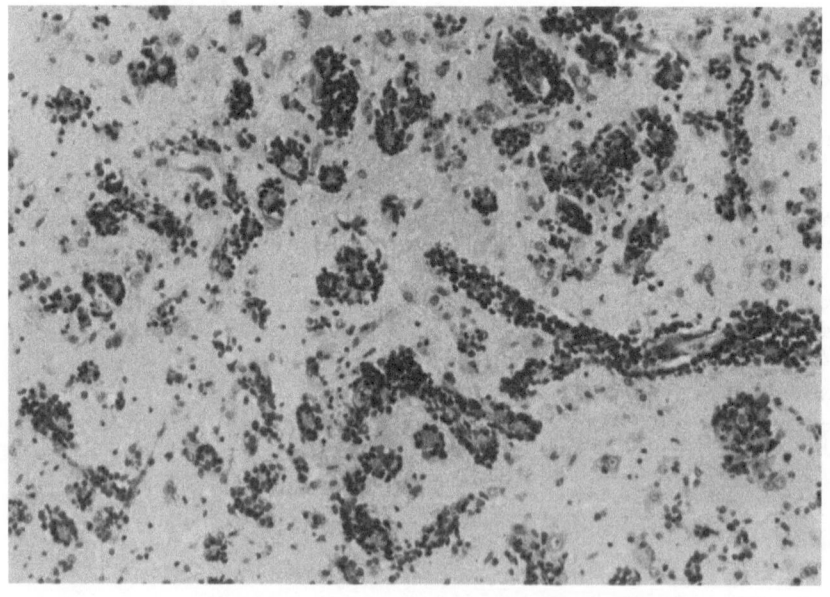

Fig. 2. The neoplastic cell infiltration of PPBS is strictly confined to the perivascular spaces of the dentate nucleus

Multiple Sclerosis as Misdiagnosis – Neurophysiological Investigations for an Objective Diagnosis of Spino-Cervical Processes

J.-P. MALIN, R. STÖLZEL, and H.-H. v. HARTROTT

Introduction

Among the various forms of multiple sclerosis (MS), we have studied the spinal variant. Differential diagnosis of this pictures of a progressive spinal syndrome (progressive parapareses or paraplegias) poses special difficulties as compared to other non-disseminated spinal diseases. Particularly the diseases which are relevant from the neurosurgical point of view, i. e. spinal tumors and the so-called cervical myelopathy associated with spondylotic lesions of the cervical spine, merit special discussion.

The importance on these questions to the neurosurgeon were illustrated by the studies of MARSHALL (12), who, at the National Hospital in London, examined 80 patients suffering from spastic paraparesis or paraplegia. In the course of this period (the study ran from 1930 to 1952) an absolutely certain diagnosis could be established in only 25 of these patients. Ten of these suffered from spinal MS, seven had a spinal tumor, three an intervertebral disc prolapse and one had syringomyelia. In 5 cases the cause of the paraparesis was demonstrated to be a cervical spondylosis. BRAIN and WILKINSON (4) have reported on the simultaneous occurrence of cervical spondylosis and MS. The difficult differential diagnosis was aided by differences in the course of the disease: The cervical myelopathy did not produce any remissions comparable to those found in spinal MS (10, 13). It is especially important to note that the clinical course of spinal meningiomas, angiomas or neurinomas can have a striking resemblance to the remissions found in MS, mainly during pregnancy (2, 3, 6, 9, 15).

Main Section

What contributions can neurophysiological investigations make towards answering questions of differential diagnosis (spinal tumor, cervical myelopathy or spinal variant of MS) as objectively as possible?

We have limited ourselves to those neurophysiological methods which are routinely applied in clinical diagnostics and have left aside any experimental methods requiring a disproportionate amount of technical facilities. The question to be examined is, therefore, to what extent electromyography (EMG) and electroneurography, i. e. the measurement of nerve conduction velocity, can be of additional help to the neurosurgeon.

1. EMG and MS

It must first be admitted that electromyography and electroneurography (ENG) do not play a role in the diagnosis of MS comparable to that of the examination of the CSF, particularly the immuno-diffusion method (11, 13).

Electromyography can provide the general criteria of spasticity and this is possible in the early stage when there might be only a discrete increase in reflex excitability. Whether this is possible in all cases must, however, be doubted. But an EMG is an insufficient basis for deciding whether MS, myelitis or a spinal tumor is the cause of the paraspastic condition (8, 16).

2. MS and Nerve Conduction Velocity

Neither the measurement of sensory and motor nerve conduction velocities nor distal latencies provide findings on which to base the diagnosis. In the ulnar nerve, HOPF found a prolongation and an increased variation of the distal motor latency in 8 out of 15 MS patients. This is in contrast to the studies of CONRAD and BECHINGER (5) who carried out measurements in the ulnar and median nerves of 68 MS patients (19 with an acute attack) and of 54 healthy persons without finding any statistically significant differences.

3. Cervical Myelopathy

Here, too, the EMG can only provide the general criteria of spasticity. If, however, there is only a lesion of individual cervical roots, the electromyographic comparison of the affected myotomes with healthy segments can help localize the area. After examining 24 cases RUPRECHT and STRUPPLER (14) described the electromyographic findings for lesions of the two lower cervical roots and were able to differentiate between a so-called "radial type" (C 7) and an "ulnar type" (C 8): The patients showed denervation processes (fibrillation, positive waves) in the affected segments. In the nonaffected segments there is a normal EMG.

In one of our patients (K. G.) who presented with the clinical picture of a cervicospinal process we were able to demonstrate signs of denervation in the segments C 4 to C 6. Air myelography then showed unusual spondylotic narrowing of the cervical canal between C 4 and C 6 in this 36-year-old patient.

On the other hand, the measurement of the nerve conduction velocities of our 8 patients with the clinical and X-ray diagnosis of a cervical myelopathy did not result in any significant pathological values, which was also not to be expected.

4. EMG and Spinal Tumors

ABBRUZESE et al. (1) examined 18 patients with spinal tumors electromyographically. There were 9 intramedullary and 9 extramedullary tumors. The investigation resulted in the electromyographical picture of a proximal lesion of the peripheral motor neuron, i. e. a rarefaction of the interference pattern, denervation potentials as well as an increased amount of polyphasic potentials. The picture was more distinct in the patients with intramedullary tumors.

Conclusions

On the basis of our experience and the relevant literature, it can be said that electromyography and electroneurography help the differential diagnosis in the following way:

1. Neurological examination and close observation of the course of the disease are the best methods for ruling out or verifying spinal MS; CSF examination must be given priority among the auxiliary methods.

2. In the diagnosis of spinal space-occupying processes simple neurophysiological investigations such as EMG and ENG do not have a diagnostic significance comparable to myelography.

3. In patients with so-called cervical myelopathy, which is so ambiguous in its symptoms, the lesion can be localized by demonstrating radicular syndromes with the EMG, before more radical methods (myelography) are used.

REFERENCES

1. ABBRUZESE, M., del CONTE, J., PASTORINO, P., SACCO, G.: EMG-findings in Spinal Tumors. 4th International Congress of Electromyography, Brussels, Sept. 1971.

2. BICKERSTAFF, E. R., SMALL, J. M., GUEST, J. A.: The relapsing course of certain meningiomas in relation to pregnancy and menstruation. J. Neurol. Neurosurg. Psychiat. 21, 89 - 91 (1958).

3. BODECHTEL, G.: Differentialdiagnose neurologischer Krankheitsbilder. Stuttgart: Georg Thieme 1974.

4. BRAIN, R., WILKINSON, M.: The association of cervical spondylosis and disseminated sclerosis. Brain 80, 456 - 478 (1957).

5. CONRAD, B., BECHINGER, D.: Sensorische und motorische Nervenleitgeschwindigkeiten und distale Latenz bei multipler Sklerose. Arch. Psychiat. Nervenkr. 212, 140 - 149 (1969).

6. HIRSCHBIEGEL, H.: Remittierende Verläufe bei Spinaltumoren. Dtsch. Zschr. Nervenheilk. 190, 74 - 82 (1967).

7. HOPF, H. C.: Leitgeschwindigkeit motorischer Nerven bei der multiplen Sklerose und unter dem Einfluß hoher Cortisonmedikation. Dtsch. Z. Nervenheilk. 187, 522 - 526 (1965).

8. HOPF, H. C., STRUPPLER, A.: Elektromyographie - Lehrbuch und Atlas. Stuttgart: Georg Thieme 1974.

9. JANZEN, R.: Differentialdiagnostische Schwierigkeiten bei multipler Sklerose. Dtsch. med. Wschr. 92, 764 - 765 (1967).

10. KUHLENDAHL, H., HIRSCHBIEGEL, H., BÖCHEM, K. F.: Die klinisch-neurologische Symptomatik der chronischen zervikalen Myelopathie vertebraler Genese. In: Wirbelsäule und Nervensystem (Hrsg. E. TROSTDORF, H. St. STENDER), S. 108 - 112. Stuttgart: Georg Thieme 1970.

11. KURTZKE, J. F.: Clinical manifestations of multiple sclerosis. In: Handbook of Clinical Neurology, Vol. 9 (eds. P. J. VINKEN, G. W. BRUYN), pp. 161 - 216. Amsterdam: North Holland Publ. Comp. 1970.

12. MARSHALL, L.: Spastic paraplegia of middle age. A clinico-pathological study. Lancet 1, 643 - 646 (1955).

13. McALPINE, D., LUMSDEN, C. E., ACHESON, E. D.: Multiple Sclerosis, 2nd edition. Livingstone - Edinburgh - London: Churchill 1972.

14. RUPRECHT, E. O., STRUPPLER, A.: Läsionen der unteren Zervikalwurzeln. Z. EEG - EMG 4, 60 - 67 (1973).

15. SCHRADER, A., WEISE, H.: Kasuistischer Beitrag zur Differentialdiagnose zwischen spinaler Erscheinungsform der multiplen Sklerose und Rückenmarkstumor. Nervenarzt $\underline{22}$, 447 - 451 (1951).

16. STRUPPLER, A., RUPRECHT, E. O.: Elektromyographie (EMG) und Elek-
troneurographie (ENG). Grundlagen und diagnostische Bedeutung.
Z. EEG - EMG $\underline{2}$, 2 - 16 (1971).

Report on 373 Patients Operated on for Meningiomas (from June 1, 1951 to December 31, 1973)

R. SATTLEGGER, M. HASCHEMI, and W. KLUG

During the period of reference from June 1st, 1951 to December 31st, 1973 a total of 373 patients were operated on for meningiomas, i. e. on mesodermal tumors originating from the Pacchionian granulations in the Neurosurgical Clinic Bochum - Langendreer.

One hundred and thirty-one (131) patients had a so-called parasagittal meningioma (attached near the sinus, originating from the Pacchonian granulations).

In 138 patients the meningioma growth originated from the area of the base of the skull, while in 104 patients the tumor was located on the convexity of the cerebral hemisphere.

The evaluation of the clinical histories and the surgical reports yielded results that well agreed with the respective medical literature. Within the group of the parasagittal meningiomas the tumor situated in the region of the so-called medial third of the sagittal sinus (71.75 %) were clearly predominant. The meningiomas located in the anterior third of the sinus accounted for 14.75 % whereas those situated in the posterior third of the sinus amounted to 13.7 % of the cases.

Among the patients with tumors originating at the base of the skull the sphenoid meningiomas prevailed and a distinction was made only between medial and lateral tumors.

In a total of 70 patients the tumor growth was located in the sphenoid bone with the point of attachment being lateral in 40 cases and medial in 30. In 34 patients the olfactory groove was the site of the meningioma and in 12 patients the tumor involved the tentorium cerebelli. Seven meningiomas were localized in the cerebellopontine angle, eight in the suprasellar region and three in MECKEL's cavity. A generalized meningiomatosis of the base of the skull was found in two cases.

The petrosal sinus was the origin of the operated tumor in a single case.

Among the 104 reported cases of so-called convexity meningiomas the tumorous growth originated in 20 patients in the region of the frontal convexity, in 60 patients at the parietal dura mater, in 21 patients the point of attachment was the temporal convexity and in only three patients the meningiomas was sited in the occipital dura.

Especially the basal meningiomas were found to affect primarily female persons. While the female sex, referred to the total number of cases (373), accounted for 64.9 % and the male sex for 35.1 % of the cases, the female patients clearly prevailed among basal meningiomas, where

111 out of 140 operated patients were women (80,5 %). Here the male sex merely accounted for 27 cases (19,5 %).

With respect to the convexity meningiomas, the females prevailed with 71.2 per cent against 28.8 % for the male patients.

Regarding parasagittal meningiomas, the female sex accounted for 64.9 % of the cases and was thus far more frequently affected than males (35.1 %). The rate of incidence showed striking differences as to age groups and localization. The parasagittal meningiomas were found to occur more frequently during the fourth and fifth decades of life, while for basal meningiomas the highest rate of incidence was in the period between the fifth and sixth decade. The convexity meningiomas had the maximum incidence rate at the average age of 50.

In establishing the mortality rate we have applied strict criteria and allowed also an extended postoperative period to be considered. All postoperative complications such as pneumonia, thrombosis, pulmonary infarction, marasmus, etc., were included in the statistics. Moreover, it must be considered that, as a result of the imperfect anaesthesia and after-care in the years from 1951 to 1960, the mortality rate is distinctly higher than it is in the following decade.

Compared with the figures reported in literature, the patients surgically treated in our clinic fall predominantly in the higher age group, especially with basal meningioma.

As emphasized by several authors, age plays a decisive role in the success of surgery, particularly with basal meningiomas. Consequently, the total mortality rate was 36.2 % for the patients operated on basal meningiomas in our clinic. The overall mortality rate of the sagittal meningiomas accounted for 26 % and that of the convexity meningiomas for 18.2 %. If we restrict our analysis to the last 10 years the mortality rate for the basal meningiomas is found to have clearly improved.

Based on relatively high patient age, the mortality rate was as low as 20 %. Furthermore, it must be borne in mind that, precisely in this decade, a major portion of the operated cases showed the tumor to originate from the medial wing of the sphenoid bone where a complete removal often proves impossible.

The vicinity of the internal carotid artery and of the basal veins plays a decisive role in the surgery of medial sphenoid meningiomas so that frequently only a partial resection can be performed.

Since the increased risk of partial resection has been dealt with extensively in literature, we wish to mention it here in passing only.

History and Symptomatology

Based on an analysis of the case histories we have tried to statistically cover those symptoms which had been apparent within a year's period prior to surgery. In the case of frontal localizations, the analysis of the case histories yielded poor results both for parasagittal and convexity meningiomas.

The more frequent symptoms such as headache and, occasionally, a change in personality were inconclusive. Impaired vision and vertigo were present in isolated cases only.

By contrast, when meningiomas originating from the medial third of the sinus were involved, motor weakness in the extremities, spasmodic fits of a focal or generalized character had developed and had been described more frequently already a year before hospitalization. An apoplectic onset had, nevertheless, been verified in six cases already a year before hospitalization, while speech defects had been manifest at least temporarily in four patients with prevalent involvement of the dominant hemisphere and relatively rapid growth of the tumor in the years prior to clinical treatment.

In the case of parietal convexity meningiomas such general symptoms as headache and dizziness also prevailed and only few patients presented local and pointer symptoms in the form of focal and generalized spasmodic fits. In the same way basal meningiomas only occasionally presented early symptoms, depending on their extension toward the anterior medial and posterior cranial fossae. Thus, when meningiomas expanded from the olfactory groove and the sphenoid bone, early visual disturbances were frequently observed over years, usually beginning in one eye. The patients were very often found indolent and prepared to accept one-sided blindness as their fate. To all appearances, this unilateral blindness develops so slowly that often only a careful ophthalmological examination is capable of establishing this early diagnosis. Olfactory disturbances were observed only in very few meningioma patients with the expansion growth involving the anterior fossa.

In the presence of considerable tumor expansion within the anterior and medial fossa and uncharacteristic psychic change was often detected as an early syndrome, whereas in the event of tumors involving the posterior cranial fossa and the transitional zone between the manifest symptoms were occasional deafness, disequilibrium, disturbances of the occular muscles and incoordination.

A protrusion of the eyeball developed as an early symptom in some sphenoid meningiomas and had been noticed by the patients themselves or other persons. These meningiomas are known to present usually inoperable involvement so that the prognosis for these patients is extremely unfavourable.

Discussion

The slow, expansive growth of the mesodermal meningiomas is unfortunately known to be characterized by taking a relatively asymptomatic course so that in the differential diagnosis of a meningioma a most thorough follow-up examination by the ophthalmologist, the otorhynolaryngologist, the internist and the neurologist in cooperation with the attending neurosurgeon cannot be dispensed with. The slightest suspicion of a possible subcranial space-occupying lesion should, in our view, prompt us to initiate extensive neuroradiological diagnostic studies.

Mainly during the last few years experience with cerebral scintigraphy was very encouraging in our clinic: As compared with an angiography of the large cerebral vessels and ventriculography, scintigraphy afford the eminent advantage of producing almost no side-effects.

The recurrency rate of our patients totalled 5.36 % (20 cases) with the medial sinus and the base of the skull showing the highest frequency (9 recurrences for parasagittal meningiomas, 10 for basal meningiomas. There was only one recurrences of a convexity process).

Review on 101 Meningiomas (1965–1973)

J. BOCKHORN

In 1965 SCHÄFER (5) reported the results of the Göttingen Neurosurgical Clinic in treating meningiomas during the time from 1938 till
1964. We may cite the summary of his paper "Recurrence Rate in Meningiomas":

"274 meningioma patients observed during a period of 25 years
are described. Females (70 % of the patients) were affected more than
twice as frequently as males (30 %). ... The base of the skull and
its vault were affected in about equal proportions. ... Recurrences
developed as quickly as only a few months up to a maximum of 17 years
after the first operation. After macroscopically complete removal
of the tumor there were only 8 % of recurrences, but after partial removal of the original tumor further treatment became necessary in 26 %
of patients".

This paper now is a report on 101 microscopically verified cranial
meningiomas treated from 1965 - 1973 (65 females and 36 males). This
female to male relation lies between that found by SCHÄFER (5) and
the observation by CUSHING (1) who found a relation of 60 : 40.
DANDY's (2) statement of the relation being 1 : 1 is not confirmed by
our series.

As a reason for this distinct dominance by females SCHÄFER (5) suggested a population-shift caused by World War II. The drift in our series
towards CUSHING's 60 :40 ratio might support SCHÄFER's view.

Even in view of the age distribution this theory of a war-induced
shift of the sex relation seems to be confirmed. In the age period
between 51 and 60 years of age - the age group that was chiefly affected by World War II - there is a considerable divergence of the
sex relation with a ratio of 29 females to six males, graphically a
depression of the curve of the male patients aged 51 to 60 years,
whereas both curves lie nearly parallel in the other age groups (Fig.1).

Different to the status found by CUSHING (1) we observed the peak of
the age curve of patients with meningiomas at the time of hospital
admission in the 6th decade. In CUSHING's series the maximum was observed in the 5th decade. The average age in our patients at the time
of admission to the hospital was 50.2 years with spreading from 16 to
70 years of age. In the female patients the average age was 49.7 years,
in the males 51.1 years. We could not detect the difference in the
average ages of females and males of about 10 years found by CUSHING
(1).

A further point we want to refer to is the distribution of these 101
meningiomas regarding the origin of the tumors. The relation is close
to 1 : 1 with slight preponderance of the meningiomas arising from

the convexity with 52 tumors to 49 tumors with origin at the cranial base (Fig. 2). This proportion corresponds in the whole with the results of ELSBERG (3) and OLIVECRONA (4) who both found a slight to distinct dominance of the meningiomas arising from the cranial vault.

CUSHING (1), on the contrary, found that meningiomas arising from the cranial base slightly exceeded in number those that underlay the convexity.

Most of the meningiomas of this series originated close to the sagittal sinus in the middle third with a total of 21 tumors (Fig. 2 a). The next frequent point of origin was the sphenoid wing with dominance of the lateral part with 14 tumors over the medial sphenoid ridge with 8 tumors, followed by the presellar area and the olfactory groove with 8 meningiomas, too (Fig. 2 b).

Additional to the above mentioned 100 meningiomas (40 arising from the base and 52 underlying the cranial vault) we found 1 tumor localized at the trigone of the lateral ventricle, i. e. with a frequency of 100 : 1. In the series of ELSBERG (3) a tumor of such localization was not reported under a total of 102 meningiomas. CUSHING (1), too, did not quote an intraventricular tumor under his more than 300 meningiomas. In OLIVECRONA's (4) series two tumors localized in the lateral ventricle were found out of 82 meningiomas.

Six of the reported 101 meningiomas were inoperable. Dependent partly on their site at the clivus or in the depth of the basal ganglia, partly on their close relation to other anatomical structures - especially to the carotid arteries, which were encased by meningiomas in several cases - removal of the tumors was not possible without danger of injuring those structures. In these - as inoperable classified - cases surgery was limited to a biopsy. In the patient with a meningioma localized in the basal ganglia of the left side only a biopsy by streotactic means was done. After knowledge of the result of the microscopical examination of the tumor the family of the minor patient could not agree to further surgery in view of eventually postoperative arising neurological disorders.

Under the remaining 95 patients the meningiomas could be removed totally in 76 patients and partially in 19 patients, whereby all tumors localized close to the sagittal sinus and suspicious of remains of the tumor in or close to the sinus were classified as "partly removed".

During the postoperative period 18 of the 101 patients died, whereby the postoperative period comprised the first four weeks after surgery. The average age of the deceased patients was found at 57.3 years with spreading from 38 to 70 years of age. Three of these 18 patients died of malacia of a cerebral hemisphere following carotid thrombosis or occlusion of a branch of the anterior or middle cerebral arteries. One patient, aged 38 years, expired following a coagulopathia after large intraoperative transfusions. In most of the patients who died during the postoperative period cardiac or pulmonary complications were found as cause of death, surely as result of the considerable age of the patients in connection with the strain and stress after surgery. Most of the expired patients were at the end of the 5th and in the 6th decade.

Out of the 101 reported meningiomas in 9 patients the further course showed recurrences of the tumors. One of these 9 patients was treated surgically for a meningioma 20 years ago elsewhere. Then a recurrence of the meningioma at the place of primary surgery occurred. The meningioma could be removed totally in a second operation (Fig. 3). In three additional patients who died three months to three quarters of a year after surgery for a meningioma the autopsy showed recurrences of the tumors. In one case even a recurrence of the removed tumor and besides that two further tumors - till than unknown and untreated - on the opposite side of the skull were found. In this last patient the treated meningioma had been removed totally, in the two other patients only a partial removal had been possible.

Altogether we found under the 9 patients with recurrences of meningiomas (c. 9 %) five patients, in whom a so-called "real" recurrence took place (Fig. 4 a), i. e. a recurrence after total removal of the meningioma at the time of primary surgery. In three patients so-called "false" recurrences were present (Fig. 4 b), i. e. during primary surgery remains of the tumor had to be left in place respectively there was suspicion that minimal parts of the tumor had not been removed. In the ninth patient who was operated elsewhere details concerning primary surgery were not available.

Finally we want to present a case, in which spinal metastases of an intracranial meningioma were found.

Case history 150/71: At the time of the first admission the 20 years old female patient has had a history of left-sided migraine for about 9 months. Bilateral choked discs, no further neurological disorders.

Radiological findings: left-sided, parieto-occipital space-occupying lesion.

After biopsy on March 24, 1964 total removal of a left-sided, parieto-occipital meningioma was carried out on April 22, 1964. No signs of malignant degeneration.

On October 20, 1969 - 5 1/2 years after primar surgery - partial removal of a meningioma after recidivation. This time on the microscopical slides increase of the rate of mitoses, therefore radiation treatment.

Nearly 1 1/2 years after the second surgery increasing spastic paraparesis with sensory level a D 8. Laminectomy at this level showed a sarcomatous degenerated meningioma that was removed subtotally.

Summary

101 meningioma patients observed during the time from 1965 - 1973 are described. With the aid of graphs the age and sex distribution as well as the distribution of the meningiomas with regard to their localization is demonstrated.

18 patients died postoperatively, in 9 patients a second operation was necessary for removing a meningioma after recurrence.

References

1. CUSHING, H., EISENHARDT, L.: Meningiomas. New York: Hafner 1962.
2. DANDY, W. E.: The Brain, pp. 501 - 517. New York - Evanston - London: Hoeber Medical Division, Harper and Row 1969.

3. ELSBERG, C. A.: The parasagittal meningeal fibroblastoma. Bull. Neurol. Inst. New York 1, 389 - 418 (1931).

4. OLIVECRONA, H.: Die parasagittalen Meningeome. Leipzig: Springer 1934.

5. SCHÄFER, E. R.: Rezidivhäufigkeit bei Meningeomen. Acta neurochir. 13, 186 - 195 (1965).

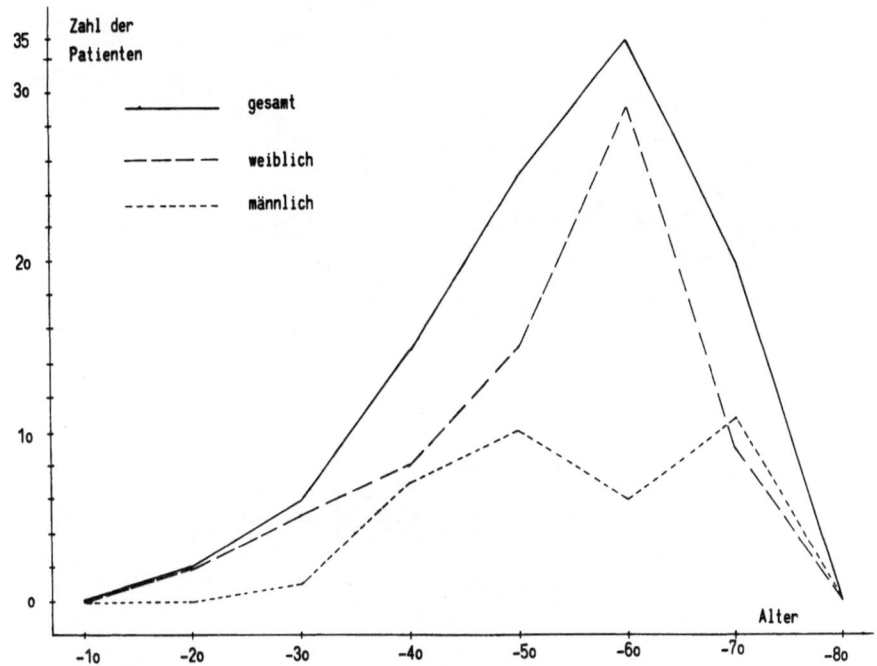

Fig. 1. Age and sex distribution in 101 patients with meningiomas

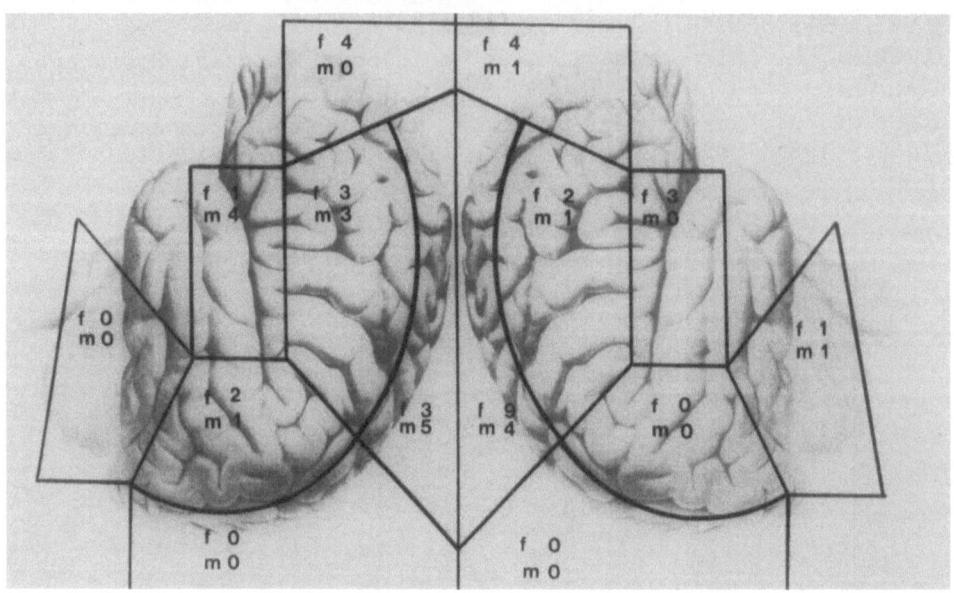

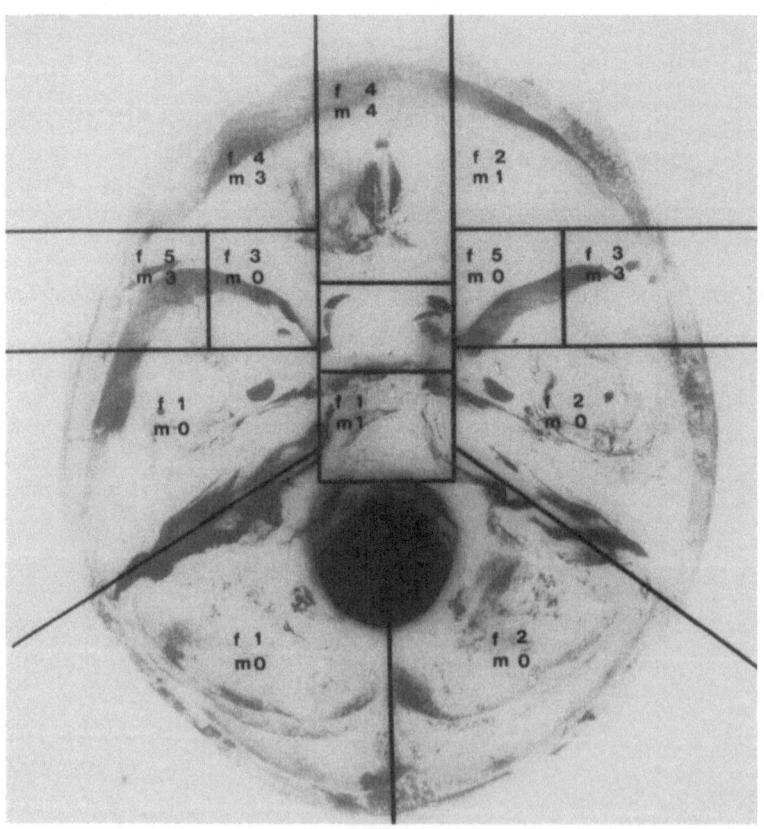

Fig. 2. Distribution of 101 meningiomas on the vault
(52 tumors, Fig. 2 a) and the cranial base; 48 tumors, Fig. 2 b)

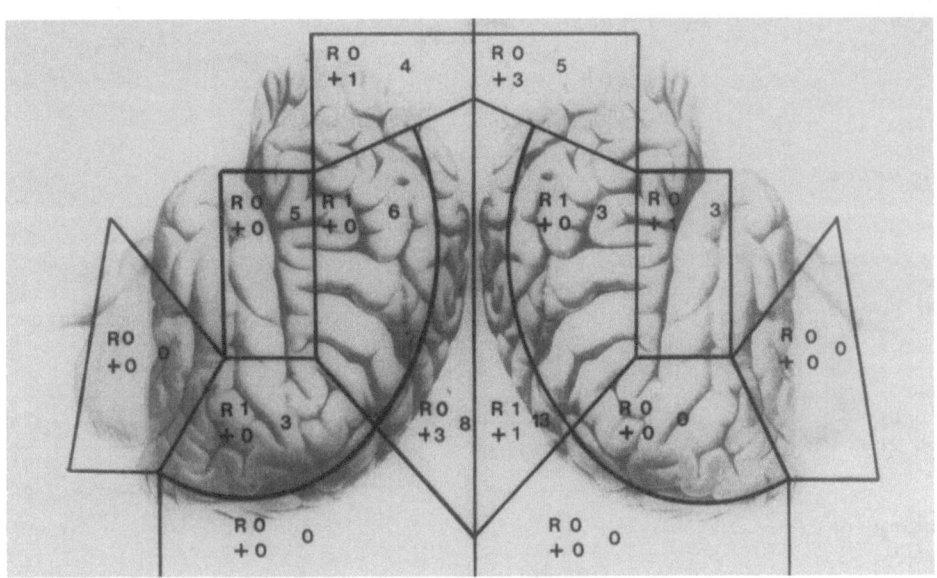

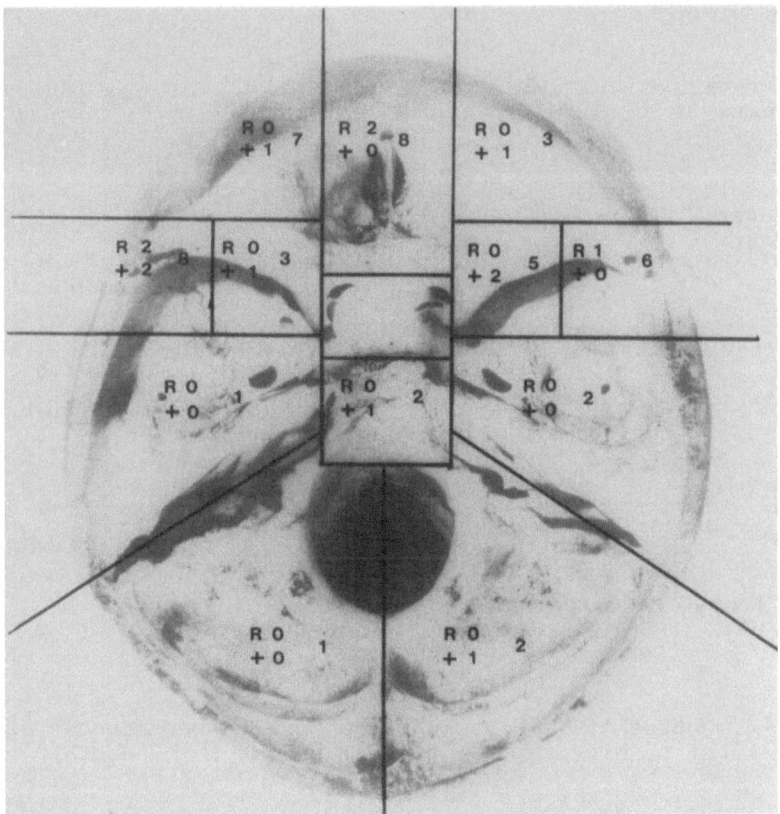

Fig. 3. Distribution of recurrences (R) and postoperative fatalities
(+) with regard to the tumor localization (see Fig. 2)

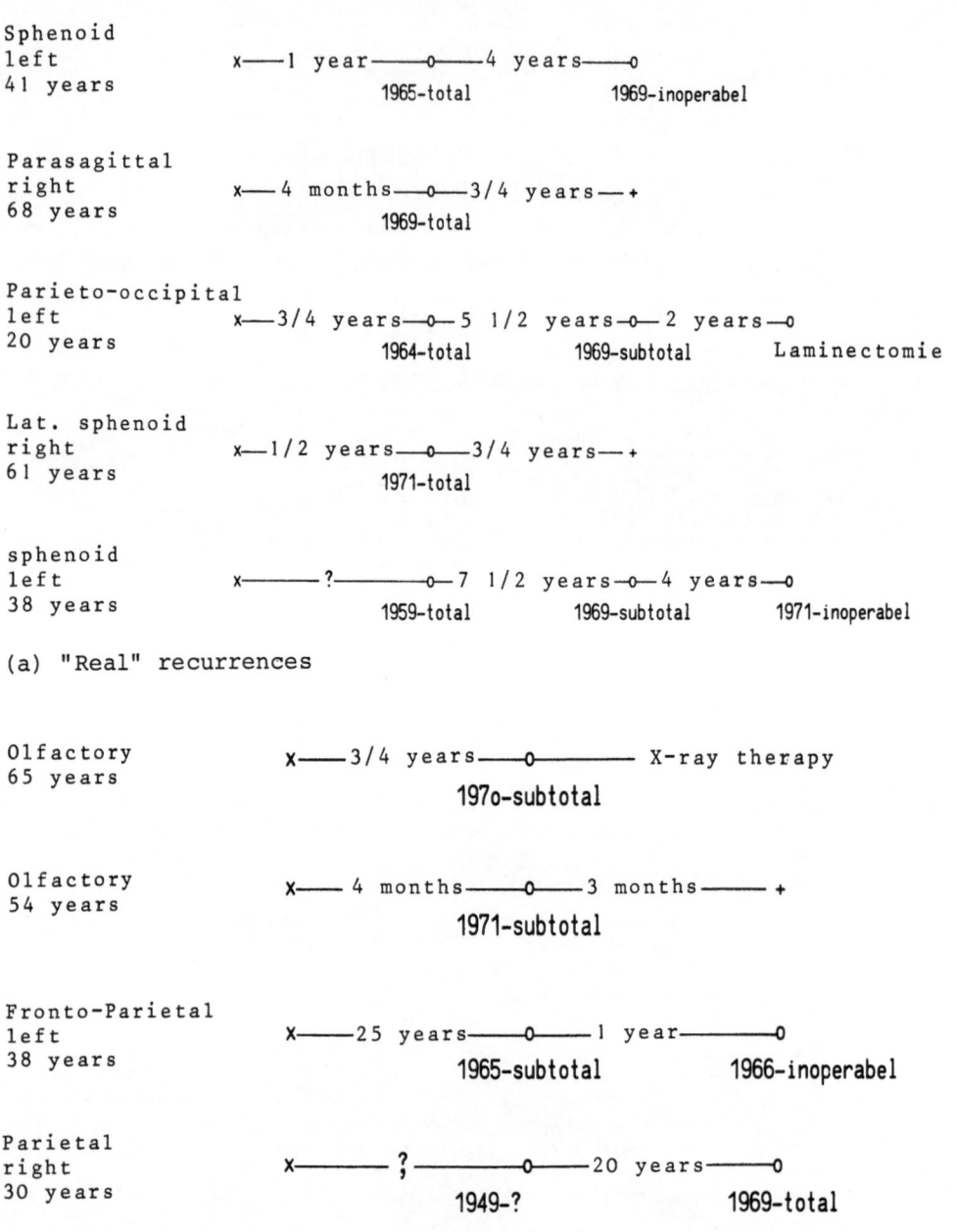

Sphenoid
left
41 years
x——1 year——o——4 years——o
            1965-total   1969-inoperabel

Parasagittal
right
68 years
x—— 4 months——o——3/4 years——+
            1969-total

Parieto-occipital
left
20 years
x——3/4 years——o— 5 1/2 years—o— 2 years—o
          1964-total   1969-subtotal   Laminectomie

Lat. sphenoid
right
61 years
x——1/2 years——o——3/4 years——+
          1971-total

sphenoid
left
38 years
x——————?——————o—7 1/2 years—o—4 years—o
         1959-total   1969-subtotal   1971-inoperabel

(a) "Real" recurrences

Olfactory
65 years
x——3/4 years——o—————— X-ray therapy
          1970-subtotal

Olfactory
54 years
x—— 4 months——o—— 3 months —— +
          1971-subtotal

Fronto-Parietal
left
38 years
x——25 years——o—— 1 year——o
        1965-subtotal   1966-inoperabel

Parietal
right
30 years
x——————?——————o——20 years——o
       1949-?   1969-total

(b) "False" recurrences

Fig. 4. Course of illness in patients with recurrences of meningiomas
(x = onset of history, O = time of surgery, + 3 death)

A Structural Study of Ossification and Calcification in Meningiomas

T. Tzonos and F. Heuck

In meningiomas of the convex surface of the cerebrum which have also infiltrated the dura, peculiar transformations of diploe's spongy tissue and spicule like formations are regularly produced on the internal as well as the external tables of the skull. These structural changes in the diploe are even more clearly evident after mazeration preparation of the bone (Fig. 1). In none of our cases have we been able to prove a purely reactive hyperostosis due to a presumably strong increase,in blood circulation but without a direct tumor invasion. It would be wrong, judging from these macroscopic pictures, to assume that a pure destruction of the skull by infiltration of meningioma tissue was taking place. Histologically and microradiographically, that is, through X-rays of bone cuts, we see clear signs of bone formation as well as degeneration. Newly formed bone tissue whose mineral content is in part incomplete is found boardering the tumor (Fig. 2). In the osteocyte lacunae lie osteocytes rich in cytoplasm with a large nucleus and sometimes vacuols. The small canals of threads of osteocytes can be clearly seen in colored thinly sliced bone sections. We do not see oesteclasts, so we must assume that osteolysis of the osteocytes has occured (2, 3). The meeting of such destructive events in juxtaposition shows a very dynamic bone renovation. Obviously, the osteocyte is capable of bringing about bone formation as well as deterioration.

Another cell, the meningioma cell, is also capable of special performances. In one of our patients with an upper thoracic paraplegia syndrome we surgically removed a stone hard intradural tumor, measuring 1,5 cm in length. Histologically we found an ossified meningioma. We also found many large osteocyte lacunae lying closely together as well as a widened demineralization (Fig. 3).

Next to this, newly formed areas of bone are seen. The picture evidences a rash transformation. It can therefore hardly be said that the tumor will die as a result of a sluggish metabolism!

The most solid impermeable bodies which are found in meningiomas are not ossified but rather calcified and of psammomatous origin. They are microscopically small, unstructured pearl sheaped calcifications formed by a protein rich product of the endothelial cells and the fibroplasts of the tumor tissue which impregnate the tumor cells (1, 4).

In my presentation of this paper I wished to show the high degree of metabolism which takes place even in seemingly "dead tissue" as the tumor ossification and calcification show. The cause of this lastly relates to the multipowers evidenced by the mesenchymal cell.

REFERENCES

1. GONATAS, N. K., BESEN, M.: An electron microscopic study of three human psammomatous meningiomas. J. Neuropath. exp. Neurol. 22, 263 - 273 (1963).

2. JUSTER, M., FISCHGOLD, H., LAVAL-JEANTET, M.: Premiers éléments de microradiographie clinique. Paris: Masson et Cie. 1963.

3. PIEPGRAS, U., HEUCK, F.: Une modification de la structure macroscopique et microscopique des os du crâne par les hyperostoses réactionelles. Exp. Sci. VIII. Symposium Neuroradiologicum. Paris 1967.

4. KEPES, J.: Observations on the formation of psammoma bodies and pseudopsammoma bodies in meningiomas. J. Neuropath. exp. Neurol. 20, 255 - 262 (1961).

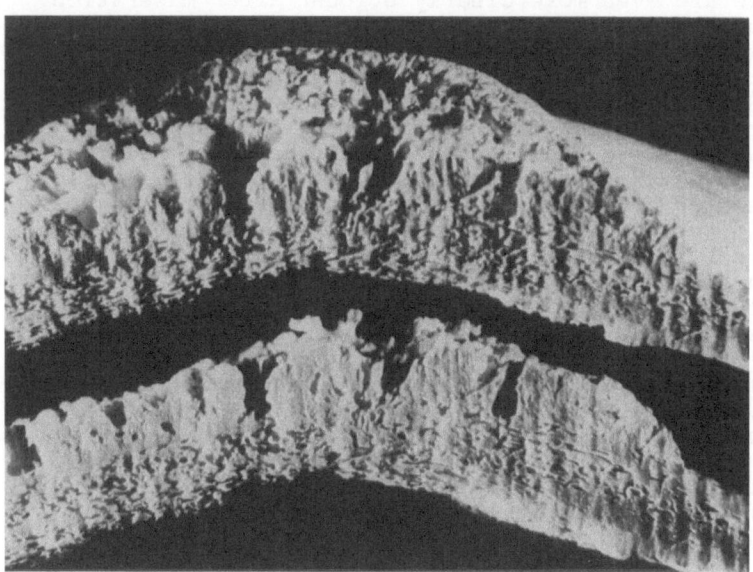

Fig. 1. Structural changes in the diploe after mazeration preparation of the bone

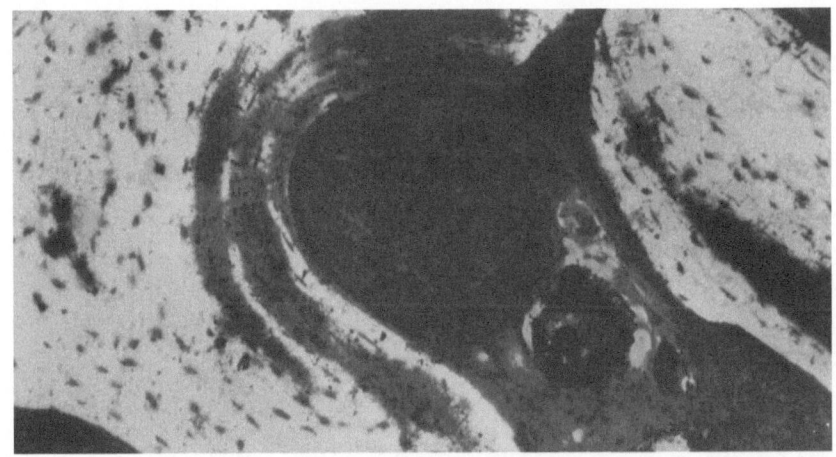

Fig. 2. Newly formed bone tissue whose mineral content is in part incomplete is found boardering the tumor

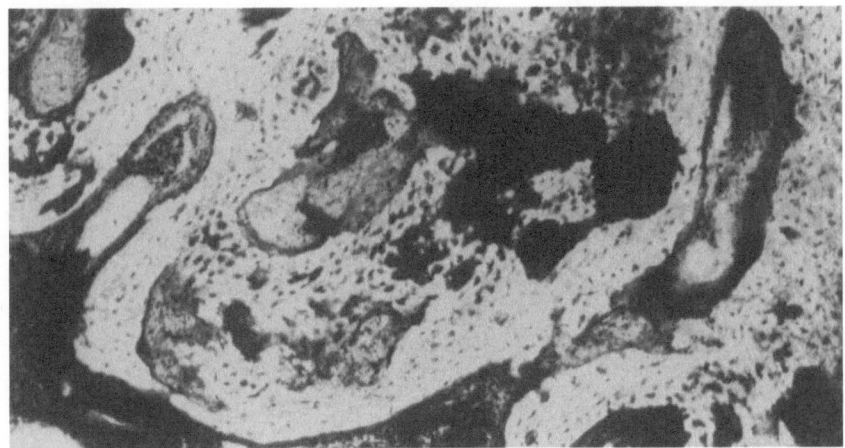

Fig. 3. Ossified spinal meningioma

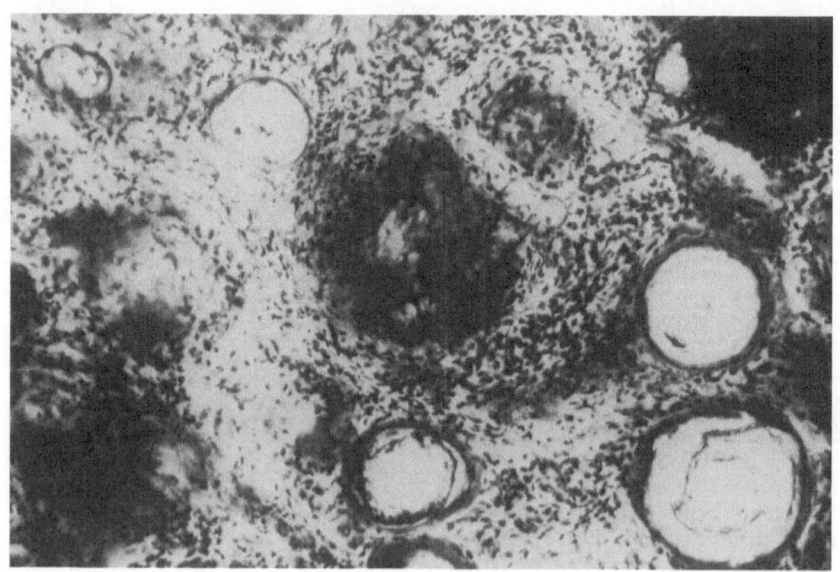

Fig. 4. Psammoma bodies in meningioma tissue

Alterations in the Bone Structure of the Skull as a Differential Diagnostic Indication of Meningioma

G. ERBS, J. MENZEL, P. GEORGI, and B. WIMMER

The scintigraphic diagnosis of tumors and other pathological alterations of the brain is based on the disturbance of the blood-liquor-border in the concerned area. Structural alterations of the capillaries in comparison to normal brain capillaries were demonstrated by electronic microscopy (6). As this pathological mechanism is the same in all brain tumors, the possibility of differential diagnosis is limited for the most part. From this point of view meningioma presents less problems than other brain tumors.

The radiopharmacon mostly used for brain scintigraphy - Pertechnetate - is absorbed very intensively and quickly after intravenous injection (1). This can be demonstrated by sequential scintigraphy of the brain with a gamma-camera. Fig. 1 shows for example a parasagittal meningioma. 2 minutes after injection the tumor is perceptible sharply circumscribed and storing intensively.

The sequential scintigraphy can be the first hint for the diagnosis. A further development in the evaluation of this method of investigation is EDP. On one side it is possible to compare impulse-rates in the tumor area with so called static scintigrams made after optional time intervals after injection. On the other side it is possible to leave the patient for a time of i. e. 20 minutes beyond the gamma-camera with a computer storing the impulses digitally in optional time steps (2, 3, 5). After the investigation the computer makes a summary picture allowing to set regions of interest around the tumor area and a correspondingly large neutral brain area, thus deriving time-activity-curves of these areas.

Fig. 3 shows a time-activity-curve derived from an area of meningioma showing the typical quick reaching of activity maximum and the following plateau or slight decrease. The fact, that some skull neighboured meningiomas show hyperostosis in X-ray examination brought us to the idea to make an investigation with bone seeking radiopharmacon in addition to the usual brainscan (4). For technical reasons ^{18}F seems to be optimal because of its high affinity to the bone as well as of its physical qualities. They allow to make both investigations - brain scan and can of the skull - at the same day. Therefore all patients suffering from brain tumor near the convexity and base of the skull were investigated during the last 6 months both, by brain scan as well as by bone scan of the skull. The perifocal storage of ^{18}F was observed only with meningioma thus far.

Fig. 4 shows a left side meningiomas of the sphenoid with a correlated hot area of ^{18}F as a sign for an intensive bone affection. The bone lesion does not always correspond with the localization of the tumor. Fig. 5 shows a circumscribed meningioma left parietal whereas the ^{18}F storing area is visible more frontally. Fig. 6 shows a tumor right frontal with intensive bone affection of the temporal bone. Especially the tumors near the skull base are sometimes difficult to diagnose. Fig. 7 shows that the presence of ^{18}F storing can help evaluate a doubtful scan.

The genesis of such bone affections is not known. X-ray examination was negative in all of the demonstrated patients. The microscopic investigation of biopsy material of the ^{18}F storing bone areas could not reveal any sign of tumor invasion or other structural alterations. Therefore we take the presence of ^{18}F accumulation in the region of the skull connected with brain tumor as further sign for meningioma without having an explanation of this pathophysiological finding.

Summary

The scintigraphic methods of differential diagnosis of meningiomas are shown. Apart from the already known characteristics of the tumor a double tracer method for the evidence of perifocal bone lesion is described.

REFERENCES

1. FIEBACH, O., SAUER, J., OTTO, H.: Die Szintigraphie im Vergleich zur Angiographie und Enzephalographie bei Hirntumoren. Röntenstr. 116, 185 - 189 (1972).

2. HANDA, J., NABESHIMA, S., HANDA, H., HAMAMOTO, K., KOUSAKA, T., TORIZUKA, K.: Serial Brain Scanning with Technetium ^{99m} and Scintillation Camera. Amer. J. Roentgenolog. 109, 701 - 706 (1970).

3. RAMSEY, G., QUINN, J. L.: Comparison of Accuracy between Initial and Delayed ^{99m}Tc-Pertechnetate Brain Scans. Journ. Nucl. Med. 13, 131 - 134 (1971).

4. RANSOHOFF, J.: Parasagittal meningiomas. J. Neurosurg. 37, 372 - 378 (1972).

5. SAUER, J.: Die diagnostische Aussagekraft der Hirnszintigraphie. Fortschr. Röntgenstr. 116, 179 - 184 (1972).

6. TAKAHASHI, M., NOFAL, M. M., BEIERWALTERS, W. H.: Correlation of Brain Scan Image and Area Counting After Scanning with Tumor Pathology. Hourn. Nucl. Med. 7, 32 - 40 (1966).

7. ZEIDLER, U., KOTTKE, S., HUNDESHAGEN, H.: Hirnszintigraphie, Technik und Klinik. Berlin - Heidelberg - New York: Springer 1972.

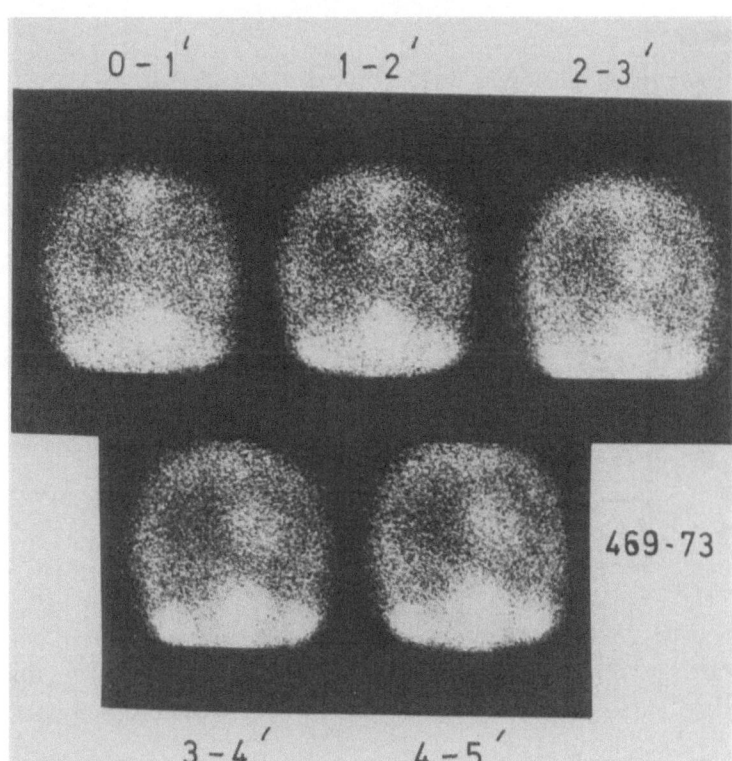

Fig. 1. Sequential scintiphotos showing tumoractivity from time of injection to 5 minutes after injection

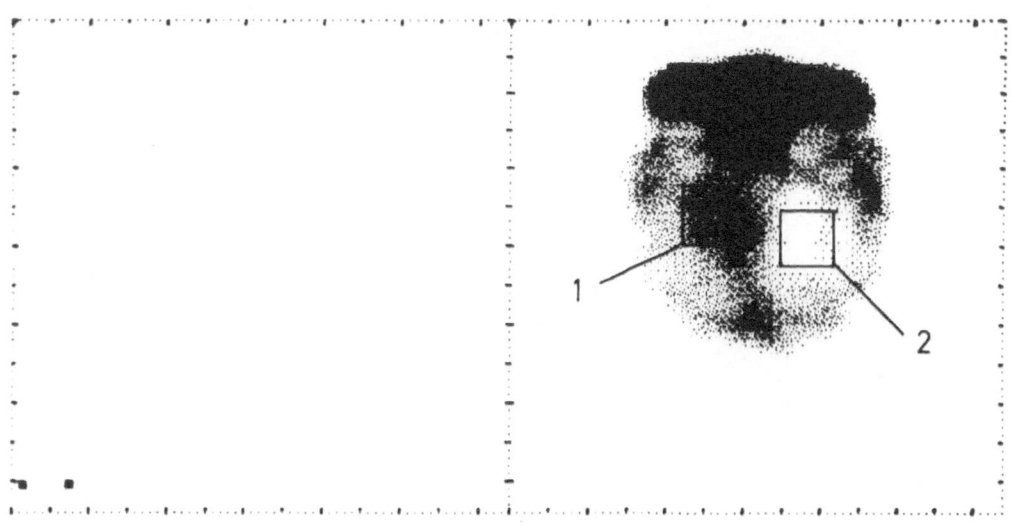

Fig. 2. Summary picture of the computer showing the regions of interest

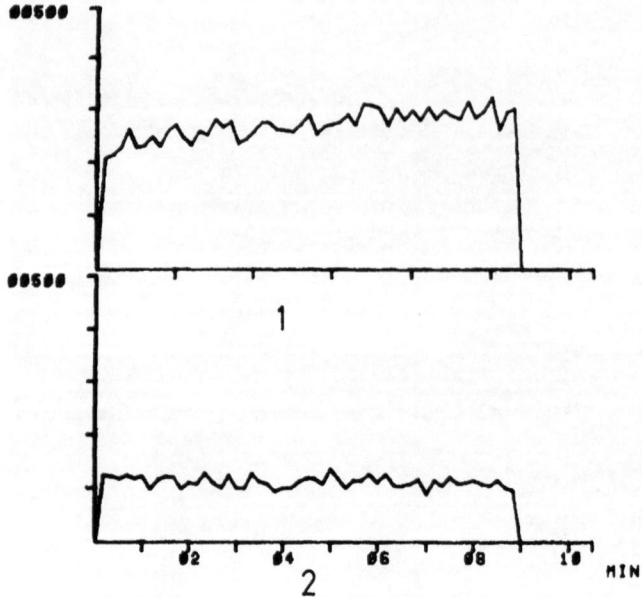

Fig. 3. Time activity curves beyond tumor (1) - and neutral brain area

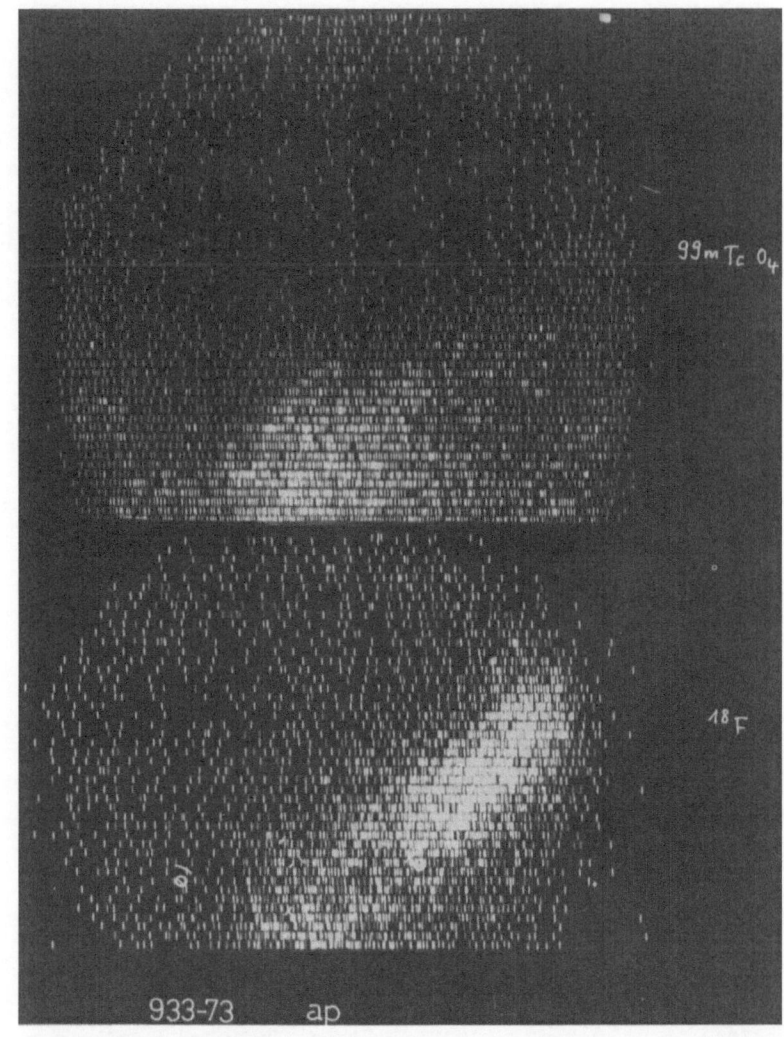

Fig. 4. Meningioma of the sphenoid with corresponding bone process.

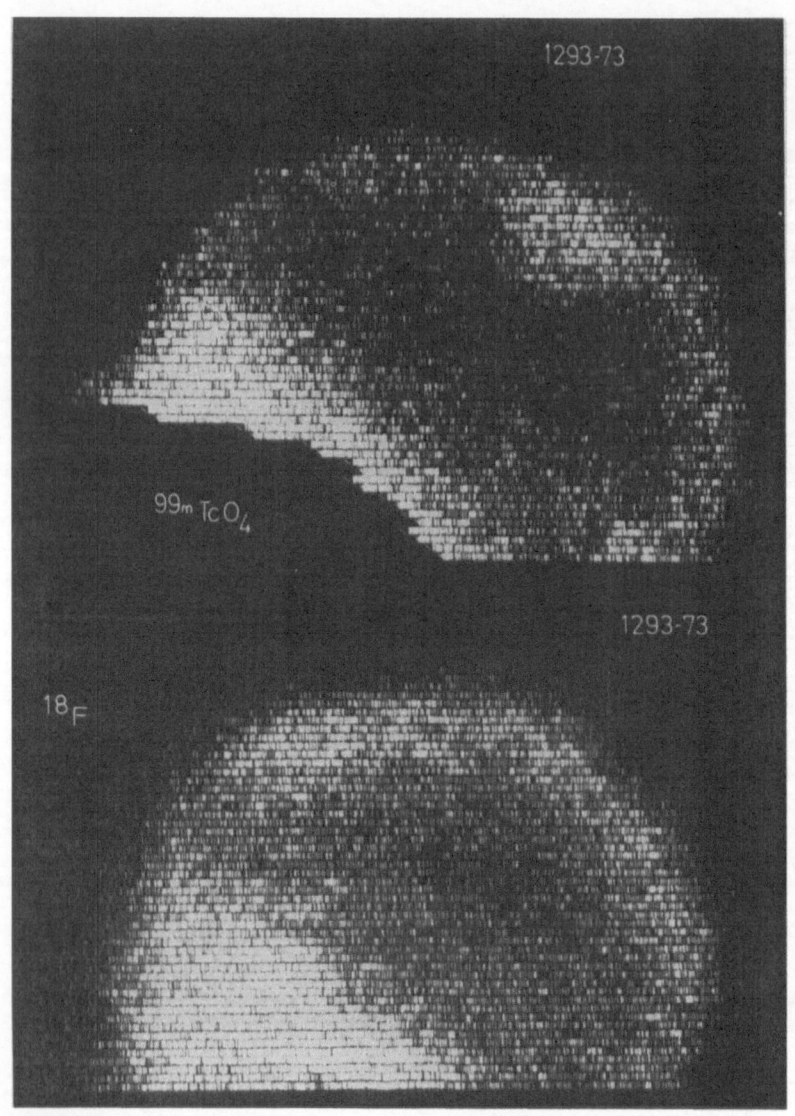

Fig. 5. Parietal meningioma with not identically corresponding bone process

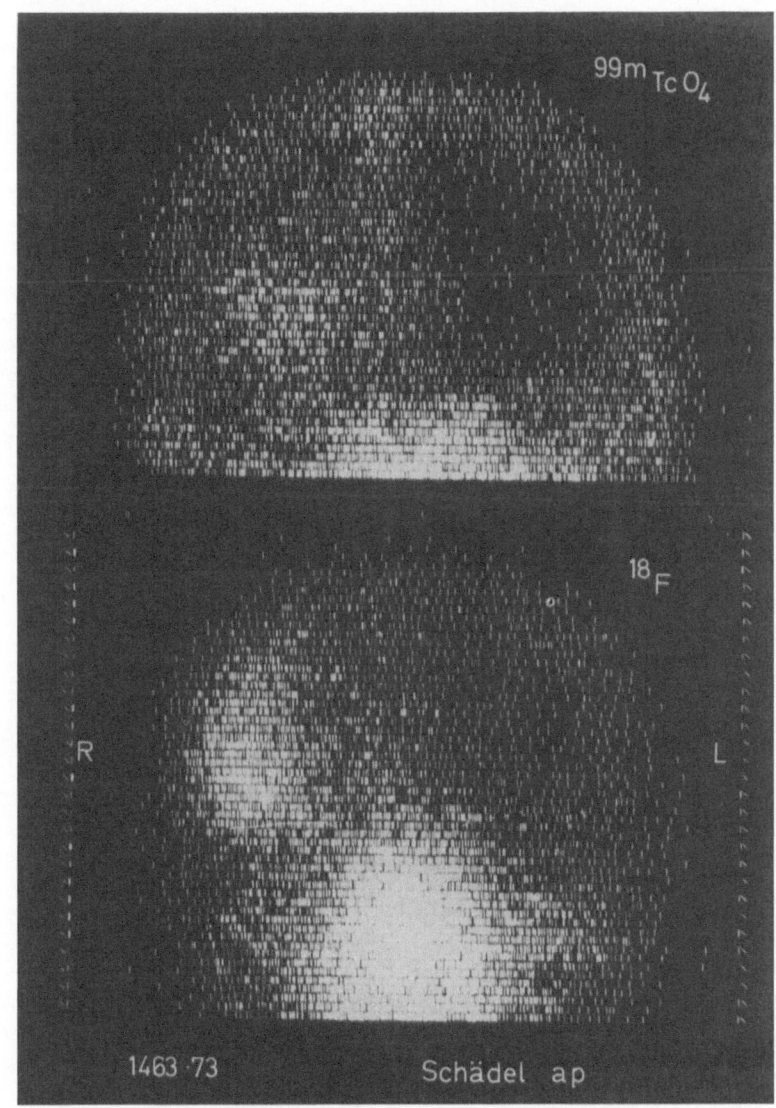

Fig. 6. Frontal meningioma with process in temporal bone

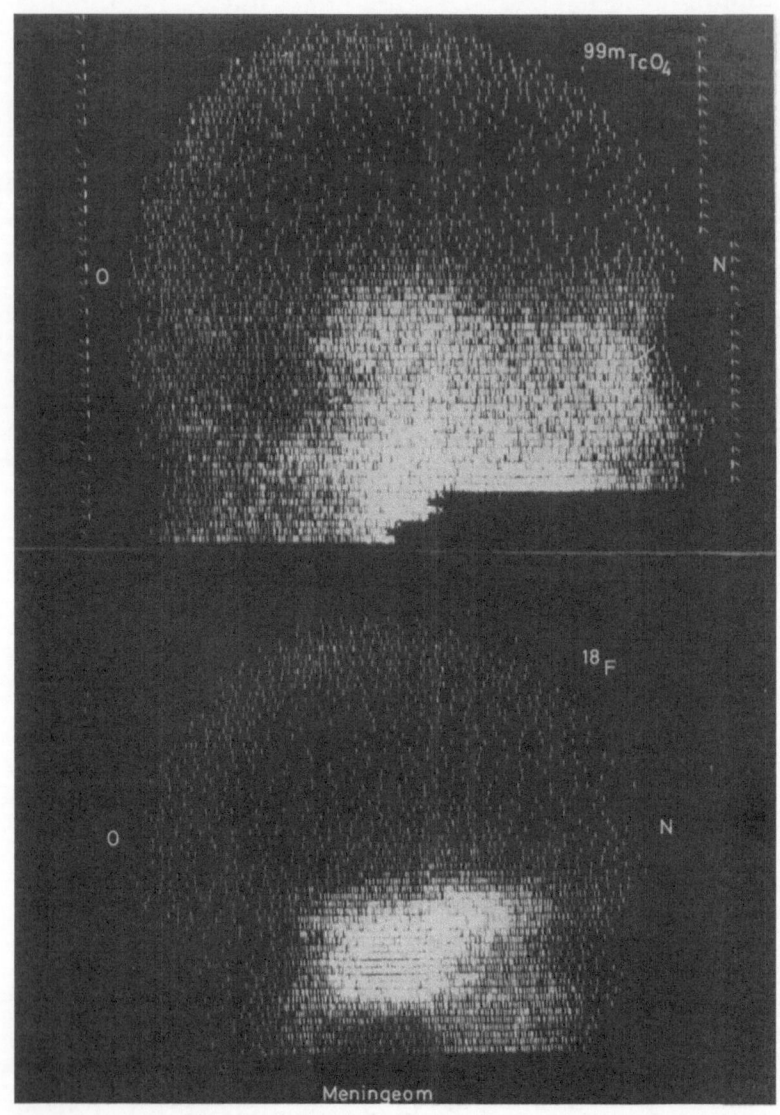

Fig. 7. Basal meningioma with lesion in base of skull

Osteomas and Meningiomas

C. Lopez-Brugos

The true fibro-osseous tumors of the cranial bones can be classified
into various groups according to KLEINSASSER and ALBRECHT (3, 4, 10).

Of the osteomas of the roof of the skull that are of interest to us
with regard to meningiomas, the cortical osteomas of the external
tabula and the large, mostly spongy osteomas of the roof of the skull
are to be considered. In contrast to the other intracranial tumors,
the meningiomas - as is well known - may also spread out far into the
cranial bones, it might even be said that they grow solely intra-
osseously. In the case of large osteomas, the operative procedure is
influenced by this fact (1, 2, 5, 6, 7, 8, 9, 11).

We propose to discuss the problems involved by reporting on several
cases.

Case 1: Mrs. B. Waltraud, aged 47

Seven years prior to clinic admission, a hard tumor which developed
slowly but steadily increased in size formed in the left frontal side
area, close beside the median line. Subjective symptoms were not complained of and only a cosmetic disfigurement existed.

On admission a tumor of hard consistence the size of a hand palm was
found on the left hair margin. No neurological disturbances were
located. During the operation, a large tumor located left fronto-
parietally that stretched across the midline towards the right, and
having the size of a child's fist, was removed.

Histology: Endotheliomatous meningioma. The decalcification of the
bone had produced an eburnized osteoma.

Case 2: Mrs. O. Juliane, aged 62

Eleven years prior to admission, the patient sustained an injury in
the left frontal side area of the trauma, without subjective symptoms.
Transfer to our clinic was made solely for cosmetic reasons.

The examination revealed left fronto-parietally a tumor the size of
a child's first, neurologically at the most a slight accentuation of
the right tendon stretching reflexes. The radiographs showed a pronounced thickening of the external tabula, in particular in the fron-
to-parieto-temporal region encroaching onto the anterior base of the
skull and the lateral orbital wall. Carotid angiography indicated an
intracranial growth. The huge tumor removed after osteoplastic trepanation proved microhistologically to be a typically structured
osteoma; the tumor with a "flower-bed-type" structure on the underside
of the dura was found to be an endotheliomatous meningioma, one of the
striking features being an invasion of the bone, i. e. the benign osteoma.

Case 3: Mrs. P. Maria, aged 44

One year prior to admission, a swelling increasing in size occurred
in the fronto-central area following a trivial injury, without subjective symptoms. In our clinic, an intracranial tumorous growth was
discovered. Trepanation revealed a palmsized tumor of the bone in the
midline area, which was completely removed. Microhistologically, an
endotheliomatous meningioma with infiltration of the medullary spaces
of the skull roof and the histologically verified osteoma was found.

Case 4: Mrs. H. Carola, aged 49

Eleven years prior to clinic admission, Mrs. H. noticed a small
swelling in the left temporal area. Six years later, a left temporal
osteoma the size of a hen's egg was removed in a non-local clinic.
The tumor started into regrowth. On the initial examination in our
clinic, she was found to have a bone tumor above the left temple the
size of a child's fist. Osteoplastic led to the removal of a large
bone tumor that was impressive for an osteoma. The underlying dura
exhibited tumorous changes on its interior. The histological diagnosis
showed the adhering tumorous tissue to be an epitheloid variant of an
endotheliomatous meningioma.

Case 5: Mrs. B. Cläre, aged 54

Four years before clinic admission a bony swelling the size of a
cherry located high on the forehead to the right, which had been
operated in a non-local clinic on the assumption that it was an
osteoma, was established. Regrowth of the tumor then occurred. Referral was made on cosmetic grounds. The examination revealed a right
frontal palm-sized swelling that extended across the median line,
without neurological disturbances. Routine carotid angiography confirmed the suspicion that a large frontal space-consuming process,
which was also intracranial, existed. Osteoplastic trepanation discovered a tumor growing in part extradurally, in part intradurally.

Histology: Fibromatous meningioma.

Discussion and Assessment

Based upon the case description from a number of patients admitted to
our clinic diagnosed for suspected "osteoma", from the observations
made on patients between admission and discharge, and from operation
results, the following points are to be made: wherever extensive
changes are present in the bones of the skull, an intracranial growth
should always be considered plus the fact that appropriate differential diagnostic measures are absolutely necessary for clarification
prior to operation (3, 4, 6, 7, 11). To the discussion the appearance
of meningiomas in these cases, we should like to contribute the view
that, apparently in these patients, an osteoma originally affected
the bone only: thus, the possibility should be considered that there
was a certain inductive effect of the osteoma on the cerebral dura
during development of the meningioma. An interesting fact appears to
us to be that all cases described exclusively involved the female sex,
and that the ages in which the disease manifested itself were between
38 and 51 years (38, 40, 44, 49, 51 years).

The localization - as is more or less typical for osteomas - was mainly to be found in the frontal region. Only in two cases was an involvement of the temporal and parietal regions demonstrable, and in one
case the base of the skull as well. The previous histories extended
over a period of several years. Only in one case had the swelling and

the subsequent thickening of the bone been noticed one year before
the operation. The patients were invariably transferred for cosmetic
reasons. Neurological and psychopathological disturbances had not
been observed.

The histological diagnosis of the meningioma parts showed an endotheliomatous character in 4 cases, and fibromatous character in one
case. No case of regrowth has come to our attention.

Summary

The simultaneous appearance of osteomas and meningiomas is reviewed.
The case is made for the necessity of a comprehensive pre-operative
examination using contrast techniques on account of frequent growth
of bone tumors - which can also be intracranial - that often present
the appearance of osteomas or osteoma-like growths.

REFERENCES

1. ECHLIN, F.: Cranial osteomas and hyperostoses produced by meningeal fibroblastomas. Arch. Surg. (Chicago) 28, 357 - 405 (1934).

2. ELLERMANN, M.: A case of monstrous osteoma on the skull. Acta
   psychiat. (Kbh) 17, 139 - 148 (1942).

3. GERLACH, J., SIMON, G.: Gutartige Primärgeschwülste des Hirnschädels. Erkennung, Differentialdiagnose und Behandlung der Geschwülste. In: Handbuch der Neurochirurgie, Bd. IV/1, S. 215 - 23.
   Berlin - Göttingen - Heidelberg: Springer 1960.

4. KLEINSASSER, O.: Pathologie der Geschwülste des Hirnschädels.
   Gutartige Formen. Handbuch der Neurochirurgie, Bd. IV/1, S. 372 -
   86. Berlin - Göttingen - Heidelberg: Springer 1960.

5. PICH, G.: Über das Osteoangiom des Schädeldaches. Beitr. Path.
   Anat. 101, 181 - 88 (1938).

6. RAND, C. W.: Osteoma of the skull. Report of two cases, one being
   associated with a large intracranial endothelioma. Arch. Surg.
   (Chicago) 6, 573 - 586 (1923).

7. RICHTHAMMER, H.: Osteoangiom des Schädeldaches. Krebsarzt 5,
   62 - 64 (1950).

8. SANCHO RIPOLL, F.: Right frontal intracranial osteoma. Rev. Esp.
   Otoneurooofthalmol. Neurocir. 29, 355 - 359. Nov. - Dec. 1971
   (Eng. Abstr.) Spa.

9. SCHWARTZ et CHEVRIER, C. W.: Cranial osteomas from a roentgenological viewpoint. Amer. J. Roentgenol. 45, 18 - 26 (1941).

10. SEEMEN, J.: Osteom des Schädeldaches. Zbl. Chir. 2331 (1936).

11. SCHUNK, H. et al: A study of meningiomas with correlation of
    hyperostosis and tumor vascul. Amer. J. Roentgen 91, 431 - 43
    (1964).

Possibilities and Limitations of Scintigraphy on Meningiomas

O. WILCKE

Meningiomas can be detected with greater certainty than other brain tumors by means of nearly all the radioisotopes currently used in tumor diagnosis. Evidently, their good detection is due to strong vascularization of meningiomas. Therefore, isotope compounds such J^{131}-albumin (RIHSA) and Tc^{99m}, which stay in the blood stream over a period of time, offer especially favourable conditions for detecting meningiomas. Clinical experience however shows that equally satisfactory results can be obtained with radioactive compounds, which remain only briefly in the blood stream and are quickly metabolized such as Hg-compounds (Hg^{197} and Hg^{203}), Bi^{206} and positron radiations As^{74}, Cu^{64} and Ga^{68} (Fig. 1). A synopsis of ample statistical studies shows that most isotopes are able to detect over 90 % of the meningiomas with varying degrees of localization. The relatively poor results in using Hg^{197} and Cu^{64} are probably attributable to insufficient methods and equipment. We observed no essential difference in the diagnostic exactness of As^{74} and Cu^{64}, taking into account the different impulse outputs due to another radiation quality. Compounds remaining in the blood stream for a long time are obliged to exclude activity originating from voluminous cerebral sinuses, so that small tumors and those next to a sinus may be overlooked.

Similar to other parenchymatous tissue, meningiomas have a much higher degree of enrichment than normal brain tissue or tumors which develop from the brain tissue and thus depend on the function of blood-brain barrier for the uptake of radioactive substance. Meningiomas, being excluded from the brain metabolism, do not depend on the blood-brain-barrier for their enrichment.

This high degree of enrichment makes good detection possible even in cases of rare localization. Fig. 2 shows the typical picture of a cerebellopontine angle meningioma and Fig. 3 a suprasellar meningioma, which was detected during the initial clinical examination. In addition, szintigraphy can provide valuable information with respect to the extent of the tumor, for instance in the case of a tentorium meningioma. Fig. 4. shows a restricted infratentorial meningioma, while Fig. 5 shows a meningioma with both infratentorial and supratentorial components.

The combination of angiography and scintigraphy provides valuable information about the kind of tumor, especially in cases of parietal and occipital tumors, where angiography can give no certain diagnosis. Fig. 6 shows the angiogram and scintigram of a left parieto-occipital meningioma. According to the angiogram, an extended process can be detected; classification or localization is, however, not possible. The scintigram with its clearly delineated enrichment gives the typical symptoms and the exact localization of the meningioma.

Szintigraphy is superior to all other clinical methods for detecting meningioma recurrences. Those regions difficult to detect angiographically show up especially clearly. Fig. 7 shows the detection of an interosseous-developed recurrence of a sphenoid-ridge meningioma. Fig. 8 shows a recurrence of a meningioma extending into the middle fossa. Of the 41 patients who were under observation for a number of years, 14 patients showed a definite recurrence, 26 patients showed a complete elimination and in one case a diagnosis was not possible, since the isotope examination took place shortly after an intercurrent subarachnoid hemorrhage.

Especially interesting from the clinical point of view is the question to what extent diagnostic-type predetermination is possible. Here differentiation from the glioblastoma is particularly difficult since glioblastomas also cause high enrichment. Frequently, however, the patterns of enrichments are different, for example more diffuse than in the case of the meningioma (Fig. 9).

A summary of the results of our 210 meningioma cases (Fig. 10), for which we have an angiogram as well as a scintigram, a X-ray picture and an EEG, shows that in 71 % of the cases, meningioma detection was possible from the scintigram. In 43 % of the cases the angiogram showed the typical meningioma symptoms and in 36 % the X-ray picture showed typical meningioma changes. In 39 % of the cases demarcation of a focus were found in the EEG. Thus, scintigraphy has proved superior to other clinical methods in differential diagnosis of meningiomas. In 97 % of meningiomas the scintigram was positiv. 29 % could not be classified or recognized by scintigram. An uncharacteristic enrichment was observed relatively often in tentorium meningiomas, suprasellar meningiomas and medial sphenoid-ridge meningiomas. Meningiomas of the convexity, including the falx and the frontal basis, showed, for the most part, characteristic enrichment.

Summary

Of all brain tumors, meningiomas can be detected scintigraphically with the highest degree of certainty. We could localize correctly 97 % of our 210 cases and classify according to type 71 %. Compared with angiographic findings, X-ray findings and EEG results, the scintigraphic findings have proved the most valuable technique for detecting meningiomas. Considering the atypical scintigraphic findings in 29 % of the cases, it is necessary to combine these findings with the other usual clinical findings.

REFERENCES

1. BOTTERELL, E. H., LOUGHEED, W. M., MORLEY, T. P., TASKER, R. R.: Use of radioactive arsenic (As[74]) in the diagnosis of supratentorial brain tumors. Canad. Med. Ass. J. 85, 1321 - 1328 (1961).

2. BRENNER, M., PIHKANEN, T. A., VOUTILAINEN, A.: Radioisotopic diagnosis of brain tumors. Ann. Med. exp. Fenn. 42, 145 - 151 (1964).

3. BRINKMANN, C. A., WEGST, A. V., KAHN, E. A.: Brain scanning with Mercury-203 labelled neohydrin. J. Neurosurg. 19, 644 - 651 (1962).

4. BUCY, P. C., CIRIC, I. S.: Value of radioactive brain scans in the diagnosis of brain tumors as compared with other methods. Acta Neurochir. (Wien) 13, 113 - 132 (1965).

5. BUDABIN, M., SIEGEL, G. J.: The anatomical correlation of the abnormal RISHA brain scan. J. Nucl. Med. 7, 128 - 139 (1966).

6. De DIVITIIS, E., MEGNA, G., TURCHIARO, G.: Aspetto complementare della elettroencefalografia e della scintigrafia cerebrale nella diagnostica dei processi espansivi endocranici. Di Clin.e Terap. Vol. XLVI/22, 1 - 8 (1966).

7. DUGGER, G. S., PEPPER, F. D.: The reliability of radioisotopic encephalography. Neurology 13, 1042 - 1053 (1963).

8. Van ECK, J. H. M., WOLDRING, M .G.: Scanning the brain with various radioisotopes. Europ. Neurol. 2, 1 - 12 (1969).

9. GOODRICH, J. K., TUTOR, F. T.: The isotope encephalogram in brain tumor diagnosis. J. Nucl. Med. 6, 5-1 - 548 (1965).

10. KUBA, J., HUSAK, V., SEVCIK, M., KLAUS, E.: Vergleich der Eigenschaften von ^{99m}-Pertechnetat und ^{113m}In-EDTA in der Szintigraphie. Röfo 112, 806 - 813 (1970).

11. LOKEN, M. K., WIGDAHL, L. O., GILSON, J. M., STAAB, E. V.: Mercury-197 and Mercury-203 chlormerodrin for evaluation of brain lesions using a rectilinear scanner and scintillation camera. J. Nucl. Med. 7, 209 - 218 (1966).

12. MUNDINGER, F., ASAI, A.: Ergebnisse der digitalen Gammaenzephalographie bei Hirntumoren; Vergleich von Wismut-206, Quecksilber-203-Neohydrin und Technetium-99 m. Arch. Psych. Zeitschr. f. d. ges. Neurol. 210, 297 - 312 (1967).

13. OJEMANN, R. G., ARONOW, S. A., SWEET, W. H.: Scanning with positron-emitting radioisotopes. Arch. Neurol. 10, 218 - 228 (1964).

14. OVERTON, M. C., OTTE, W. K., BEENTJES, L. B., HAYNIE, T. P.: A comparison of Mercury-197 and Mercury-203 chlormerodrin in clinical brain scanning. J. Nucl. Med. 6, 28 - 37 (1965).

15. PLANIOL, T.: Gamma-Encephalography after ten years of utilization in neurosurgery. Progr. Neurol. Surg. Vol. I, 93 - 147 (1966).

16. RASMUSSEN, P., BUHL, J., BUSCH, H., HAASE, J., HARMSEN, A.: Brain scanning - cerebral scintigraphy. Act. Neurochir. 23, 103 - 119 (1970).

17. RHOTON, A. L., EICHLING, J., TER-POGOSSIAN, M. M.: Comparative study of Mercury-197 chlormerodrin and Mercury-203 chlormerodrin for brain scanning. J. Nucl. Med. 7, 50 - 59 (1966).

18. ROBERTS, D. J., BASILIE, J. X. R.: Clinical evaluation as a neurodiagnostic procedure. Geriatrics, Vol. 23, 91 - 97 (1968).

19. SCHENCK, P., KLAR, E., PIOTROWSKI, W.: Der Nachweis von Hirntumoren mit konventioneller Scanner-Methodik und Szintillationskamera. Therapiewoche 33, 1149 - 1155 (1967).

20. SKLAROFF, D., POLAKOFF, P. P., LIN, P. M., CHARKES, N. D.: Cerebral scanning with radioactive chlormerodrin (neohydrin). Neurology, Vol. 13/1, 79 - 85 (1963).

21. SWEET, W. H., ARONOW, S., BROWNELL, G. L.: External localization of intracranial lesions with radioactive isotopes. Schweiz. med. Woch. 92, 1545 - 1550 (1962).

22. WENDE, S., SCHULE, A., MARX, P.: Die neuroradiologische Diagnostik der Meningiome. Radiologe 9, 26 - 31 (1969).

23. WILCKE, O.: Die Bedeutung der Szintigraphie im Rahmen der neurochirurgischen Tumordiagnostik. Act. Neurochir. 23, 285 -295 (1970).

24. WILCKE, O., FROWEIN, R. A.: Meningiomas. In: Handbook of clinical Neurology.

25. Zum WINKEL, K., PIOTROWSKI, W., KLAR, E., SCHEER, K. E.: Nachweis und Lokalisation von Hirntumoren mit Radioneohydrin. Act. Neurochir., Vol. XIV/1 - 2, 105 - 125 (1966).

26. WITCOFSKI, R. L., MAYNARD, C. D., ROPER, T. J.: A comparative analysis of the accuracy of the Technetium-99m pertechnetate brain scan: Followup of 1.000 patients. J. Nucl. Med. 8, 187 - 196 (1967).

27. YAMAMOTO, Y. L., FEINDEL, W., ZANELLI, J.: Comparative study of radioactive Chlormerodrin (neohydrin) tagged with Mercury-197 and Mercury-203 for brain scanning. Neurology Vol. 14/9, 815 - 820 (1964).

28. ZEIDLER, U., KOTTKE, S.: Hirngeschwulstnachweis durch Szintigraphie. Dtsch. Z. Nervenheilk. 196, 63 - 84 (1969).

Isotop	Number of meningiomas	+	-	%+	Authors[+]
RISHA	283	263	20	93	1
Hg^{197}	33	25	8	76	2
Hg^{203}	71	69	2	97	3
Hg^{197} or Hg^{203}	162	148	14	91	4
Tc^{99m}	118	114	4	97	5
Tc^{99m} or Hg^{203}				83	6
Bi^{206}				96	7
In^{113m}	8	8		100	8
As^{74}	123	116	7	94	9
Cu^{64}	62	48	14	77	10
As^{74} or Cu^{64}	210	203	7	97	11

1. BUDABIN (1966), v. ECK (1969), PLANIOL (1967), WENDE (1969)
2. OVERTON (1965), RHOTON (1966), ZEIDLER (1969)
3. v. ECK (1969), FAUST (1965), DUGGER (1963), BRINKMANN (1962), BRENNER (1964), DIVITIIS (1966), SKLAROFF (1963), OVERTON (1965) z. WINKEL (1966), MUNDINGER (1967), RHOTON (1966), ROBERTS (1968)
4. ZEIDLER (1969), GOODRICH (1965), LOKEN (1966), BUCY (1965), YAMAMOTO (1964)
5. RASMUSSEN (1970), WITCOFSKI (1967), SCHNEIDER (1967), SCHENK (1967), ZEIDLER (1969), KUBA (1970)
6. MUNDINGER (1967)
7. MUNDINGER (1967)
8. KUBA (1970)
9. BOTTERELL (1961), SWEET (1962), OJEMANN (1964)
10. SWEET (1962), OJEMANN (1964)
11. WILCKE (1974

Fig. 1. Results of meningioma diagnosis by application of usual isotopes

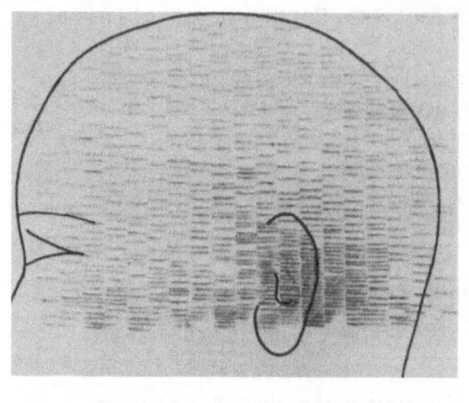
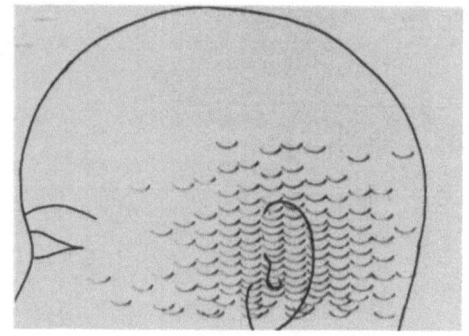
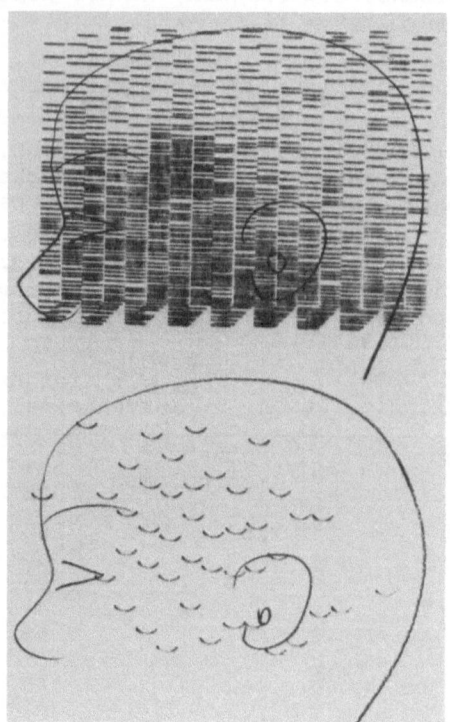

Fig. 2. Szintigram of a cere-
bellar-pontine angle meningioma

Fig. 3. Szintigram of a suprasellar meningioma

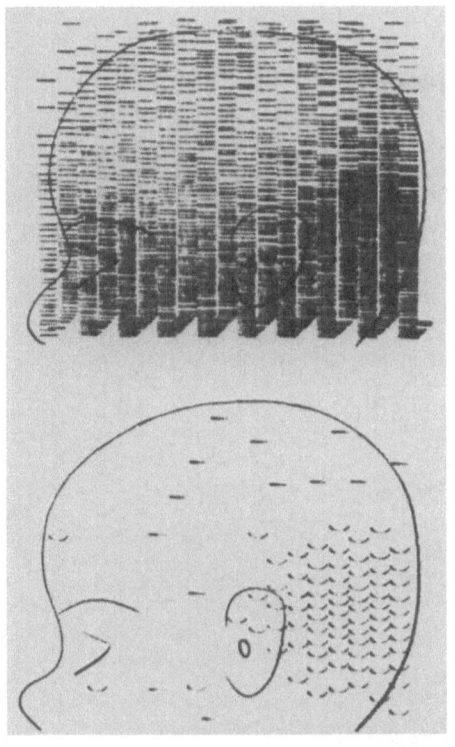

Fig. 4. Szintigram of an
infratentorial tentorial
meningioma

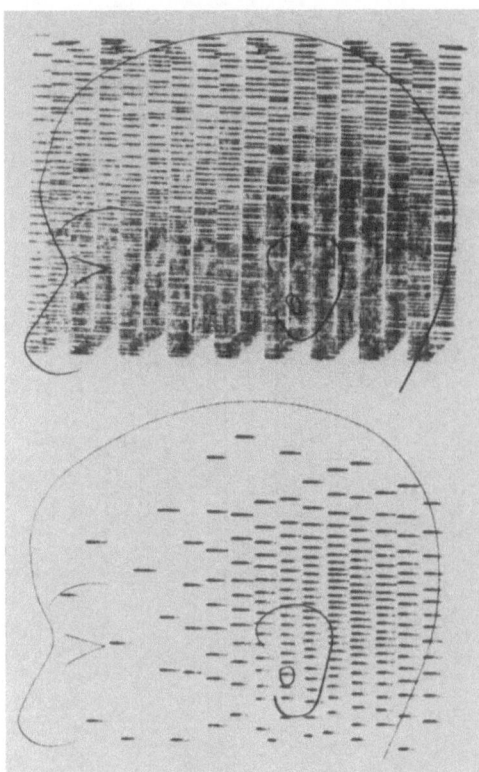

Fig. 5. Szintigram of a supra-
and infratentorial developed tentorial meningioma

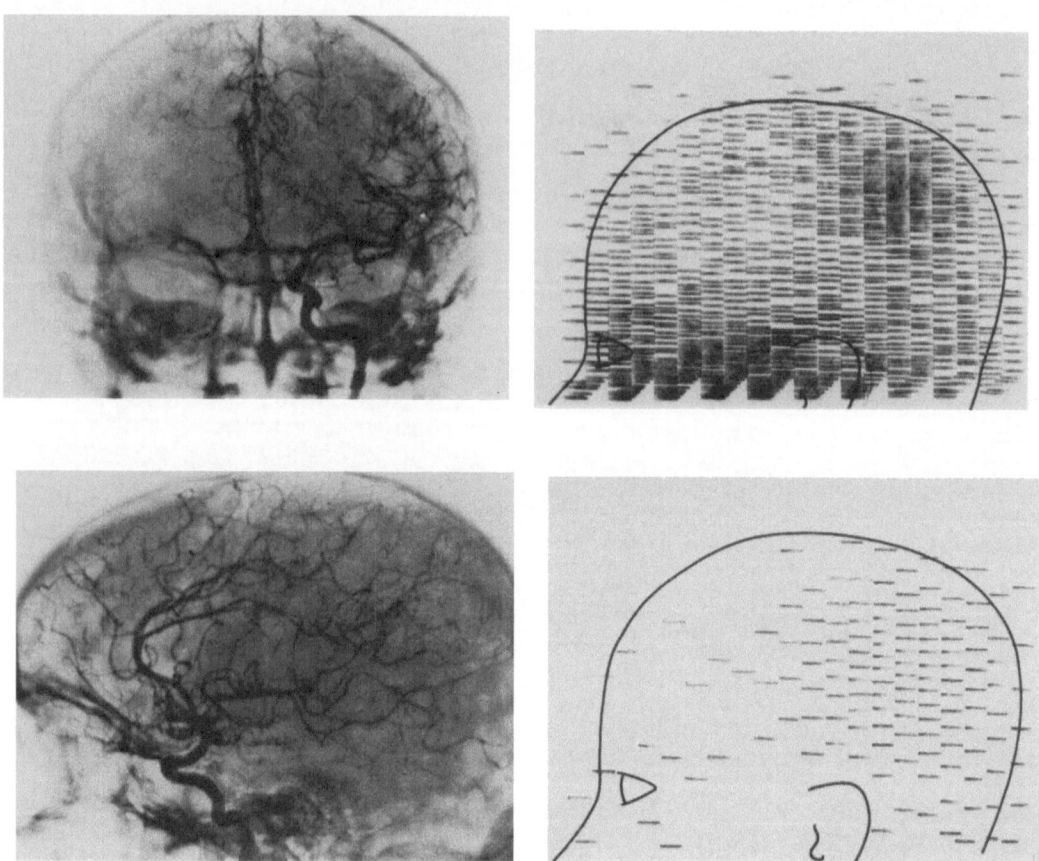

Fig. 6. Angiogram and Szintigram of a parietal meningioma

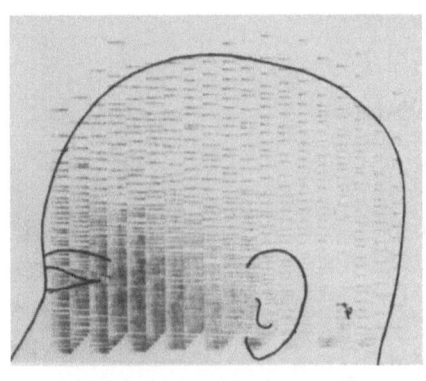

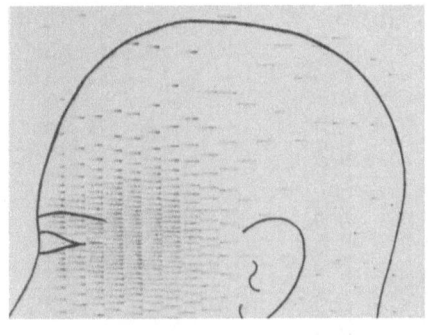

Fig. 7. Recurrence of a interosseus-developed sphenoid-ridge meningioma

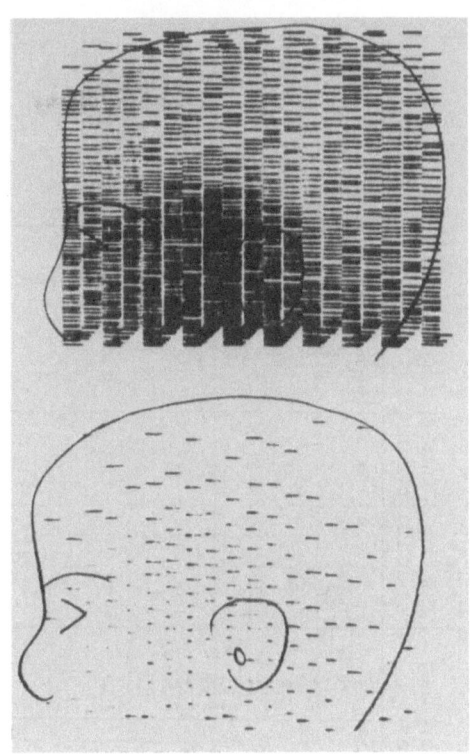

Fig. 8. Recurrence of a para-sellar meningioma

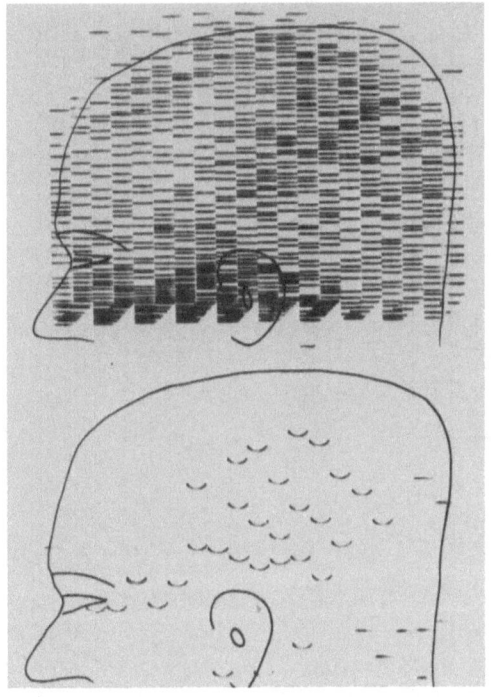

Fig. 9. Szintigram of a parietal glioblastoma

Localization	Σ	Isotop. Scan Mening. specif.	uptake	neg.	Angiography Mening. specif.	Tumor signs	neg.	X-Ray Mening. specif.	Tumor signs	neg.	EEG focal signs	Dys-rhythm.	neg.
Convexity	44	35	9	-	21	22	1	15	9	20	26	8	10
Sphenoid-ridge	43	26	14	3	14	27	2	26	11	6	18	14	11
Parasagittal	38	33	4	1	18	19	1	8	9	21	20	10	8
Falx	23	22	1	-	13	10	-	5	11	7	6	13	4
Suprasellar	12	3	8	1	4	6	2	4	4	4	-	6	6
Olfactory	12	10	1	1	9	3	-	8	2	2	4	5	3
Intraventricular	3	1	2	-	1	2	-	-	1	2	1	2	-
Tentorium	18	5	13	-	5	13	-	2	8	8	6	10	2
Cerebellopontine angle	13	10	2	1	4	4	5	5	4	4	1	5	7
Cerebellar convexity	4	2	2	-	1	3	-	1	1	2	-	3	1
Σ	210	147	56	7	90	109	11	75	60	75	82	76	52
%		71	26	3	43	52	5	36	28	36	39	36	25

Fig. 10. Comparative test of szintigram, angiogram, X-ray and EEG-findings in 210 cases of different localizated meningiomas

Value of Joint Neuroradiological and Angioscintigraphical Investigation of Meningiomas

E. Deisenhammer, B. Hammer, and A. Gund

According to the studies of ZUELCH the endotheliomatous meningioma shows a regular vascular network with giant capillaries and sinusoidal vessels. The angiomatous meningioma is characterized by especially enriched vessels. Only the rarer fibromatous meningioma contains a rather meager vessel network. Hence, the angiography almost always produces a characteristic delineation of the tumor vessel (4, 8, 9, 10, 11, 12). Accordingly, the diagnosis of the meningioma is especially suitable for the application of neuroradiological and nuclearmedical methods, with a view to providing maximal preoperative information for the neurosurgeon about the localization, type and size of the operable tumor.

Material and Methods

With this aim, we ran the following tests supplementary to the normal clinical investigations of 50 operatively or autopsically proven cases of meningiomas:
48 brain-scans (Tc 99m - Pertechnetat)
48 general angiographies through puncture of the common or internal carotid artery (a. car. comm. or a. car. int.)
23 isolated serial angiographies of the external carotid artery (a. car. ext.)
20 angioscintigraphies (I 131 - Macroaggregates) of the a. car. int.
26 angioscintigraphies of the a. car. ext.

The varying types of the 50 meningiomas were:
10 falx meningiomas,
 7 parasagittal meningiomas,
10 hemispheral meningiomas,
 7 lateral meningiomas of the sphenoid wing,
 5 medial meningiomas of the sphenoid wing,
 7 frontobasal meningiomas,
 4 meningiomas of the posterior cranial fossa.

Results

The investigations gave the following results.

1. Brain Scanning: They were positive in 47 cases and questionable in one basal infratentorial meningioma.

A meningioma can be positively located by a brain scan, the area showing as an intensive, sharply defined enrichment of the nuclid. On the other hand, the differential diagnosis is conjecturally only of use in typical localizations, for example, a falx meningioma.

2. The General Angiography: This ensured localization of the tumor in 43 cases (89,5 %). By a flatly growing tumor and a parasagittal parietal meningioma the area was only indecisively marked. In a falx meningioma of the middle third, a frontobasal meningioma, and a meningioma of the cerebellopontine angle, the findings were not pathological. The differential diagnosis of more or less typical pathological vessels was successful in 34 out of 48 cases, that is, 68,7 %.

3. The Isolated Angiography of the A. Car. Ext. gave the correct diagnosis in 20 out of 23 patients, by virtue of demarcation of typical pathological vessels (86,9 %).

2 meningiomas of the middle of the sphenoid wing were without pathological findings, and the results were unusable in one case of a poorly vascularized falx meningioma.

4. The Angioscintigraphy was carried out in 20 patients by injection of the particles in the internal carotid artery. In 10 cases, no activity was observed in the tumor position, and in 4 cases of the basal meningiomas, a moderate enrichment of the particles was noted. The results in 6 cases were unclear or appeared without pathological findings. The particles were also injected 26 times in the external carotid artery. In 18 patients, we found a highly concentrated, clearly defined particle capture. In 4 cases, the results were unusable; in one meningioma of the medial sphenoid wing, 2 frontobasal meningiomas, and one poorly vascularized falx meningioma were no pathological findings.

Discussion

The value of the investigations lies less in the single test, but much more in a combination of the results. The diagnostic problems and the possibility of misinterpretation in one can be compensated for by the other method. Thus, the meningioma or tumor area, predominantly supplied from the interna, can be detected, as we know, by a general angiography. However, the predominant part of the tumor gets its vascularization from the a. car. ext. circulation, at least in as much as the tumor is connected with the dura.

Only in a few cases, the contrast medium, which is flowing off through the a. car. ext. in case of a communis puncture, is large enough to allow delineation of the tumor vessels. Only in the area of the base of the skull the meningeal branches come predominantly from the branches of the a. car. int., ophthalmica or lacrimalis.

Tentorial meningiomas are partly supplied by the tentorial artery of BERNASCONI and CASSINARI. Thus, in c-ses of basal meningiomas and meningiomas of the posterior cranial fossa, the pinpointing of the tumor is occasionally successful over the a. car. int.. But, at least in cases where the general angiography does not lead to a definite enough localization of the tumor, an angiography of the a. car. ext. is necessary.

Additional information can be gained from an angioscintigraphy with macro-aggregates. According to whether the particles are injected into the vessel leading to the tumor or not, one finds either particle capture or negative localization of the tumor.

Demarcation from the glioma is possible because of the different vessel behaviour of the two types of the tumors (2).

A synopsis of the individual investigations of all the patients produced a high percentage of correct preoperative type-diagnosis. These could be stepwise improved in 30 multiply investigated meningiomas by the additional methods as follows.

With a general angiography alone   21 cases - 70,0 %
with an additional a. car. ext. angiography   25 cases - 83,3 %
with a final angioscintigraphy of the a. car. ext.   27 cases - 90,0 %

As already mentioned, the plotting of a meningioma above the a. car. ext. circulation is dependant, in a characteristic way, upon the tumor localization (3). These characteristics can be still better elaborated by an angioscintigraphy.

Cortical supratentorial meningiomas (parasagittal, hemispheral and lateral sphenoid wing meningiomas) behave in the same manner (Table 1). They receive their blood supply from the branches of the a. car. external; only secondarily are those of the a. car. int. tapped (4). Localization is made possible for all types by a brain-scan and a general angiography, but a characteristic vessel pattern is only found in 50 - 80 % of the cases. The angiography of the a. car. ext. shows the tumor circulation in any case, hence accordingly the angioscintigraphy of the a. car. int. a cold area, that of the a. car. ext. a massive particle capture.

Table 1. Localization and type diagnosis in 24 cortical supratentorial meningiomas

Method	Cases	Localization in	Type diagnosis in
Brain scan	23	23 = 100 %	-
General angiography	22	22 = 100 %	15 = 60 %
Angiography of the external carotid artery	10	10 = 100 %	10 = 100 %
Angioszintigraphy of the internal carotid artery	6	6 = 100 %	6 = 100 %
Angioszintigraphy of the external carotid artery	10	10 = 100 %	10 = 100 %

Falx meningioma (Table 2) could be localized by means of a brain-scan for sure, the general angiography gives a demarcation only in 70 %.

The angiography of the a. car. ext. was in 7 of 8 cases successful, the angioscintigraphy of the a. car. int. gave in 3 of 4 cases a negative location, that of the a. car. ext. in 5 of 8 a particle capture.

Still less uniform are the results from the basal meningiomas (Table 3). Medial sphenoid wing meningiomas were only localized in 4 out of 5 cases through a general angiography, after the angiography of the a. car. ext., now in 2 out of four. The angioscintigraph of the a. car. ext. gave particle capture only in 3 out of 5 cases. By frontobasal meningiomas, the angiosctintigraphy of the a. car. ext. failed, that

Table 2. Localization and type diagnosis in 10 falx meningiomas

Method	Cases	Localization in	Type diagnosis in
Brain scan	9	9 = 100 %	-
General angiography	10	9 = 90 %	7 = 70 %
Angiography of the external carotid artery	8	7 = 87,5 %	7 = 87,5 %
Angioscintigraphy of the internal carotid artery	4	3 = 75 %	5 = 62,5 %
Angioscintigraphy of the external carotid artery	8	5 = 62,5 %	5 = 62,5 %

of the a. car. int. produced a cold area twice, and once a capture.
The localization of pathological vessels was angiographically possible
in 5 cases above the ophthalmic artery, but only once above the a.
car. ext..

Table 3. Localization and type diagnosis in 12 basal meningiomas

Method	Cases	Localization in	Type diagnosis in
Brain scan	12	12 = 100 %	-
General angiography	12	11 = 91,6 %	8 = 66,6 %
Angiography of the external carotid artery	5	3 = 60 %	3 = 60 %
Angioscintigraphy of the internal carotid artery	9	5 = 55,5 %	5 = 55,5 %
Angioscintigraphy of the external carotid artery	8	3 = 37,5 %	3 = 37,5 %

Meningiomas of the posterior cranial fossa respectively the tentorium
(Table 4) occupy a special position. They could be differentially
diagnosed by means of a general angiography, but the demonstration
of the tentorial artery of CASSINARI and BERNASCONI is not, however,
specific for the meningioma.

All other methods gave unusable results. The brain-scan was successful in locating 3 out of 4 cases.

Summary

In order to increase the accuracy of the preoperative diagnosis of the
tumor-type 50 meningiomas of different location were, when possible,
thoroughly investigated with brain-scan, general angiography, isolated
external carotid artery angiography, angioscintigraphy of the internal

Table 4. Localization and type diagnosis in 4 meningiomas of the posterior fossa

Method	Cases	Localization in	Type diagnosis in
Brain scan	4	3 = 75 %	-
General angiography	3	2 = 66,6 %	2 = 66,6 =
Angiography of the external carotid artery	O	O	O
Angioscintigraphy of the internal carotid artery	1	O	O
Angioscintigraphy of the external carotid artery	O	O	O

and external carotid artery. Through a synopsis of the given results, it was possible to correctly predict the preoperative diagnosis of the tumor type in 90 % of the cases. The influence of the localization of the meningioma on its ability to be located above the branches of the external or internal carotid artery as well as by negative location or particle capture in the angioscintigraphy is discussed.

REFERENCES

1. BERNASCONI, V., CASSINARI, V.: Un segno carotidografico tipico di meningioma del tentorio. Chirurgia 11, 586 - 588 (1956).

2. BERGMANN, H., BÖCK, F., BRENNER, H., HÖFER, R.: Shuntvolumenbestimmung mit radioaktiven markierten Albuminpartikeln zur Differentialdiagnostik der Hirntumore. Fortschr. Rö-strahlen 115, 348 - 357 (1971).

3. DETTORI, P., BRADAC, G. B., SCIALFA, G.: Selective angiography of the diagnosis of supra-tentorial meningiomas. Neuroradiol. 1, 166 - 172 (1970).

4. GUND, A.: Was vermag die Serienagniographie über die Hirndurchblutung bei raumbeengenden Prozessen, insbesondere Meningiomen, Glioblastomen und arteriovenösen Hämangiomen auszusagen? Dtsch. Z. Nervenheilk. 181, 593 - 601 (1961).

5. GUND, A.: Die Hirnzirkulation im Bild der schnellen Serienangiographie unter normalen Verhältnissen und bei raumbeengenden Prozessen. Paracelsus-Beihefte. Wien: Hollinek 1966.

6. GUND, A.: Die arteriellen Zuflüsse angefärbter Hirntumore im Serienangiogramm. Acta neurochir. 19, 233 - 240 (1968).

7. MINGRINO, S., PISTOLESI, G. F., FRASSON, F., MERLI, G. A.: Selective angiography of the external carotid and its branches by catheterization of the superficial temporal artery. Acta neurochir. 24, 225 - 236 (1971).

8. TÖNNIS, W., SCHIEFER, W.: Zirkulationsstörungen des Gehirns im Serienangiogramm. Berlin - Göttingen - Heidelberg: Springer 1959.

9. WICKBOM, I.: Angiography of the carotid artery. Acta radiol. Suppl. 72 (1948).

10. WICKBOM, I.: Angiographic determination of tumor pathology. Acta radiol. 40, 529 - 546 (1953).

11. WICKBOM, I., STATTIN, S.: Roentgen Examination of Intracranial Meningiomas. Acta radiol. 50, 175 - 186 (1958).

12. ZÜLCH, K. J.: Biologie und Pathologie der Hirngeschwülste. In: Handbuch der Neurochirurgie, Bd. III (Hrsg. H. OLIVECRONA, W. TÖNNIS), S. 391 - 455. Berlin - Göttingen - Heidelberg: Springer 1956.

Angiographic Aspects in Parasagittal Meningiomas

A. WALKENHORST

In the evaluation of angiograms of parasagittal meningiomas operated on by us, the question was asked as to whether there was sufficient information present to enable a parasagittal meningioma of the dural sinus angle to be differentiated angiographically from a meningioma of the falx cerebri (5).

In connection with the blood supply to the sections of the brain in question it should be recalled that the medial region of the hemisphere and the "edge" of the medio-lateral transitional area of the frontal lobe as well as the medial and parasagittal parts of the parietal lobe obtain their blood supply through branches of the anterior cerebral artery. In the case of the lateral regions located directly alongside the "edge" of the medio-lateral transitional area the blood supply is effected via the middle cerebral artery. This might well be the explanation for the multiple supply being effected via the anterior as well as the middle cerebral arteries, particularly in the case of parasagittal meningiomas. The medial and parasagittal regions of the occipital lobe are supplied by the anterior and posterior cerebral arteries (1, 2, 4).

Generally speaking, important progress has been made in the diagnosis of tumor types since the introduction of serial angiography, thus permitting for the first time the complete staining of tumors (3, 6, 10, 11, 12).

Of the meningiomas operated on at our Clinic since May, 1951, 132 were located parasagittally. During the present evaluation 17 cases had to be left out of consideration since it was not possible to decide with certainty on the basis of the operation report whether it was actually a parasagittal meningioma of the dural sinus angle or whether it might be classified as a convexity meningioma. Of the 114 parasagittal meningiomas evaluated, 79 were found to be parasagittal meningiomas of the dural sinus angle and 35 to be falx meningiomas. One of the criteria for classifying a falx meningioma was that the point of attachment actually was in the falx as seen during the operation. It was furthermore demonstrated that the falx meningiomas were always covered by brain, if only to a minor extent. The further classification depended on whether the meningiomas were situated in the anterior, middle or posterior third parts of the sinus (8).

On examining the angiograms it became apparent that all falx meningiomas, whether located in the anterior or middle third part obtained their blood supply exclusively from branches of the anterior cerebral artery, and that a falx meningioma in the posterior third part obtained its blood supply additionally from the posterior cerebral artery. No involvement of the externa circulation was demonstrable in any of the cases.

The major part of the 79 parasagittal meningiomas of the dural sinus angle revealed a multiple blood supply (58 cases) from branches of the anterior cerebral artery and the middle cerebral artery; in 14 cases, the anterior cerebral artery was involved exclusively, and in 4 cases it was the middle cerebral artery. An additional involvement of the externa circulation, very frequently arranged in the form of a radiate star, was demonstrated in 77,2 % of the cases. The parasagittal meningiomas of the dura sinus angle were found to be subsequently richer in blood vessels than the meningiomas of the falx. Where there was an involvement of the externa circulation it was observed that the middle meningeal artery was usually hypertrophied. We did not carry out selective angiography of the external carotid artery (9). Perhaps this should be recommended for the future. In this event there might be a possibility of demonstrating a still greater involvement of the externa circulation. Furthermore, a better demonstration of the externa vessels, and hence also of the arterial tributaries in this area is to be expected.

In the lateral angiogram a distinct basal-convex bowing of the arteria pericallosa in the regional sections was to be seen in 29 of the 35 falx meningiomas. With increasing duration of the illness from one year onwards it was observed that this bow became increasingly pronounced. It is to be expected that the size and location of the tumor depends on whether the point of attachment to the falx is situated nearer to the superior or the inferior longitudinal sinus. Sometimes surprise is occasioned by the frequently considerable bowing in relation to the (relatively small) size of the tumor. Local oedema must be taken into account (7). Retrospectively, we are unable to make any binding statement on this.

As regards the parasagittal meningiomas of the dural sinus angle, in almost 50 % of these cases an arborization of the middle cerebral artery with partial caudal displacement was demonstrated in the lateral angiogram.

Summarizing, it can be stated that in the case of parasagittal meningiomas in the patients treated by us, a falx meningioma was as good as excluded if, in addition to the tumor staining present in many meningiomas of various locations, the angiogram revealed that the tumor was receiving its blood supply from branches of the middle cerebral artery, or that an involvement of the externa was present. A distinct basalconvex bowing of the arteria pericallosa in the regional sections in the lateral angiogram might be regarded as an adequate indication of this type of tumor. By way of qualification it should be observed, however, that one should not fall into any possible error here, since we did not carry out any selective angiography, namely, in these cases, of the external carotid artery. Falx and tentorium with more complex supply systems require selective angiography, since it may be that multiple vessels are involved.

REFERENCES

1. CLARA, M.: Das Nervensystem des Menschen. S. 772. Leipzig: Joh. Ambr. Barth 1953.

2. FERNER, H., KAUTZKY, R.: Angewandte Anatomie des Gehirns und seiner Häute. In: Handbuch der Neurochirurgie. Bd. 1. Berlin - Göttingen - Heidelberg: Springer 1959.

3. GROTHE, W.: Das Meningiom im Serienbild. Zbl. Neurochir. 15, 31 - 38 (1955).

4. GUND, A.: Die arteriellen Zuflüsse angefärbter Hirntumoren im Serienangiogramm. Acta Neurochir. _19_, 233 - 240 (1968).

5. HAAR, H., TIWISINA, Th.: Die angiographische Differentialdiagnose des parasagittalen und des Falx-Meningioms. Fortschr. der Rö-Strahlen _77_, 653 - 661 (1952).

6. LINDGREN, E.: Röntgenologie einschließlich Kontrastmethoden. In: Handbuch der Neurochirurgie, Bd. II, S. 141 - 144, S. 180 - 181. Berlin - Göttingen - Heidelberg: Springer 1954.

7. MERREM, G.: Die parasagittalen Meningiome. Acta Neurochir. _23_, 203 - 216 (1970).

8. OLIVECRONA, H.: The surgical treatment of intracranial tumors. In: Handbuch der Neurochirurgie, Bd. IV/4, S. 125 - 142. Berlin - Heidelberg - New York: Springer 1967.

9. SALAMON, G., GUERINEL, G., COMBALBERT, A., FAURE, J.-J., GUIDI-CELLI, G.: Etude artériographique de meningiomes intracraniens. Correlations radioanatomiques. Ann. Radiol. _12_, 661 - 679 (1969).

10. SCHIEFER, W., TÖNNIS, W., UDVARHELYI, G.: Die Artdiagnose des Meningeoms im Gefäßbild (Unter besonderer Berücksichtigung der Serienangiographie). Dtsch. Z. Nervenheilkunde _172_, 436 - 456 (1955).

11. TÖNNIS, W.: Die Bedeutung der Serienangiographie für die Artdiagnose der Großhirngeschwülste. Acta Neurochir. Suppl. III, 153 - 170 (1955).

12. TÖNNIS, W.: Diagnostik der intracraniellen Geschwülste. In: Handbuch der Neurochirurgie, Bd. IV/3, S. 39 - 46, S. 338 - 347. Berlin - Göttingen - Heidelberg: Springer 1962.

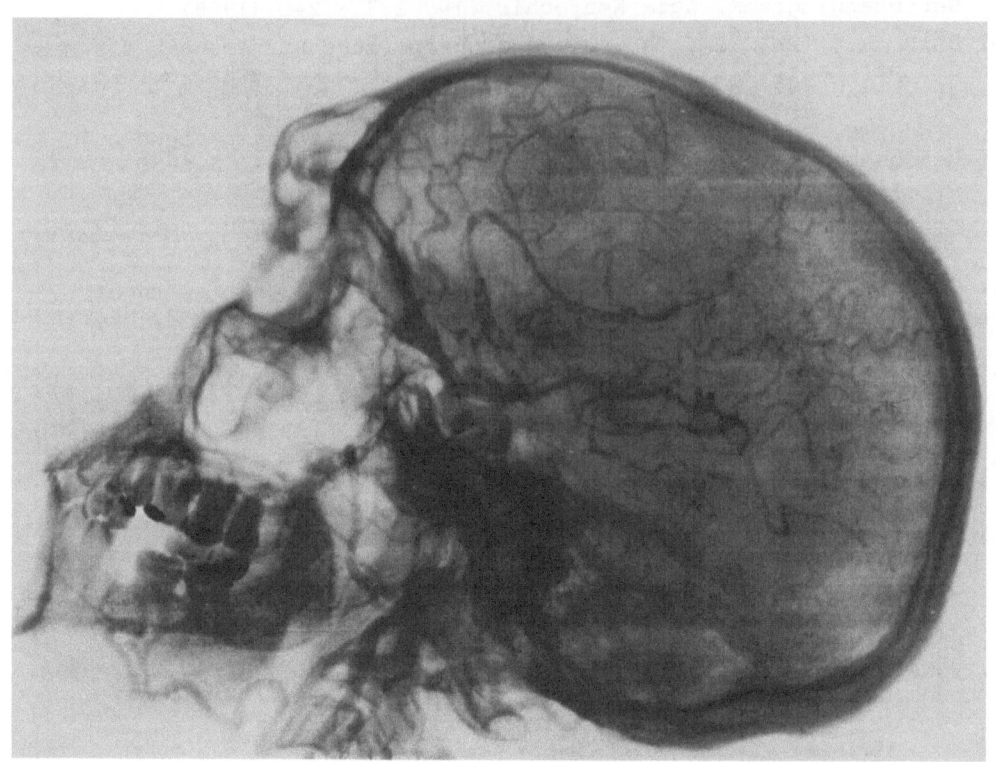

Fig. 1. N. F. 43 years old, Op. Feb. 14, 1953. Falx meningioma with
basal convex bowing of the arteria pericallosa

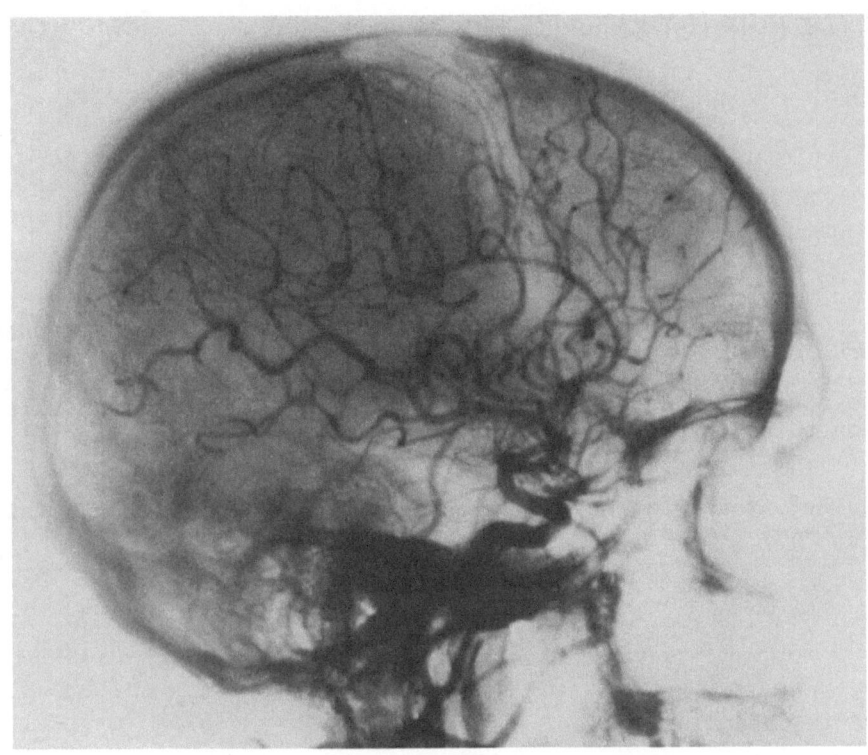

Fig. 2. K. W. 29 years old; Op. Oct. 22, 1971. Parasagittal meningioma
(dural sinus angle) with arborization of the middle cerebral artery
and involvement of the externa

Angiographic Aspects in Meningiomas of the Posterior Cranial Fossa

M. NADJMI, M. RATZKA, and G. MOISSL

On reviewing the cases already published, CUSHING and EISENHARDT (2) were in doubt as to whether the low percentage of meningiomas of the posterior fossa in relation to all other meningiomas could represent their real incidence. - Numerous later reports confirmed this impression to be true (Table 1).

Table 1. Meningiomas of the posterior fossa in relation to all cerebral meningiomas

Author	Meningiomas of the posterior fossa in relation to all cerebral meningiomas	%
FASIANI	11 : 236	4,6
CUSHING and EISENHARDT	23 : 295	7,7
OLIVECRONA	88 : 803	10,8
WÜRZBURG 1967 - 1974	18 : 140	12,9

According to all series which are reported here (1, 5) about 13 percent of all cerebral meningiomas are localized in the posterior fossa. We can really expect to find this incidence - not calculating a certain number of cases which are so far advanced and in such poor condition that a diagnosis cannot be made.

The very slow increase of uncharacteristic clinical signs at the beginning of the disease - such as neck- and headache, the subjective impression of an unsteady gait or mental alterations delay the onset of diagnostic measures. When neurological defects are evident, whether these are cranial nerve symptoms, disorders of the motor or sensory systems or ataxia, the tumor has reached such a volume that it cannot be missed by the following diagnostic investigations.

In only one third of the cases does the plain skull X-ray film show bone alterations. These are generally found in the basiocciput and clivus, the tip of the pyramid of the petrous bone and the porus acusticus internus (6). - Local bone destruction in all cerebral meningiomas is to be expected in 63 % of the cases (3).

Formerly ventriculography or encephalography were the most important among the contrast studies. The typical findings are deforming of the fourth ventricle and displacement of the aqueduct. Today angiographic investigations are performed in all cases before ventricular visualization. Only from the angiograms can we make some statements about

the nature of the process and even about special problems of location.

Therefore, the most important improvement from the diagnostic point
of view is increasing the rate of positive tumor signs in the angiograms.

By demonstrating smaller meningeal arteries not only by selective
measures but also in routine angiograms, some advance has been reached.
These meningeal branches originating from various sources will be seen
in different cases of increased vascularization for instance of the
tentorium - they were found in five of seven cases of tentorium meningioma (4).

Our patient group from the years of 1967 to 1974 consists of 18 meningiomas of the posterior fossa, seven of them localized at the tentorium, 4 in the cerebellar hemispheres, 4 at the clivus, and 3 at the
ponto-cerebellar angle.

In one case even during operation, it could not be decided whether
the precise site was at the tentorium or the falx, 2 meningiomas of
the falx were broadly attached to the tentorium und supplied by tentorium vessels, and in the angiograms they had the appearance of tentorium meningiomas. Diagnosis had been made with routine angiographic
investigations without selective methods, in most cases followed by
encephalography or ventriculography. All cases were operated and the
diagnosis was confirmed by histological investigations.

In the following figures showing angiographic examples, we will demonstrate the various sources of blood vessel supply in meningiomas
of the posterior fossa.

The first most instructive figure demonstrates a meningioma of the
tentorium (Fig. 1). There is a large tumor stain and seven different
arterial branches are involved with the blood supply. We can recognize
a branch coming from the middle cerebral artery, one from the posteri-
or cerebral artery, the others coming from the upper cerebellar artery,
from tentorial branches of the cavernous region of the internal carotid artery, from a posterior branch of the middle meningeal artery and
the internal occipital artery of the external carotid artery, and from
the posterior meningeal artery of the vertebral artery.

The other figures (Figs. 2, 3, 4) show meningiomas of diverse sites
with only small or completely lacking tumor stain but with the typical
space-occupying effect on the vessels, and in addition to this we can
see meningeal branches only from two or three different sources or one
meningeal branch alone. Only in a single case were we unable to find
any meningeal branches, and we do not find the same high rate of
"BERNASCONI-Artery", perhaps caused by a low incidence of internal
carotid artery punctures.

In clinically suspicious cases where we cannot find a tumor stain
with the first angiographic study by chance, we perform "four-vessel-
angiography" making studies of retrograde arteriography of the
brachial artery from the right and left side and a common carotid
artery angiogram of the left side. Proceeding in this way raises the
chances of demonstrating one of the typical meningeal vessels of the
tumor or getting a tumor stain. Only if the filling of the brain arteries is not good or contrast is poor do we prefer special methods
like puncture of the external or internal carotid arteries or the
vertebral artery. It may also be very useful to try special technical

methods in selected cases such as angiotomography to see a latent tumor stain or to elaborate the angiograms, for example by making subtraction pictures or adding pictures of different phases of circulation to improve the reliability of the diagnostic statements.

REFERENCES

1. CASTELLANO, F., RUGGIERO, G.: Meningiomas of the Posterior Fossa. Acta Radiol. (Stockholm) Suppl. 104 (1953).

2. CUSHING, H., EISENHARDT, L.: Meningiomas: Their Classification, Regional Behaviour, Life History and Surgical End Results. Springfield/Ill.: C. Thomas 1938.

3. GOLD, L. H. A., et al: Intracranial Meningiomas. A retrospective Analysis of the Diagnostic Value of Plain Skull Films. Neurology (Minneapolis) 19, 873 (1969).

4. KRAMER, R., NEWTON, T. H.: Tentorial Branches of Internal Carotid Artery. Amer. J. Roentgenol. 95, 826 - 830 (1965).

5. MORELLO, G., PALEARI, A.: I meningiomi della fossa cranica posteriore. Chirurgia (Milano) 4, 239 (1949).

6. RUSSEL, J. R., BUCY, P. C.: Meningiomas of the posterior fossa. Surg. Gynec. Obstet. 96, 183 (1953).

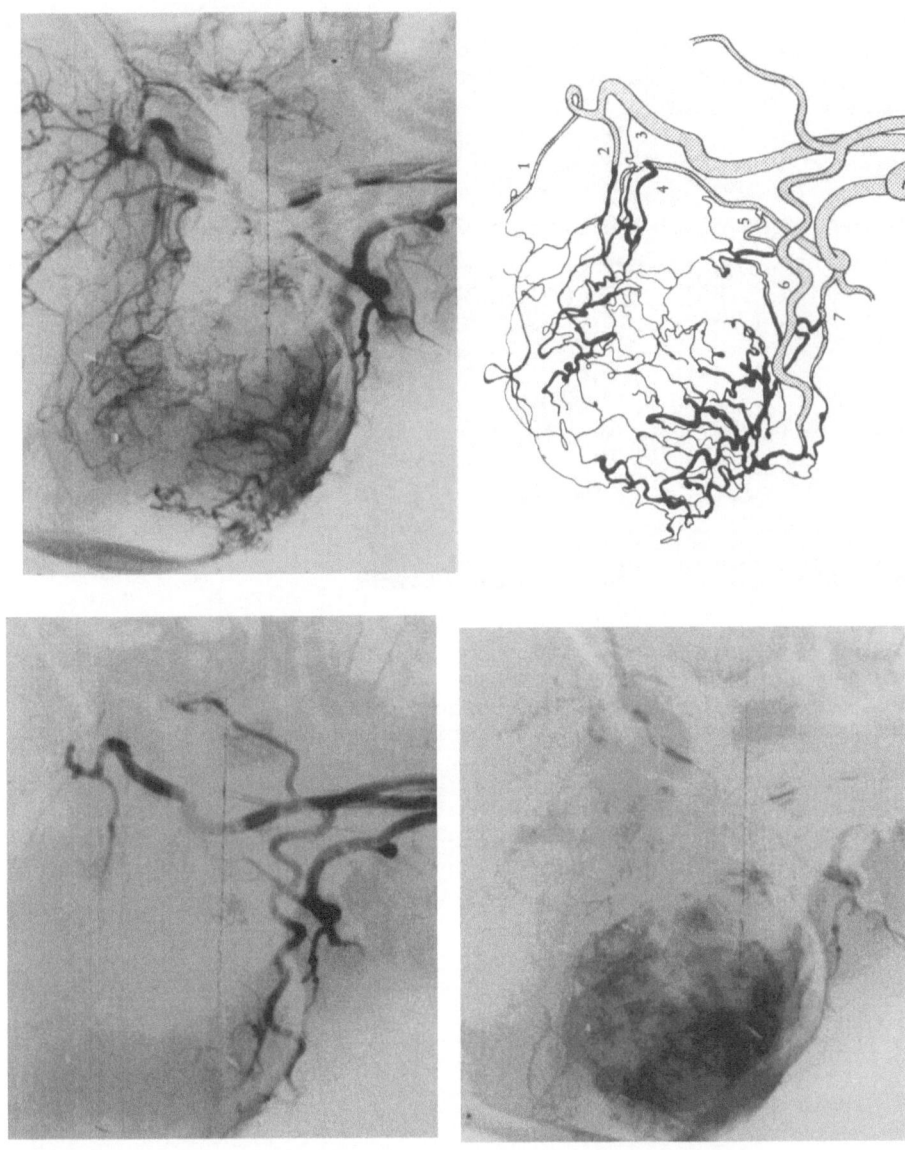

Fig. 1. Tentorium meningioma. Large tumor stain with blood supply from various arterial branches

1 branch of the middle cerebral artery
2 posterior cerebral artery
3 meningeal branch of the internal carotid artery (BERNASCONI)
4 superior cerebellar artery
5 posterior branch of the middle meningeal artery
6 intern occipital artery from the external carotid artery
7 posterior meningeal artery

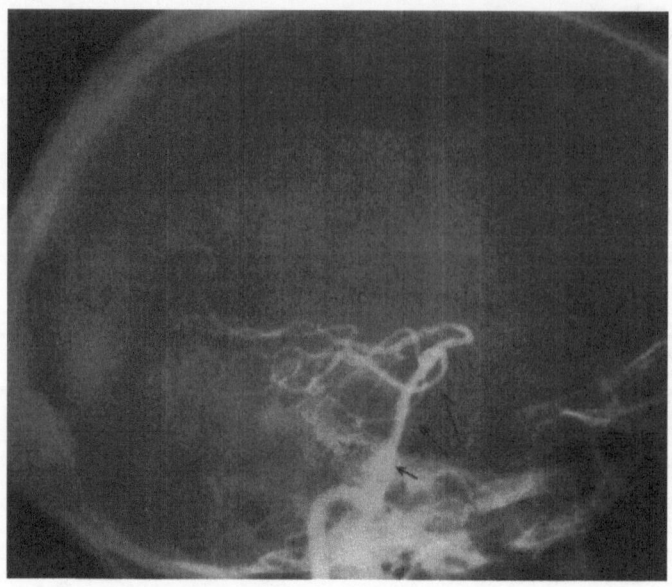

Fig. 2. Clivus meningioma
typical space occupying effect
retrograde arteriography of the left brachial artery
without demonstration of meningeal arterial branches

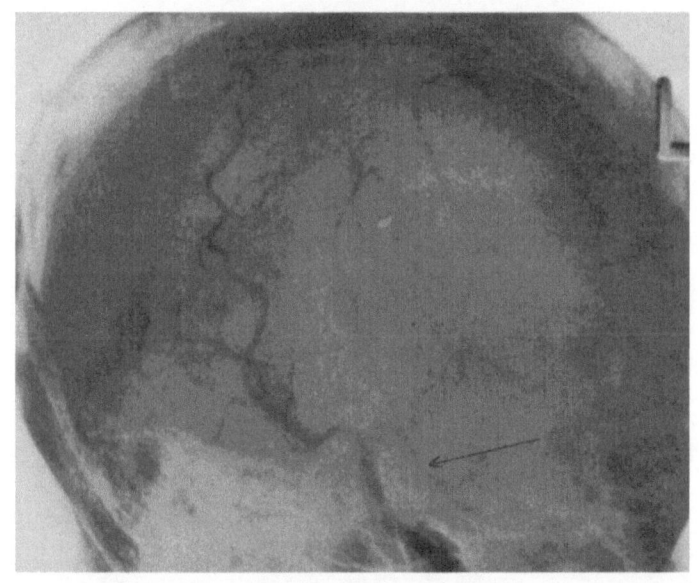

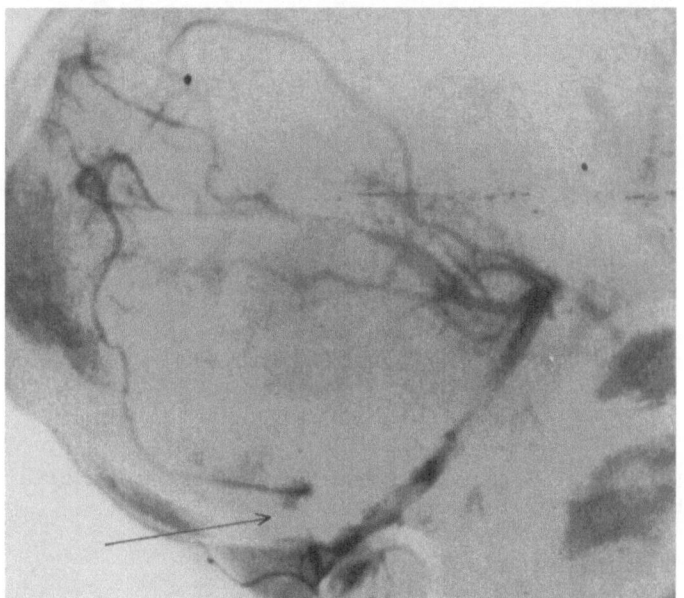

Fig. 3. Tentorium meningioma
very long meningeal branch from the vertebral artery with small tumor
stain

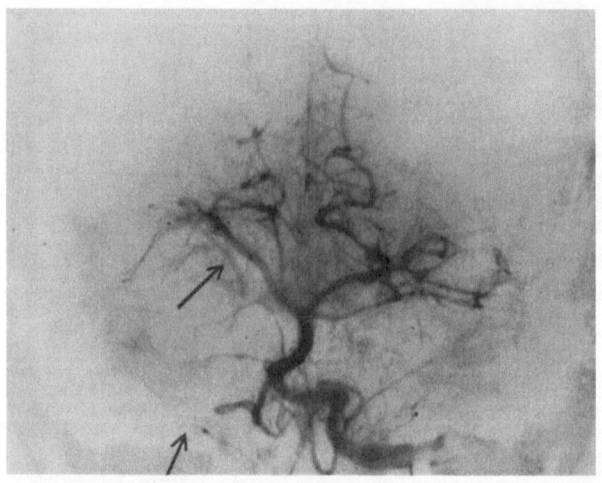

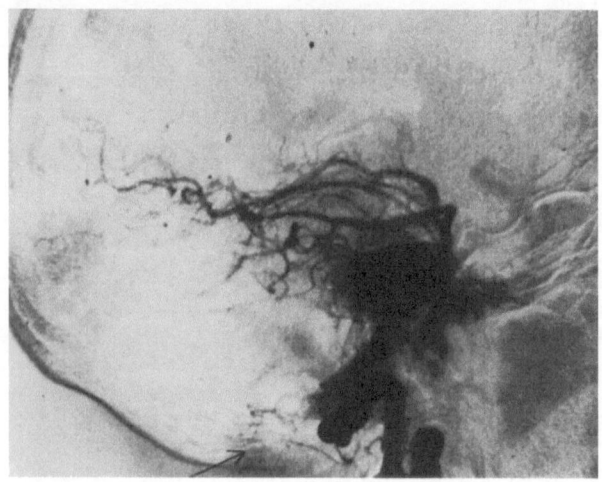

Fig. 4. Meningioma of the right pontocerebellar angle; meningeal branch from the vertebral system

Intra- and Postoperative Consequences Resulting from the Postoperative Tendency to CSF-Hypotension after Meningioma Removal

P. C. POTTHOFF

In an evaluation of 1563 postoperative lumbar pressure measurements in 411 patients with hemispheric space-occupying lesions - including 131 meningiomas - during the first nine postoperative days, a tendency to postoperative CSF (cerebrospinal fluid) - hypotension could be demonstrated for the group of 31 precentral-parietal meningiomas (2, 3). This postoperative tendency to CSF-hypotension was pronounced between the 3rd and 7th postoperative day, and was prevalent in cases of medium-sized circumscribed meningiomas of about 5 cm in diameter (3).

CSF-hypotension may - *clinically* - induce prolonged somnolence or inactivity and disturbing headache, and - indicating a reduction of intracranial, and therefore the brain's own tamponade pressure - it may *locally* - induce an e-vacuo-haemorrhage at the tumor resection site. Besides, it is still an unsolved question if certain brain tumors - including meningiomas - due to their specific tissue properties, may contain or produce fibrinolytic agents (1) to a sufficient degree to cause a haemorrhagic diathesis. At least, haemorrhagic tendencies have been observed in major and prolonged neurosurgical tumor operations, and may be demonstrated in the thrombelastogram (Fig. 1).

To counteract the intermingling tendencies to CSF-hypotension and to evacuo and/or fibrinolytic haemorrhage with operations of circumscribed, medium-sized meningiomas - especially of the precentral and parietal convexity - the following consequences should be adopted and precautions taken:

I. For Intraoperative Management

1. Increased cerebral perfusion volume (by transfusion of blood and plasma *before* major blood losses);

2. systemic haemostasis (by antifibrinolytic/haemostatic medication during the operation if local haemostasis becomes difficult with increased bleeding tendency from the brain parenchyma);

3. marking with tantalum powder
   a. of the tumor resection site,
   b. epidural ("rallye stripe"),
   (to allow tracing of intracerebral or epidural postoperative haemorrhage by simple X-ray without angiography);

4. sufficient number of dural stay sutures (to prevent dural collapse and extradural haematoma);

5. osteoplastic trepanation (replacement of bone flap to prevent excessive collapse of brain tissue). -

II. For Postoperative Management

1. Increased perfusion volume (to forego postoperative CSF-hypotension);

2. restraint from osmotherapy (sorbitol or mannitol only in cases of proven elevated intracranial pressure, not as a preventive measure);

3. surveillance for postoperative haemorrhagic diathesis (including laboratory analyses of haemostatic mechanisms and - dependent thereon - possibly antifibrinolytic/haemostatic medication);

4. X-ray controls of the skull (showing positional constancy or changes of intracerebral or epidural tantalum markings);

5. flat position of patient in bed (head not elevated above the level of right cardial atrium during the first two or three postoperative days).

All these precautions only concern patients with circumscribed medium-sized meningioma of the precentral and parietal convexity, removed without major trauma to the cerebrum and without evidence of intraoperative reactive brain edema, and these precautions are directed against possible CSF-hypotension and local postoperative haemorrhage. Meningiomas of the same precentral and parietal localization that render *exceptions* from the above precautions (and include therapeutic aspects as in glioma patients, i. e. major attention for critical elevation of intracranial pressure) are

1. meningiomas of large size (above 8 cm in diameter) with major resection trauma to the brain (causing increased postoperative brain edema),

2. meningiomas of critical relation to draining veins, sinus and falx (disturbed venous drainage may induce critical local edema),

3. meningioma en plaque,

4. multiple meningiomas,

5. invasive meningioma (for the same reasons as with 1. and 2.).

In conclusion, the intra- and postoperative aspects of medical-neurosurgical treatment for meningiomas of the convexity - within the triad of osmo- and oncotherapy and haemostasis - tend predominantly towards a prevalence of oncotherapy and haemostasis, and to a restriction of osmotherapeutic activity (Fig. 2).

REFERENCES

1. KRAUS, H.: Fibrinolytic Properties of Different Brain Tumors. In: Proceedings of the German Society for Neurosurgery, Vol. 1 - 2, pp. 232 - 238. Amsterdam: Excerpta Medica 1971. (Further bibliography on cerebral haemostasis see same volume of same congress).

2. POTTHOFF, P. C., SCHULZE, W., SCHMIDT, K.: The Course of CSF-Pressure after Operations on Hemispheric Brain Tumors. International Congress Series. Excerpta Medica 193, 72 - 73 (1969).

3. POTTHOFF, P. C.: Liquorunterdruck nach Meningiom-Operation. Arch. Psychiat. Nervenkr. 215, 62 - 74 (1971).

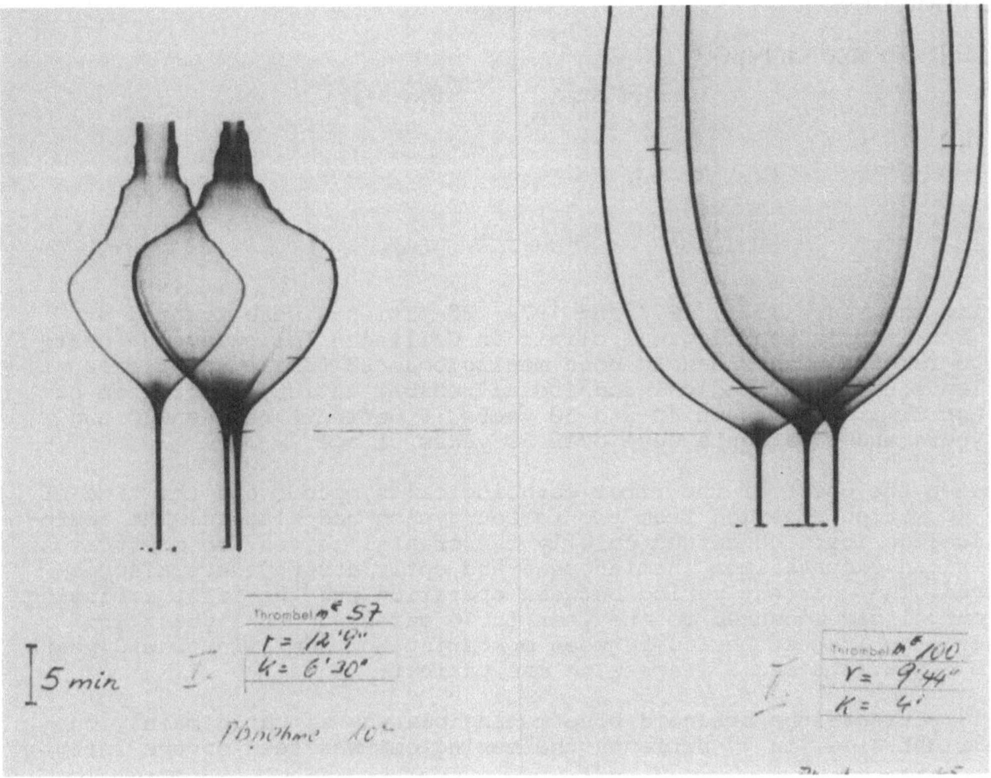

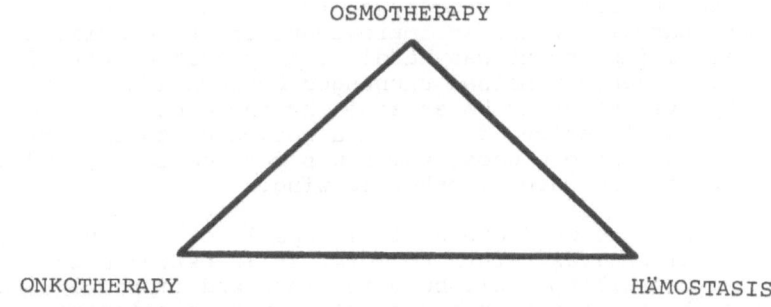

Fig. 1. Thrombelastograms during operation of a large bi-parietal transosseous falx-sinus-meningioma (F. F., male, 17.4.40): First measurement 30 minutes after beginning of the operation, second measurement after 2 hours, and 15 minutes after haemostyptic medication: Thrombelastogram normalizes after initial deficiency in spite of prolonged and major meningioma operation through haemostyptic medication

OSMOTHERAPY

ONKOTHERAPY   HÄMOSTASIS

Fig. 2. Triad of systemic medical-neurosurgical therapy after major brain operations (see text)

Post-Operative Rehabilitation of Patients with Sphenoid Bone Meningiomas

O. LEITHOLF and G. KISCH

During the years 1971, 1972 and 1973 28 patients were treated at
Dr. Schmieder's neurological clinic in Gailingen following the operative removal of a sphenoid bone meningioma. 23 female and 5 male
patients underwent medical and social rehabilitation, 14 of whom had
an age limit of between 40 and 50 years, 6 patients between 30 and
40 years and 8 patients were over 50 years of age.

Between the onset of the first pathological symptoms and the time of
the operation a period from two to four years had elapsed. The neurological deficits concerned chiefly the cranial nerves. In most cases
one-sided exophthalmos, hemianopsia and optic atrophy were also observed. The shortest period between operation and the first admission
to our clinic amounted to one year in 10 cases, up to 2 years in 5
cases; the longest period between operation and admission was 8 years
with 2 patients and 9 years with one patient.

In 17 patients the sphenoid bone meningioma was situated mainly on
the right side, in 11 patients the meningioma was seen on the left.

As stated above with 18 patients, cranial nerve signs, i. e.visual impairment was the main symptom on admission to the clinic. In addition,
the pathological signs were dominated by a hemiplegia in 7 patients,
aphasia in 5 patients and hemihypesthesia in 2 patients. In 17 patients an accompanying mental change could be observed with secondary
brain deficiency. Simultaneously, 8 patients were reported to have
focal or small epileptic seizures, while generalized convulsions did
not occur in any of the observed cases.

As a result of physiotherapy, occupational therapy, work therapy and
psychological training (mainly memory and concentration exercises),
17 patients could leave the clinic considerably improved. In 4 patients the result of treatment could be described as being very good.
The recovery referred chiefly to the mental change, the aphasia and
the hemiparesis, while an improvement of the cranial nerve defects
and visual impairment was hardly ever possible. With 7 patients the
medical evidence remained unchanged between admission and discharge.
The improvement could be attained by those patients who underwent
early rehabilitation, i. e., in a period up to 2 years after the operation, and by those whose tumor was not too large, and above all was
situated in the lateral sphenoid wing.

Of the patients who were still incapable of working prior to admission,
8 could afterwards return to work. In 12 patients the already existing
working capability could be maintained and improved through rehabilitation. 5 of our patients came already as pensioners for treatment,
i. e. had applied for a pension in 3 cases. In one case steps for
finding work were taken with positive results. In the other cases

this was superfluous. 20 patients came to our clinic for the first time, 6 patients for the second time, and 2 patients for the third time. The average length of stay and treatment amounted to 8 weeks.

It has been shown that patients after an operative removal of a sphenoid bone meningioma are particularly suitable for medical and social rehabilitation if the meningioma is localized laterally and does not exceed a certain size. Also the post-operative treatment should be introduced as soon as possible after the operation, at least however within a period from one to two years.

This short survey about the post-operative rehabilitation of patients with sphenoid bone meningiomas seemed to us particularly suitable to show the possibilities of after-care and rehabilitation of patients who allowed especially good opportunities for comparison because of the constant and well-defined localization of the tumor, and the similar neurological and psychological symptoms.

Cliniconeurological Development of Spinal Lesions under Hyperbaric Oxygenation Treatment (HO)

K.-H. HOLBACH, H. WASSMANN, K. L. HOHELÜCHTER, D. LINKE, and B. ZIEMANN

Experimental research has established in numerous instances that hypoxia of the spinal cord is one of the major facts causing functional disturbances and, finally, irreversible damage to the spinal cord. In this context, hypoxia may, for instance, be caused by circulatory disturbances in the spinal cord itself, by trauma, or by a compressive lesion. To this date, we have applied hyperbaric oxygenation treatment to four cases of compressive lesions of the spinal cord, thus treating hypoxia while at the same time avoiding any hypoxic damage to the spinal cord.

Case Histories and Methods

In cases 1 and 2 (Fig. 1) compression of the spinal cord was caused by partially perforated prolapses of cervical discs, the prolapses protruding far into the spinal canal. In case 3 (Fig. 2) we have an arachnitic adhesion surrounding the upper cervical region of the spinal cord, the latter being pallid and clearly tumefied. In case 4 a large arachnoid cyst was compressing the lower thoracic region of the spinal cord. After both cervical prolapses had been surgically removed a Brown-Sequard syndrome remained in case 1, while in case 2 a left-sided convulsive tetraparesis remained. In case 3 both tetraparesis and partial plegia showed no tendency to improve after surgery. The same applies to the paraplegia of the legs manifest in case 4.

In this situation we applied hyperbaric oxygenation (HO) to those four cases, each receiving a course of treatment consisting of 15 individual treatments lasting for 35 to 40 minutes at a pressure of 1.5 atmospheres. In order to establish the effects of HO treatment as well as to register any changes in their neurological condition the patients were examined before, during, and immediately after each treatment.

Results

During the course of HO treatment all cases showed subjective as well as objective improvement of previous motor deficiencies, sensory deficiencies being less obviously affected (Table 1). All improvements were clearly observeable immediately after HO treatment but would often partially recede after a few hours. However, improvements in the patient's condition caused by HO never receded completely between two HO treatments. Therefore, in the course of HO treatment grave neurological disturbances would recede to a large extent. Improvements were especially marked during the first part of a series of treatments.

Table 1. The recovery of motor and sensory functions at the end of the treatment with 15 courses of HO given to each case

Case	Cause of spinal cord (SC) lesion	Symptoms before treatment with HO	Recovery following treatment with HO Motor functions	Sensory functions
♂, 57 y.	Cervical disc protrusion C 4/5	Brown Sequard S. with hemiplegia	Definite, able to walk and move the arm	Slight
♂, 68 y.	Cervical disc protrusion C 3/4 and C 5/6	Severe tetraparesis l. > r. with sensory disturbances	Definite, able to walk and move the arms	Slight
♂, 65 y.	Adhesions and edema of upper SC	Severe tetraparesis with partial plegia	Definite, able to walk and move the arms	Definite
♀, 49 y.	Arachnoidal cyst of thoracic SC	Paraplegia	Slight, not able to stand	Slight

263

We were also able to obtain qualitative results demonstrating the improvement of the supply of oxygen to the spinal cord under HO treatment (Fig. 3). We obtained these results by measuring simultaneously the pO_2 values of the arterial blood as well as of the spinal fluid. We were able to show that, together with a marked increase in the arterial pO_2 value, the spinal fluid pO_2 will rise to about 4 times its original level and will remain above the arterial pO_2 value for as long as 15 to 20 minutes after return to normal respiration.

Although we are not in a position to use spinal fluid pO_2 values as a basis from which to determine the pO_2 values of the affected spinal cord, we may assume that the spinal pO_2 will increase considerably and that the supply of O_2 will, therefore, improve markedly.

In view of our favourable findings we can conclude that HO constitutes an effective additional treatment in a variety of spinal lesions, especially if they should coincide with circulatory disturbances or hypoxia.

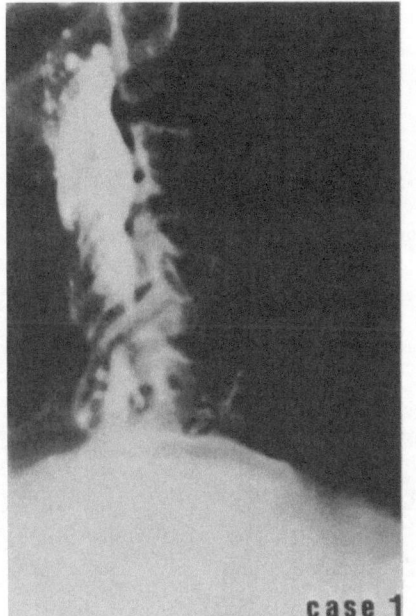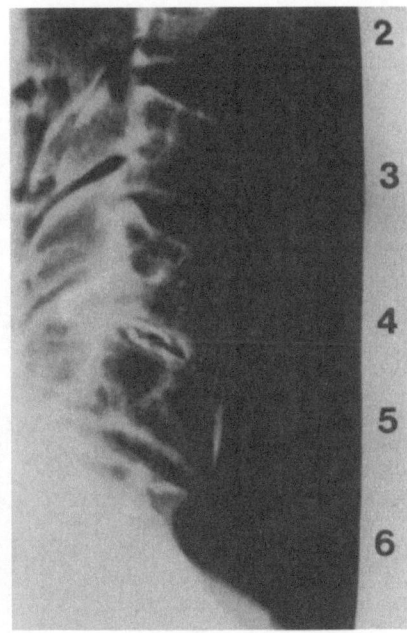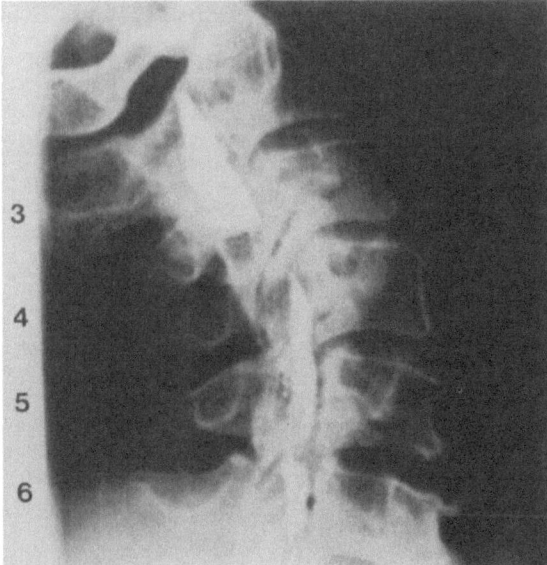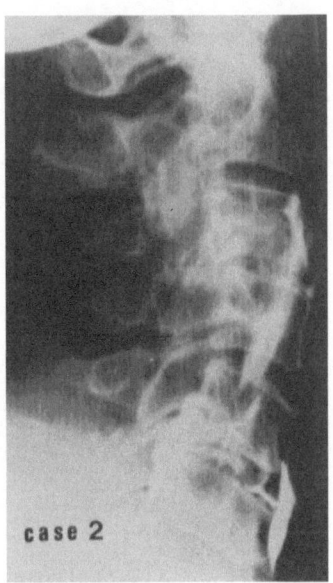

Fig. 1. The myelograms and discograms show the extensive dorsal protrusion of the cervical discs in case 1 between the 4th and the 5th, in case 2 between the 3rd and 4th and also between the 5th and 6th vertebral body

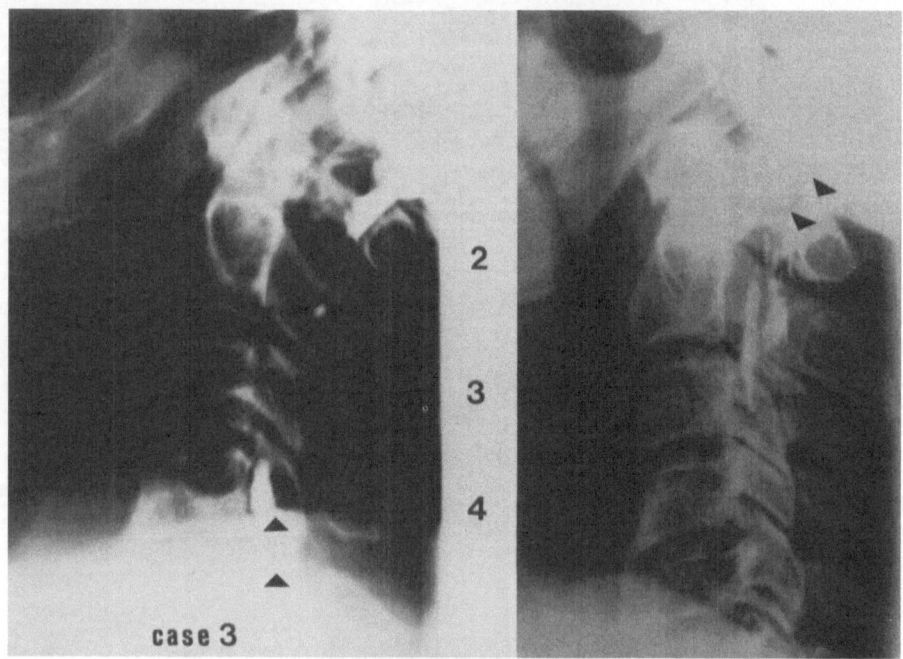

Fig. 2. The myelogram reveals a large space occupying lesion of the cervical SC between the 2nd and the 4th vertebral body

pO$_2$ in Spinal Cord Lesions

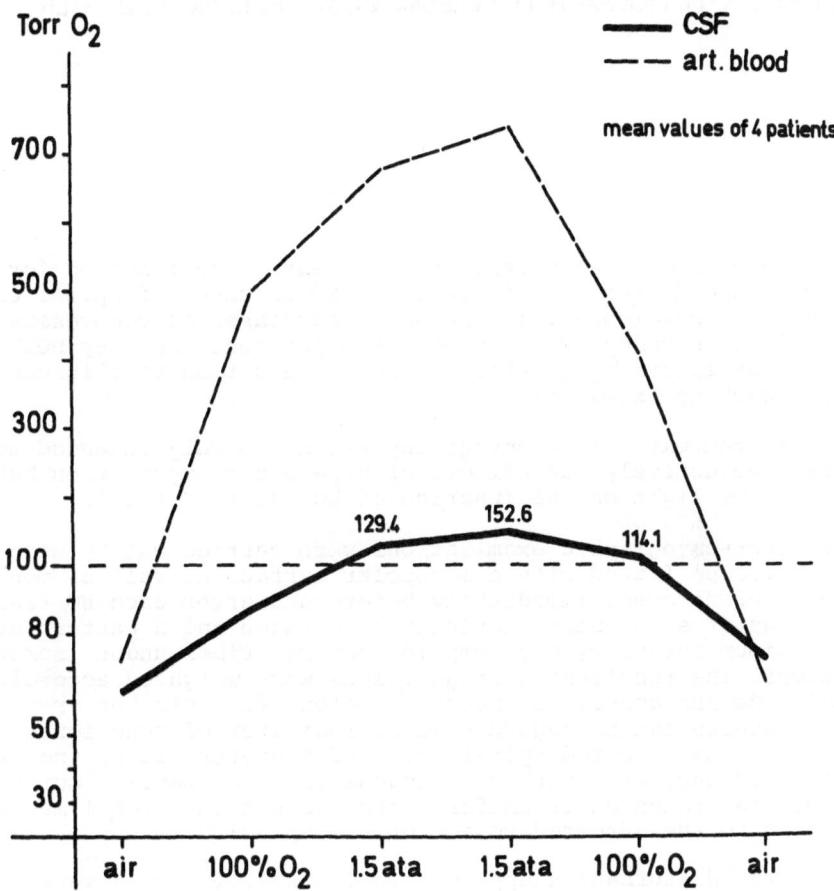

Fig. 3. Simultaneous measurements of pO$_2$ in art. blood and in CSF during 4 different courses of HO given to 4 patients

Electromyographic Surveillance of Hyperbaric Oxygenation Treatment (HO) of Spinal Lesions

D. LINKE, K.-H. HOLBACH, H. WASSMANN, and K. L. HOHELÜCHTER

Since electromyography represents a nearly ideal method for establishing the degree of efficiency of HO in cases of spinal cord lesions, the development of the same four cases of compressive spinal cord lesions under HO treatment (see previous paper by HOLBACH et al.) underwent electromyographic control in addition to cliniconeurological check-up examinations.

In this context, electromyography was not merely intended to demonstrate objectively the effects of hyperbaric oxygenation but also to throw some light on the function of HO therapy itself.

All electromyographic examinations were carried out by means of an oscilloscope fitted with a monopolar surface as well as monopolar needle electrodes. Immediately before and after each HO treatment, recordings of spontaneous activity were taken and a pattern of activity at maximum intensity was compiled several times under isometric conditions. The resultant average values were weighted according to the amplitude and density of muscular potentials. Figures arrived at in this fashion can be regarded as an indicator of functional alterations in the affected spinal cord and therefore as an indicator of the efficiency of hyperbaric oxygenation. We compiled our values from recordings taken under uniform conditions from several muscles belonging to the affected region of the spinal cord.

The motor disturbances apparent in cases 1, 2, and 3 were caused by a damaged corticospinal tract. Since the muscular potential recorded after nerve stimulation in case 4 was low, we concluded that the main source of disturbance was the second motoneuron.

Figs. 1 and 2 show the electromyographic pattern of the triceps muscle before and after treatment with hyperbaric oxygenation.

In all four cases an obvious increase in the density of voluntary activity patterns was recorded after each HO treatment. This shows that the recruiting of motor units improved rather than the impulse frequency of discharging motoneurons.

The incidence of improved recruiting of motor units after HO was not uniform in all sets of muscles observed but tended to concentrate on some muscles rather than on others.

Improvements, however, were not concentrated consistently on some groups of muscles, such as flexors or extensors, distal or proximal muscles, or those of the upper or lower extremities.

A comparison of the average amplitude levels of voluntary activity of sample muscles recorded after several consecutive HO treatments in cases 1 to 3 reveals a marked improvement especially after the first few initial treatments (Fig. 3).

Improvements obtained after HO treatment will often recede after a few hours. They will not, however, recede to the initial level before the onset of the next HO treatment. Subsequent HO treatments frequently carried the level of improvement beyond the previous peak. Therefore, a graph of the increase of muscular potential amplitudes recorded during a course of treatment of HO represents a polygonal curve with an upward trend.

In agreement with cliniconeurological findings these results show that HO caused appreciable increases in the function of the nerve structures concerned. Since any functional improvement of this nature is concomitant with an increased formation of electric potentials which again necessitates an increased energy supply, we may safely conclude that HO treatment improves cytometabolism. This improvement very probably takes the form of a decrease in anaerobic metabolism balances by a corresponding increase in aerobic or oxydative metabolism which is capable of supplying the nerve cells with a greater amount of energy for functional and regenerative purposes.

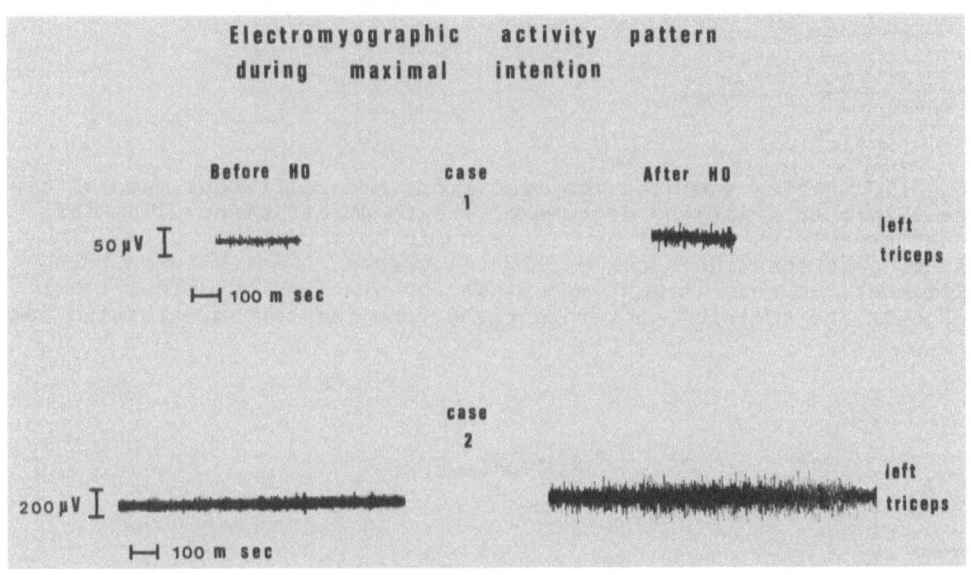

Fig. 1. Immediately before an individual treatment the m. triceps of case 1 showed a pattern of voluntary activity with amplitudes ranging from 10 - 20 uV. After treatment we found a pattern of activity displaying amplitudes ranging from 20 - 40 uV.

Immediately before an individual treatment the left m. triceps of case 2 showed a pattern of activity with amplitudes ranging between 40 and 100 uV. After treatment we found a pattern of activity displaying amplitudes ranging between 180 and 300 uV

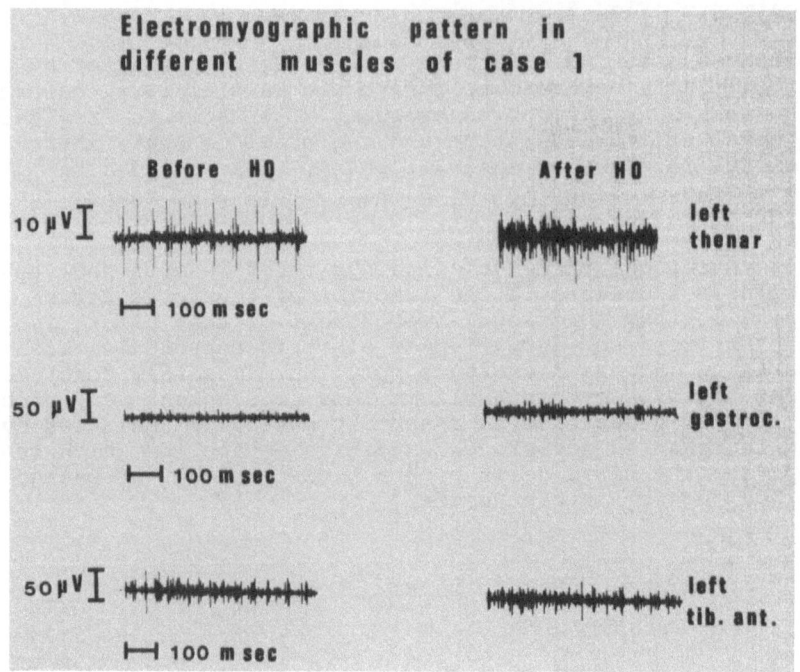

Fig. 2. Comparing the data compiled from three different muscles of
case 1 we obtain varying degrees of treatment efficiency. The left
thenar clearly shows that new motor units have been recruited. The
left m. gastrocnemius shows a slight increase in activity pattern
amplitudes, whereas it was impossible to establish any significant
change in the activity pattern derived from the left m. tibialis ant.

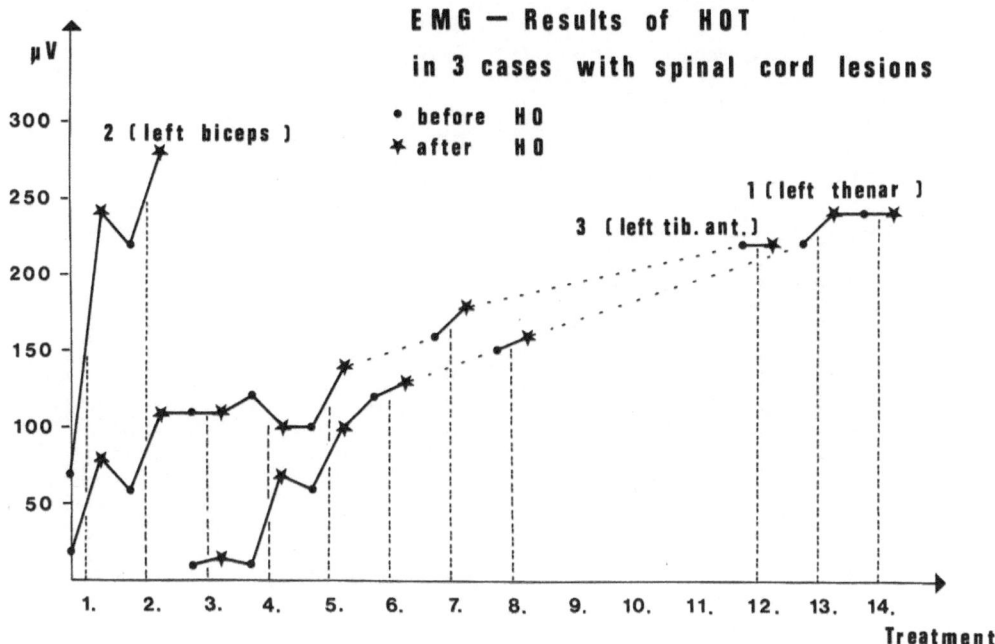

Fig. 3. Comparison of the average amplitude levels of voluntary activity of sample muscles recorded after several HO treatments. Note the marked improvement after the first few treatments

Forensic Problems in Neurosurgery

The Doctor's Liability in the Field of Neurosurgery

M. REICHENBACH

I do not suppose that your society has casually taken the decision to
have a paper on the subject "The doctor's liability in the field of
neurosurgery" presented at its 25th annual meeting. The question as
to whether liability cases are on the increase has been asked time
and again during the last few years. In my view this question can be
answered neither with a clear "yes" nor with a flat "no".

Liability means one's obligation to compensate any damage inflicted
on another person. As a rule, the liability for damages originates
from the various legal regulations, from a contractual commitment or
from a wrongful act. The obligation to make good a damage devolves
predominantly on those who have caused the damage by culpable negligence. Those who disregard the usual care required in their business
act with culpable negligence.

If the question is to be answered as to whether the physician today
exercises less care in his work than in the past in terms of actions
and omissions, and whether he more frequently caused damage by culpable negligence, I would not give an affirmative answer on the grounds
of my personal experience.

However, it is undeniable that in Germany, too, the doctor's liability
has for some time been receiving increasing attention both in legal
and medical literature, and even more so in radio and television pro-
grammes aimed at the lay public. A consequence of this is that, undoubtedly more claims for damages are being made against physicians
today than in the past. But this certainly does not imply that they
are justifiable in any individual case.

The topic "The doctor's liability in the field of neurosurgery" which
I was requested to deal with, as well as the results of the inquiries
held at neurosurgical clinics on the problems concerned, and the resulting questions that are of special interest to you prompt me to
make it plain from the outset that there exists neither a special
"neurosurgical medical liability", nor a specific liability of the
neurosurgeon for iatrogenic damage. Like any other specialist or
general practitioner, the neurosurgeon is liable for damages only in
the cases established by law. But there is no doubt that in neurosurgery there are a number of particular aspects to be considered.

As a result of inquiries involving lawyers and doctors, SCHWEISSHEIMER
in 1966 and 1968 compiled records of the incidence of lawsuits and
complaints about certain specific medical events occuring as part of
a doctor's normal activity. This prompted me to examine in 1969, the
nature of the errors which the doctors in Germany are reproached with.
A total of 1840 cases with at least 2330 demarcatable and subsumable
complaints were analyzed.

The material I investigated was subdivided into clearly lineated case groups in terms of treatment, diagnosis and examination. It was not surprising to find that the reproach of alleged error in treatment prevailed. Startling, however, was the relationship to the other two groups. Faulty treatment accounted for some 75 % compared with 15 % for alleged diagnostic errors and roughly 3,5 % for errors made during an examination.

Among the cases provided by you it is also the complaint about errors of treatment that prevails. From the investigation of my case material it emerged that half of all the complaints made were associated with injections and operations, whereas the complaints covered by the questionnaire referred almost exclusively to post-operative sequelae. In this contect, I also wish to state very clearly that the neuro-surgical clinics and departments contacted abstained from classifying complaints not directly related to their specialized field, as falling under the sphere of responsibility of the general practitioner.

The limited time available to deal with this subject makes it impossible to discuss in detail the specialized surgery of the central nervous system or proximal areas.

Apart from this it would basically not be possible to do so, since alleged errors made in a specialized medical field or during specialized operations, or during examinations involving a certain specialized method cannot be assessed summarily, or in a generally binding manner. Whether a pathological allegedly harmful change, a lack of improvement or a deterioration of a pathological condition or a complication occuring after a medical measure can be causally attributed to the attending doctor and, if so, whether the physician was guilty of culpable negligence by failing to provide the usual standard of care required in his business, can only be appraised by experts and decided upon by the lawyers from case to case, supported by a full, in-depth knowledge of the facts and of the medical course of treatment.

In this context let me briefly deal with some important aspects, especially that of the activity of the medical assessors when physicians are sued for damages irrespective of whether settlement is made in or out of court.

In 1954 PERRET, my former superior and predecessor, stated that undoubtedly many a decision of the courts would have been different if the judge had been advised by the medical witness in a manner more clearly understandable to a lawyer. In 1964, in my paper entitled "Sources of error in the judgement of doctor's liability claims" I pointed out that, in principle, no court decision is made without hearing one or more physicians and medical witnesses. Consequently, the result and content of a court decision hinge on the expert opinion of the medical witnesses on whose assistance the judge also has to depend. Yet in isolated cases it has occurred that decisions have been made against the unanimous opinion of the medical witnesses. All these remarks still apply today.

The medical witnesses are asked questions that are phrased in a more or less haphazard manner to give an expert opinion as to the causality between the actions and omissions of the accused physician and the alleged bodily injury. They are equally requested to state whether culpable negligence is involved. It would appear quite obvious that the medical witness would prefer to deal with the problem of causality. After all, this question is prevalently linked with scientific and medical problems. Experience, however, shows to our surprise that in practice the reverse usually occurs. Often the medical witnesses make comprehensive comments on whether and why the physician on trial failed to use the care required in his business, or that, and then why not, this was not the case. The much more important question of causality that should be explored with priority does not receive the attention it deserves.

Frequently no comments are given at all. If comments are made on the causality relationship they are often unequivocal, not understandable for those who have to make the decisions, i. e. predominantly for the lawyer, and by no means indicate whether or why such a causality relationship must be accepted or rejected from the medical viewpoint.

If I correctly interpret the results of the questionnaire campaign with regard to the medical facts which are only hinted at - and to the alleged fault in the sense of neglecting to undertake something (an operation or another measure) or in taking faulty action (an operation), in cases in which there is no causal relationship between the alleged bodily injury and the action of the neurosurgeon or his assistants may well account for a considerable portion. However, if no causality exists, the questions of negligence need no longer be explored. With regard to this particular consequence I wish to recommend to potential providers of expert advice that they pay added attention to the appraisal of the question of causality.

On reviewing the material of the last 10 years, I, too, find complaints referring to intracranial operations and various complications, to slipped disc surgery leading to paraplegia, cardiac arrest, death due tu cardiovascular failure, to embolism of a mesenteric artery with undetected perforation of the small intestine, to a cauda equina syndrome, nerve root injury and paralysis of the peripheral nerves. However, the lesions to the central nervous system caused by surgery are not fewer in number than complaints about damage following injections or punctures in the neighbourhood of the central nervous system, although these latter are not exclusively or predominantly directed against neurosurgeons. A series of complications developed for example after paravertebral injections. After peridural anaesthesia, myelography and suboccipital puncture, various neurological complications have been observed. What strikes me, is the fact that in the answers given in the questionnaires no sequelae were mentioned as having developed after angiography, sequelae which frequently occur in my case material.

Taking into account the numerous questions of your inquiry, let me now add some fundamental, and I hope, practice-related comments on the problems linked with the physician's duty to inform the patient about his condition. In numerous liability claims the plaintiff accuses the doctor of "malpractice" without giving concrete details of the basis of the claim. Such claims are mostly motivated by the discontent with the results of treatment in a variety of different respects, but not infrequently by a misunderstood, confusing or even an ill-considered remark made by a colleague providing after-treatment. An allegation of "malpractice" does not a priori justify a claim for damages, for not every "malpractice" is the consequence of a culpable action, just as the omittance of the care required in the course of usual business cannot or need not necessarily be called "malpractice". The term "malpractice" is irrevelant legally, and therefore it is better to avoid it. In disputes associated with liability claims made against the physician it is often possible readily to show that the damage has not been caused by culpable negligence or that there is no proof of negligence. In such cases the plaintiff resorts to the allegation that the practitioner failed in his duty to provide him with full information about his case. However, a medical intervention without indication and without consent, with the latter requiring sufficient briefing on the nature and risks of the procedure to make it legally binding constitutes an unlawful bodily injury even when carried out as a medical measure. However, if it can be established that the briefing of the patient was not satisfactory and that, as a consequence, the procedure was unlawful, it is no longer of relevance that damage has been inflicted and that the practitioner acted in breach of his duties. So we can see that these legal points of view are decisive for a possible justification of liability claims which were first based on alleged "malpractice" and subsequently dropped because the rules of the art of medicine had not been violated and no culpable negligence was imputable to the doctor, simply because finally a breach of the doctor's duty to brief the patient on his condition must be assumed or even established.

Just as there are no generally accepted rules - decisions are to be made on the details of each individual case - that establish whether a specific complication was caused by the culpable action of a physician, there are likewise no generally binding rules governing a doctor's obligation to brief his patient concerning a specific medical procedure. Here again all depends exclusively on the facts of an individual case as to what extent the doctor is under obligation to inform his patient about the character of and hazards involved in a planned operation. In my view, we should be wary of laying down any set of rigid rules or drawing up catalogues concerning a doctor's duty to brief his patient. Such an approach would or could do more harm than good in each individual case since members of the legal profession are only all too willing to comply with such regulations without subjecting the case to closer examination and to regard them as a medical "law" susceptible to extended application.

The general criteria laid down in a recent decision of the Supreme Federal Court of Germany of February 12th,1974 on the purpose of the doctor's obligation to brief his patient by and large on the nature and risks of an intervention and at least on what action is planned for him must nowadays be regarded as generally accepted. The above mentioned court decision deals with the doctor's obligation to brief the patient in connection with a peridural anaesthesia for a non-urgent stomach operation with ensuing paraplegia alleged to have been caused by culpable negligence for which no evidence existed.

A physician is duty bound by a particularly urgent obligation to instruct the patient in the event of non-urgently and non-vitally indicated interventions, with the demands of the obligation to instruct the patient being most stringent in cosmetic surgery. The law also insists on a more detailed instruction of the patient, also in diagnostic procedures (e. g. angiography) in contrast to therapeutic measures, when the latter are chiefly intended to eliminate an acute state of disease. More detailed information has to be given to the patient on rather more drastic diagnostic measures, whenever other possible examination methods are available but have not been fully utilized, even though such alternative procedures cannot be expected to provide the same significant findings as the more radical diagnostic examination. In accordance with the comments contained in the Supreme Federal Court decision of February 12th,1974 it would appear to be unimportant whether the contracting partner of the patient (head physician or surgeon) instructs the patient personally or whether one of his assistants (senior physician, interns etc.) performs

the task. The instruction must be given to the person who has to give
the legally binding consent for the operation to be carried out. The
problem of the doctor's obligation towards the patient's dependants
results usually from a confusion with the "medical pledge of secrecy".

Concrete information about the doctor's obligation to instruct the patient in neurosurgery and an answer to most of your questions about
this point is, in my opinion, contained in a decision of the Federal
Supreme Court of June 22nd, 1971. This decision deals with the requirements to be satisfied by the doctor in instructing the patient himself
or his legal representative in conjunction with a planned diagnostic
examination, i. e. a cerebellar arteriography with puncture of the
vertebral artery.

As, on account of the symptoms which a sixteen-year-old girl presented,
a brain tumor was suspected, cerebral arteriography was planned. The
mother of the patient (her father was dead) signed prior to the operation a form saying: "I herewith confirm that I am agreeable to the
filling with air of the cerebral spaces (encephalography), arteriography of the brain, myelography, to an insulin electro or cardiazol
permeation treatment to be carried out on my daughter".

After a carotid arteriography first on the right and 3 days later on
the left side it was planned to perform arteriography of the vertebral artery 4 days later. When the puncture was attempted, a large
effusion of blood occurred so that the injection had to be interrupted.
On the next morning the patient was found to be suffering from a hemiplegia of the left side.

The question of causality between the medical act and the hemiplegia
was not resolved by the regional court of appeal, which at first re-
pudiated the accusation. All the courts concerned with the case ruled
that there was no evidence of culpable negligence.

There was no need to examine the claim that a consent of the almost
17-year old patient was required in addition to that of her mother,
because it appeared inadmissible to assume negligence if the clinic
or the attending doctors had not shared this opinion.

However, the Federal Court took the view that the consent of the
mother to carry out the intervention fell short of meeting the requirements of effectiveness established by law.

The Federal Court stated that an informed consent of the patient or
his legal representative requires that the person concerned be fully
informed as to the nature of the intervention.

When the courts required the prior instruction of the patient it is
with the intention to create these prerequisites. The patient should
be informed about the intended intervention in a manner commensurate
with his level of understanding so that he knows more or less what
he is agreeing to. Such objective instruction may, under certain
circumstances, also include a hint as to the possibility of uninten-
tional sequential damage attendant upon the intervention and not reliably avoidable by the exercise of medical skill, damage more or less
likely to occur, but not readily evident to a layman on account of
the nature of the intervention.

In the case underlying the sentence, one has to assume from the evidence presented that the question asked by the mother as to which of
the measures listed in the form would be taken had been answered eva-

sively by the defendant who said that all these measures were inter-connected. Also the question as to whether the planned treatment might be associated with an element of risk, was unreservedly denied. As a result of her lack of medical knowledge, the patient's mother had been unable to form an opinion of the individual measures mentioned.

The Supreme Federal Court emphasizes that the mention of remote complications is imperative whenever the intervention does not warrant definite expectations of healing or even the saving of the patient's life. In this context the Court pointed out that the Supreme Judge's findings are no longer dependent upon rigid percentages of the un-desired incidents observed so far but that it would be disquieting to belittle the possible hazards of such an operation simply because 186 cases of vertebral angiography had been carried out without com-plications in the hospital concerned.

It must be said, however, that even a diagnostic measure might acquire serious urgency with respect to the prospects of healing which the diagnosis may reveal.

In the present case there was a definite possibility that the sus-pected tumor would be accessible to surgery. Even in such a situation the pros and cons of a procedure must be explained in an appropriate manner in the course of instructing the patient because particularly in such instances, the medical layman usually cannot be expected to have an immediate appreciation of the situation. With regard to the way in which the patient is to be informed about the risk of possible incidents, a wide margin can be given to the physician's discretion. If the procedure of the arterial filling had been explained so vivid-ly that she would have been able to judge the intervention as a rather serious one, then the true reference to the long series of complica-tion-free cases would have been sufficient. However, by no means would it have been admissible flatly to deny the explicit question as to whether anything might go wrong.

The scepticism or even aversion exhibited by a large number of phy-sicians with regard to the problems associated with the physician's obligation to tell the patient the truth about his condition mainly originates from the difficulties lawyers and physicians experience in communicating with one another. The physician feels himself to be hedged in by legal regulations which he deems restrictive on his free-dom of action and basically obstructive to his desire to help and heal, both in general and in a particular individual case. He fears that the information of the patient could prompt him not to subject himself to necessary and mostly complication-free medical measures, and thus to reject the existing possibilities of healing.

The instruction of the patient is a must for legal reasons, but is also probably indispensible for medical reasons as well, provided the patient is prepared to recognize the necessity of proposed mea-sures. It is not necessary that the instruction given to the patient be viewed merely from the legal point of view, it can also be affirm-ed on a strictly medical basis and deemed justifiable, too. By strip-ping the medical obligation to tell the patient the truth about a planned procedure, of its legal relevance, it may also be easier for the physician to find the right words in his talk with the patient. Formalized consents are not enough, however, well-meant and well-phrased they might be. Nor is it sufficient to describe a medical measure to the patient in technical terms, which he will hardly ever understand. In your medical work it is certainly also of decisive importance for you to know that particularly the central nervous system, the brain and the spinal cord are absolutely unknown, almost mystical subjects to a normal patient. The layman's knowledge about bone nailing is certainly better than his knowledge about a cerebral ventricle drainage, hypophysectomy or an operation for a slipped disc.

The frequently heard demand that the patient should say what he wants to know and indicate what he wants explained to him leaves out of account the fact that most patients do not dare ask questions either because they think the gap between themselves and the doctor is insurmountable or because they do not feel they would be able to cope with such a talk intellectually, or because they have no idea what they should ask.

It was a lawyer (Bockelmann) who once requested the physician to adhere to the so-called golden rule with regard to their obligation to instruct the patient on his case. According to this rule, one should not expect another to endure what one does not wish to have to endure himself. Consequently, a physician should not expect the patient to endure what he would not like to have happen to himself were he the patient.

In connection with the problems of the doctor's duty to instruct his patient, the legal aspects stand to the fore. Medical actions are subjected to these within the legal framework and are assessed in the light of legally founded norms developed by jurisdiction whenever claims for damages are made. This principle holds despite the fact that the particular activity of a doctor as a surgeon and the special doctor/patient relationship make it difficult, if not impossible, to press the medical activities into rigid norms and to use them as a yardstick in measuring the medical result.

The requirement of medical care and especially those involving the doctor's obligation to instruct the patient have certainly been tightened by law. The fact that, as result from my analysis of 2,330 complaints about physicians, simple actions of the medical routine, complications in connection with injections, burns and heat injuries, nervous disturbances following therapeutic interventions, particularly in patient positioning for surgery, falls in connection with medical manipulations and finally blood sampling prevail as opposed to complications associated with differentiated procedures, such as special undertakings withing the scope of actual surgery, points to human shortcomings rather than to inadequate skill or knowledge. To learn the lessons from these very facts, even if my comments may have been commonplace to some of you, then you should at least view these problems in a new perspective.

Malpractice Liability in Neurosurgery

H. KROPPEN

This subject cannot be discussed comprehensively and exhaustively in the time available to me today. Nor is it possible to give to this paper a specific slant applicable to the area of neurosurgery. The principles governing medical malpractice are equally applicable to all medical specialties. Under these conditions the present paper cannot do more than provide a rough picture, somewhat like a wood engraving, of the generally applicable principles of malpractice law, based in particular on the presently existing legal precedents.

We speak of malpractice liability when a patient sues a physician for damages resulting from physical injury caused by erroneous treatment or failure to provide treatment on the part of the physician.

As a rule a suit for damages against a physician will be based on the provisions on damages for unlawful acts in accordance with Section 823 of the German Civil Code (Bürgerliches Gesetzbuch). This section provides that damages shall be paid by anyone who "unlawfully, with premeditation or through negligence, caused injury to life, limb or health of another person".

In examining whether damages are due from an unlawful act a lawyer will proceed in a certain sequence by subdividing this provision of the law into its components:

Are the facts of an unlawful act in evidence, or, more precisely speaking: did the physician commit an act which resulted in injury to the patient?

If so, was the physician's act unlawful or was the physician acting with justification?

If this is answered in the affirmative, too: did the physician act wrongfully, i. e. with negligence or premeditation?

The physician will be liable for damages only if every single one of these conditions has been satisfied.

Consequently, we must first examine whether there is factual evidence of an unlawful act. This will be the case if any action on the part of the physician resulted in bodily injury. The physician's action can also consist of an omission such as omitting a necessary physical examination, necessary treatment, necessary referral to a specialist, etc. Bodily injury is defined not only as an operation performed on the body; rather, bodily injury may be any worsening of the patient's physical condition, and this includes even slight pain or merely nausea or weakness on the part of the patient. Moreover, bodily injury will have been caused when the patient's condition is not worsened but remains the same or is even improved, provided that the patient's bodily integrity has suffered interference, i. e. that only certain examinations have been made or radiation treatment given. It is already seen from the preceeding information that there must be a cause-and-effect relationship between the action or omission of the physician and the bodily injury that was caused. Where the bodily injury, regardless of type, has not been caused by the physician's behaviour but was due to any cause other than the physician's behaviour, the physician cannot be held liable because the so-called liability-substantiating causality between the physician's behaviour and bodily injury has not been established. Consequently, in order to show grounds for liability at all, the physician's behaviour must have been an indispensable condition for the bodily injury caused. However, if any indispensable condition of this type would constitute grounds for liability, this might lead to an insufferable expansion of malpractice liability. Consequently, in civil law - unlike the more extensive equivalence theory of criminal law - the cause-and-effect relationship which is relevant with respect to the liability has been limited by the so-called adequacy theory. This provides that only that condition shall be significant which has an adequate relationship to the result. Any cause - in this case: the physician's behaviour - will be eliminated as a causative condition if, as a result of its general nature, it was insignificant to the injuries received, causing it only as a result of a quite exceptional chain of circumstances which is beyond all probability. This means that the physician's behaviour which is to be judged must be such as to cause the bodily injury under normal circumstances, not merely under specific, peculiar, improbable conditions which would not be taken into consideration under the normal course of events. Consequently, those circumstances will not be taken into consideration which, although an indispensable condition for the injury, have caused it only as a result of an unfortunate chain of events. Therefore, it is not a purely statistical or percentage improbability which is considered because this would involve the expectation of injury, although with low probability. In medical malpractice there is bound to be almost always an adequate causality of the type to provide grounds for liability. There is greater significance in the problem of an adequate chain of events within the scope of causality to provide grounds for liability which I shall discuss below.

Consequently, we can state that any medical examination or treatment measure which represents only the slightest interference with the patients's bodily integrity will be material fact of a bodily injury and hence material fact of an unlawful act.

However, in order to provide grounds for liability on the part of a physician the additional condition must be satisfied that the physician acted unlawfully when he performed the actions in question.

In principle the law assumes that any act which is part of material fact is also unlawful; in that case it is said that the unlawful nature of the act is indicated. Hence, the practical examination must determine whether the physician had justification for the bodily injury which has been determined to be a material fact. The physician's treatment, that is the bodily injury, will be justified if it took place with the effective consent of the patient. This consent can be effective only if it was preceeded by comprehensive information to the patient which in turn will be lawful only if it is based on an examination of the patient. Consequently, the effective consent of a patient is the basic prerequisite for considering the physician's actions justified. Treatment without the patient's consent will be grounds for damages even if the physician was not guilty of malpractice (Federal Supreme Court Insurance Citations 1960, page 57). However, it should be mentioned in passing that any examination of the injury caused must include the question as to whether the patient suffered injury at all when treatment which had not been approved by the patient was in fact successful.

In principle the patient's consent will be necessary for any treatment measure, even every-day or routine treatment. Medical practice often violates this requirement, for instance where the physician asks his patient to turn around and performs an injection without further discussion, where he performs radiation treatment and the like. The assumption that the patient has sufficient confidence in his physician to follow his judgement is justified only under exceptional circumstances where the patient has stated this expressly and without ambiguity in the sense of a general power of attorney. However, as a rule there will be reservations with respect to the effectiveness of such a general power of attorney under the aspect that this must have been preceeded by such comprehensive information, which we shall discuss later, that the patient is fully aware of the consequences of such a general consent. On the other hand the patient's consent need not be declared expressly; rather, it will frequently result from circumstances and from the patient's overall behaviour, as the Federal Supreme Court (Neue Juristische Wochenschrift 1961, p. 261) found in deciding a case where a patient knew that the physician felt it was indicated to place a pin to correct a thigh fracture and suffered the preparations for the operation without any objection. From this failure to voice any objection the physician was justified in concluding the patient's consent.

The situation becomes problematic in all those instances where the patient's consent cannot be obtained because the patient cannot express his will.

Where the patient has a legal guardian for his personal affairs (in the case of minors this will be the parents, the guardian, or the custodian) it will be necessary apart from great emergencies, that a guardian be appointed by the local magistrate's court to decide on the patient's consent (Federal Supreme Court 29, p. 46). If the emergency is such that the patient's consent or that of his legal guardian, or that of a guardian appointed by the court is no longer possible, a necessary medical intervention will be lawful without consent provided that the physician may assume that consent would be given. In making this decision the physician may assume that the patient would agree to medical measures which are absolutely necessary. In case of doubt the physician will be required to learn the patient's presumable intentions by questioning the patient's nearest relatives. Of course, where the situation endangers the patient's life the physician will not be required to make further inquiries. The Federal Supreme Court has held in the question as to whether consent of a minor will suffice or whether that of his parents will be required must be judged under the principle whether the minor, considering his mental and moral maturity, is able to understand the significance and consequences of the act of medical intervention and of granting his consent thereto (Federal Supreme Court 29, p. 33). This decision was given in the case of a thyroid operation on a 20 year old man.

However, the prerequisite for effective consent is always that the patient or any other person authorized to grant consent is at least aware of the significant features of the type, significance and possible consequences of the medical intervention which is contemplated

(Federal Supreme Court 29, p. 176; Neue Juristische Wochenschrift 1963, p. 393). This means that the physician must adequately inform the patient. It is especially this point which often gives rise to differences of opinion so that a majority of medical malpractice suits centers on this problem of adequate information to the patient. Adequate information includes, first, information on the type of treatment contemplated which, however, need not be described in every detail. In addition, the physician must also explain to the patient the side effects of the treatment and advise as to the typical hazards which must be expected under the present state of the art in medicine and science. The scope of this information may be smaller if the danger is more remote and if the danger to be feared is less significant with respect to the consequences which would result if the treatment were not performed. Where the patient as the result of his education - doctor, medical student, nurse - is better able to understand the nature of the medical intervention, the possible hazards and the side effects, the information provided by the physician need not be as thorough as in other cases.

The duty to inform the patient also exists in those cases where the possibility can be expected that the patient would refuse consent to necessary treatment if he were given exhaustive information. However, the duty to inform the patient terminates where to provide the patient with such information would result in a serious hazard to the patient's life or health or where the success of the treatment could be considerably endangered (Federal Supreme Court 29, p. 46; p. 176; insurance law 1956, p. 406). In these cases the physician may take those measures which are in the patient's objective interest and his presumed general intent. To learn this intent may require consultation with the nearest relatives in the individual instance.

A special subject in this connection are those cases where an extension or change of a planned operation turns out to be necessary only during the operation, or where complications of any type are encountered.

In the latter case it will always involve complications which are not necessarily involved in the medical intervention but where on the basis of medical experience it must be expected that they will occur, such as major hemorrhages, heart or circulatory failure etc. Here the physician can base his judgement on the result desired by the patient, regularly assuming that the elimination of these complications will be approved by the patient.

The true cases of extending or changing the scope of an operation, however, are different:

1. The necessity or even the possibility of a change or extention in scope was recognized even prior to the operation. Here the general principles applicable to any medical intervention must be applied, meaning that the patient be informed of the recognized possibility of extention of scope including any hazards or side effects, followed by the patient's consent and then by the proper execution of the operation. Even where the diagnosis is still uncertain to the physician or where the diagnosis can be acquired only on the basis of the operation itself, the patient must be informed so that he will give the physician the required consent.

2. If the change in the operation plan is not medically indicated but is based upon an erroneous evaluation of the situation during the operation, such additional operative action will constitute grounds

for malpractice so that the general principles of medical malpractice apply. The decisive aspect with respect to the physician's liability is whether this malpractice was wrongful or not.

3. The legal situation is also clear in the case of premeditated unauthorized treatment where the physician deliberately disregards the patient's opposing will. Here it is insignificant whether the physician was guilty of malpractice; the decisive aspect is that the patient's consent was lacking. The Federal Supreme Court (Federal Supreme Court, Neue Juristische Wochenschrift 59, p. 2299) has provided the precedent in this respect: the patient's physician and a specialist consulted as an associate at the request of the patient who suffered from an eye ailment had jointly established a plan for treatment for the injured eye. Deviating from this plan which had provided for conservative treatment, the patient's physician in the absence and without the knowledge of his colleague performed vitreous suction which resulted in blindness.

This type of case, however, also includes those instances where the operator erroneously and with negligence performs an operation on the wrong organ. Example (Frankenthal Circuit Court, Neue Juristische Wochenschrift 55, p. 1113): a patient is admitted for operation with the physician's diagnosis "left-sided hernia". The operator failed to recognize the hernia on the left side and operated on an incipient hernia which he had diagnosed on the right side ("soft inguinal region"). After the patient's discharge his physician again diagnosed a hernia on the left side so that another operation was necessary. The court held that the first operation constituted unlawful bodily injury.

4. Moreover, we must cite those cases where the extension or change of the operation planned had not been contemplated by the physician but should have been recognized as necessary if the physician had exercised care. This is almost always due to poor examination techniques, inadequate examination techniques or a malpractice diagnosis so that the fact of malpractice can be already established in the examination stage. In the event of inadequate or faulty examination it follows that the patient cannot be informed adequately so that his consent, although it may be formally given, will be ineffective because the patient was unable to recognize the consequences of his consent as a result of inadequate information. However, it should be noted that the wrongful erroneous diagnosis alone constitutes grounds for damages. In addition the precedents often hold that the lack of consent which was due to the wrongful diagnosis may be used as an auxiliary argument. However, that the latter consideration is insignificant and that it is important to consider all the possibilities which may result during an operation, based on medical experience, is shown by the following case: a patient had consented in the operative removal of a tumor of the uterus which had double the size of a fist. During the operation it turned out that due to adhesions its removal was possible only by removing the entire uterus. The physician performed the extended operation. The Federal Supreme Court held that the operation constituted unlawful bodily injury, but not in that the total removal itself was unlawful, since the physician could have assumed that the patient would consent to it, but rather the fact that the physician had neglected to acquire the patient's consent to the extended operation as a possibility which had to be foreseen.

5. What shall the phycician do in those cases where a necessary extension or change of the operation plan could not be foreseen prior to the operation even when exercising due care, meaning that the

physician was not guilty of wrongful malpractice up to his discovery
during the operation? The problem here is what a physician must do in
order to avoid liability.

If the extension of scope or change in the operation is absolutely
necessary to avoid a direct hazard to the patient's life the physician is not only justified but even required to take the measures
necessary to avoid such hazards unless he is expressly aware that the
patient's intentions are opposed. For the patient, and this should be
noted here, is not required to let himself be treated, healed or to
allow his life being saved.

When the extension of scope is not required to prevent a hazard to
life but to avoid significant danger to health the physician will also be authorized to extend the scope of an operation. Where an acute
danger of slight damage to health exists the physician must weigh the
risk of the extended scope of the operation against the consequences
of omission, again basing his decision on the presumable intentions
of an intelligent patient.

The situation becomes doubtful where the extension of scope or change
is absolutely necessary but where no acute danger is involved. Again
the law resolves this case on the basis of the provisions governing
agency of necessity by focusing on the true interest and the real or
presumable intentions of the patient. The Federal Supreme Court (Federal Supreme Court 29, p. 46) assumes in this case that "a patient
seeing his physician or going to a hospital to seek assistance for his
ailment will often be prepared to consent to medical intervention of
certain scope which is a prerequisite for regaining his health". As
a result, cases have been decided in the physician's favor where, on
the occasion of an abdominal operation a diseased appendix was to be
removed and the scope of the operation changed to include the necessary removal of a gall bladder. The greater the scope of a necessary
operation of which the patient was not advised the less can the physician presume that the patient would grant his consent, for instance
in the case of the operative removal of a breast or the total removal
of a uterus. Yet the criteria used in legal precedents, "reasonable
interest" and "presumable intentions of a reasonable patient" provide
the physician with relatively great scope. Where the extension of
scope of an operation is not very great so that organs of great importance are not involved, a "reasonable patient" will not normally
demand that the suture first be closed and the patient awakened from
his anesthesia in order to be operated again after obtaining his consent. Another aspect of a certain significance may be what operative
procedure will cause the greater treatment cost to the patient. In
addition, any change or expansion of scope of an operation plan are
not allowable if there is a possibility of achieving a cure by some
other means.

Consequently, the treatment or operation must be based on the patient's consent, preceded by adequate information provided by the
physician. That this information in turn can be proper only after
the physician has adequately examined the patient would certainly
not require explanation. However, this examination in turn requires
the patient's consent and explanations as to the type of examination,
its hazards and possible consequences. Of course, the requirements
to be imposed here will be the greater the more complicated the examination technique and the greater the intervention into the patient's physical integrity as a result of the examination. Consequently there is no principle at any stage of treatment which would justify the physician to do anything necessary in his medical judgement

on the basis of the treatment contract and his patient's confidence
alone.

Individual problems on the subject of justification or consent, especially as to who is required to obtain information and consent, shall
be discussed at the end of this paper.

In any event the patient's consent will never extend to the point
where it can cover any measure on the part of the physician which is
not within the state of the art. Of course the patient will not agree
to any axamination or treatment which are not in accordance with the
rules of medical art. In the event of malpractice, therefore, it will
be a foregone conclusion that it is never justified by consent. An
exception would apply only in the case where the physician, because
conventional treatment methods have failed to yield results, advises
the patient that he intends a treatment measure not within the state
of the art and the patient does consent to this specific case.

Where the legal examination up to this point has established that
material fact of bodily injury does in fact exist which is not justifiable and, consequently, unlawful, the next point to be investigated
is whether the physician is culpable in causing this unlawful bodily
injury, meaning that he must bear responsibility for the injury. A
person is responsible for premeditated or negligent actions, and here
only the latter case is of interest. The law provides that a person
will be negligent if he neglects to take due care required in every-
day business activities. This means that the law uses an objective,
abstract criterium, that of due care necessary in every-day business
affairs, for which a few principles exist - primarily the recognized
rules of medical standards - but which in the final analysis must be
determined by the peculiarities of the individual instance. It should
be emphasized that the law does not speak of usual care but of the
necessary care so that the physician cannot use the usual care of his
field as the yeardstick when this would be equivalent to generally
widespread carelessness.

Therefore, the examination of responsibility must center on the due
care which must be exercised by the physician and which is in part
established through the recognized rules of medical practice, a violation of which would constitute malpractice. The question as to when
malpractice is established when a physician has taken the necessary
care, cannot be answered with general applicability even through a
lengthy statement. As we have it so often, it depends on the individual case. Therefore, we shall cite only a few, necessarily quite
general principles established through legal precedents. A physician
will not act wrongfully if he uses conventional treatment recommended
in the textbooks and he will be covered even if he adheres to a minor-
ity opinion, provided that it is supported by important representa-
tives of medical science. It is required of the physician that he
has studied the applicable medical literature. Consequently, he will
violate his requirement to exercise due care if he decides on a
dangerous method of treatment because he is unaware of treatment
possibilitiés involving a lesser risk which have been discussed in
professional circles. On the other hand, he is also required to select
that treatment which promises the best success, and here it may be
necessary to weigh the risk against the chances of success. The physician must support his diagnosis by examinations such as X-rays and
laboratory tests which are required under the yardstick of due care.
Of course, here as in other possibilities of medical malpractice the
requirements imposed on the physician's care must not be excessive;
rather, a type of relatively principle applies here. The primary

criterium is that which appears reasonable and possible in order to safeguard the patient's interest, not that wich is customary. Even where it is not customary in wide circles of the medical specialty concerned to take certain precautionary measures, this will not necessarily constitute justification for the individual physician to neglect such care, too. Carelessness will remain carelessness even if it is practiced by an entire profession. Carelessness in most instances is also the cause for leaving a foreign body in an operation wound. For the physician is required to take all reasonable care to prevent such an occurence. This can be accomplished by preventing the instruments required for the operation from disappearing in the operation wound, by recording the number of instruments in order to verify their presence prior to closing the wound, etc. In individual instances this may be practically impossible in the case of very difficult operations, of unforeseen complications and the like. In that case the requirement of "bookkeeping" must take second place to the specific necessary measures of the operation. As a result there are a number of precedents where it was held that leaving foreign bodies in an operation wound must not necessarily be medical malpractice; rather, it depends on the special circumstances of the individual case such as nature and size of the foreign body and the events of the operation (thus the legal principle established by the Federal Supreme Court in LM No. 1 on Sec. 276 (Ca), German Civil Code). On the other hand the physician is not allowed to neglect a safety measure simply for the reason that this measure would involve a certain inconvenience or loss of time. This applies even where the measure in question is not usually practiced because of such inconvenience or loss of time (Federal Supreme Court Volume 8, p. 138).

Malpractice can also be established when a physician or a hospital arrive at the limits of their therapeutic capabilities in the treatment of a patient, be it because quite specialized skills are unavailable, be it because specialized examination or treatment facilities are not available, and where, in spite of being aware of this fact, the patient was not transferred to an appropriately equipped physician or hospital but his treatment was continued. Similar to medical malpractice is a violation of the supervisory duties which are imposed on the physician with respect to his subordinate medical and non-medical personnel. Here the physician in charge must convince himself through regular spotchecks that these persons operate properly and in accordance with the state of the art in medical science.

In summary, let me repeat this: the physician will be liable for damages only if he has committed an unlawful act - in this case bodily injury -, if he acted unlawfully, that is without justification, and if he is responsible for this unlawful act because he bears the responsibility. Only when these three prerequisites are satisfied can teh doctor be required under Section 823 of the German Civil Code "to pay damages to the other person".

What is covered by the concept of injuries for which the physician must pay damages? The physician is required to pay damages only for those injuries which have a certain causative connection with the act of which he is accused. I already outlined in the first part of my paper that the first requirement is a causative connection between the physician's behaviour - the erroneous or omitted treatment - and the direct violation of a legal right - the bodily injury. An example: the extraction of a tooth, which in itself was required but omitted results directly in the painful inflamation of the tooth in question. This step in the chain of causality is considered grounds for liability. The physician could have avoided to initiate the causality chain which is grounds for liability so that it can be held against him. The examination of this stage of the chain of causality was practically the entire subject up to this point of the present paper. However, the bodily injury resulting from it is only the first, direct result of injury with which may cause additional injury such as the necessity of another operation, additional loss of earnings, additional treatment cost, reduction of earning capability and the like. The patient can demand damages for these secondary injuries only if another causative connection exists between the first resulting injury - bodily injury - and the additional damages claimed, that is the so-called liability-supporting causality. The responsible person will be liable for these additional consequences of injury which are included in the overall injury as a result of liability-supporting causality even if he did not cause these additional consequences directly, meaning that the second stage of the once initiated chain of causality was unavoidable.

However, liability on the grounds of liability-supporting causality cannot be stretched to cover infinite scope. It would go too far to hold the physician responsible even for completely unforeseeable, atypical consequences purely due to fate which result from his infringement. The precedents and the existing law impose limits, at least in civil law, on the basis of the so-called adequacy theory. This rule of the adequacy of cause allows only that behaviour as grounds for the consequences of injury which appeared generally suitable to objectively cause the injury at the time of the infringing action; or, expressed in the negative: the injury which resulted must not have been beyond the bounds of all probability. The Federal Supreme Court in part modified these principles in holding that additional considerations must be applied: the court limited the causative connection in that considerations of reasonable cause must be applied. The court held that the limit must be determined to which it is reasonable for the responsible person to accept liability for the consequences of an act under reasonable evaluation of the circumstances (Federal Supreme Court Vol. 3, p. 261; Vol. 18, p. 286; Koblenz Circuit Court, Insurance Law 1959, p. 541).

Two examples shall be cited to demonstrate this boundary: if a patient suffering from an accident injury is admitted to a hospital, infected with influenza there, and dies from the influenza infection, his death will be the adequate consequence of the bodily injury sustained (Reich Supreme Court Vol. 105, p. 264).

Second Case

The physician performing treatment at first falsely diagnoses muscular cramps and lockjaw after the extraction of a tooth and takes the appropriate treatment. As a result an abscess in the cheek which was actually present is treated too late. It is only after opening this abscess that indications are found for an abscess of the brain which is is fact found to exist. In this case the Federal Supreme Court (Bundesgerichtshof, Insurance Law 1965, p. 583) held that there was no causality between the wrongful diagnosis and the development of the brain abscess but rather that this involved the regular process of an illness which could not be avoided.

The foregoing shall suffice as a brief review of malpractice liability within the scope of the "unlawful act". It should be emphasized that the physician will become liable only if all the prerequisites mentioned up to this point have been met. Of course, this is still subject to a great variety of individual problems, some of which I shall discuss now.

One important problem in a malpractice suit is regularly the question as to the burden of proof, that is the question who must prove that the prerequisites required for liability have been met. In principle the victim must prove both, the action which caused the injury, that is the physician's wrongful behaviour, and the causality of this wrongful behaviour with respect to the injury sustained. However, there are exceptions to this rule, especially in malpractice law.

These concern, first, the application of the principles of the so-called "proof of apparent guilt". These provide that, initially, prima facie, it is considered adequate proof that the facts in evidence typically indicate that the material fact concerned would be established under general experience. It is then up to the opposite party to disprove this by substantiating the facts proving the serious possibility of an atypical course of events, casting doubt upon the prima facie evidence. If the opponent succeeds in this undertaking, prima facie proof will be discarded and the party on whom the burden of proof rests, that is the victim, must then furnish his proof by some other means. In malpractice law the principles of apparent proof are applicable in two types of situations:

1. The physician is guilty of an error in medical treatment which, based on medical experience, will typically cause the injury sustained. If this is the case, it is presumed that causality exists between the established treatment error and the injury sustained.

2. Following medical treatment an injury is sustained which, based on medical experience, would be typically due to a wrongful treatment error. In that case it is presumed that a treatment error on the part of the physician did cause the injury sustained.

Examples: A patient is placed in the same hospital room with another patient suffering from scarlet fever and contracts the disease (Reich Supreme Court Vol. 165, p. 336). If a physician gives an unknown patient a highly effective intravenous injection of morphine without first examining the patient for any illness where the application of narcotics or at least their intravenous application is subject to reservations, the prima facie conclusion will be justified that an injury sustained was due to the failure to perform an examination (Federal Supreme Court, Neue Juristische Wochenschrift 1959, p. 1583). If a patient during dental treatment swallows an injection needle, the principles of apparent proof allow the conclusion that the dentist was at fault (Federal Supreme Court Vol. 8, p. 135).

The situation becomes even more difficult for the physician when the case is such that the burden of proof is reversed. We speak of a reversal of the burden of proof if it is not the victim who must prove the wrongful violation of his rights and its causality but rather that the presumably guilty party must prove that erroneous and wrongful actions did not in fact cause the injury sustained. In malpractice law the precedents assume such an inversion of the burden of proof with respect to the actions that caused the injury, when a physician wrongfully committed a gross error in treatment which was such that the actually sustained injury of the patient could have been caused by it. In that case the physician bears the full burden of proof to show that the injury was not due to his error.

It will be easier to furnish proof if the physician obtained a written statement from his patient to the effect that the patient was adequately informed and granted his consent. In many instances a printed form alone will not suffice for this purpose since the statement, especially in the case of very serious operations, must show the detail in which information was given to the patient and on which the patient's consent was based, if such a statement is to have any value at all. This means that the statement should also include the aspect that the physician pointed out possible serious side effects and hazards or the possibility of an extension of the operation plan, including the nature of this possible extension. The patient's relatives, however, will be involved in this duty on the part of the physician only where it is one of the cases mentioned above where the patient's consent cannot be obtained or where the relatives are the patient's legal guardians.

Problems with respect to the boundaries of the physician's duties and, hence, the scope of his liability, will arise where several physicians are involved in the arise where severeal physicians are involved in the treatment.

Where several physicians treat a patient, each independently in his own specialty, each of these physicians must perform the examination with respect to his specialized area and must inform the patient as far as his specialty is concerned. Where these physicians treat the patient consecutively, for instance referral from the family doctor to a specialist, the latter cannot depend on the family physician's findings where they fall into his specialty, while, inversely, the general practitioner can normally accept the findings of a specialist. Where an operating team under the direction of one physician is involved, each member of this team will act independently and in his own responsibility as far as his specialty is concerned, but the overall responsibility must be borne by the head of the team who is liable not only fro the proper composition of the team, the careful preparation of the operation plan, and the effective control of the interaction of all persons involved in the operation, but is also responsible to see that the required information is given to the patient on each partial aspect of the operation and that the patient's full consent has been obtained.

One special legal problem may arise with respect to the liability of the anesthesist. The fact that anesthesiology in its present form is a relatively new science and that, moreover, there is a shortage of anesthesists everywhere, explains that fixed rules with respect to anesthesists do not yet exist. It would transcend the scope of the present paper to even mention all the ramifications and boundary problems involved here. I shall merely mention this: If a hospital has an anesthesiology department headed by an anesthesiology specialist who is responsible for the pre-operative, operative or post-operative anesthesiology care of a patient, it will be in his own responsibility to take care of all the medical functions arising in his specialized field. The operating surgeon cannot give him any directives. Moreover, the anesthesist bears the sole responsibility for the proper coordination of the operation program with the other specialist. Even where the anesthesiology specialist present during the operation is not the head of the anesthesiology department but one of the subordinate medical members of that department, he will not be subject to directions from the surgeon.

If the anesthesiology specialist advises against an operation from the point of his specialty but the surgeon still performs that operation because he judges that the risk of not operating is greater than the anesthesia risk, the surgeon will have to bear the responsibility.

Where a certain operation requires a specially trained anesthesist or special anesthesiological equipment, and where neither are available at the hospital in question, this deficiency cannot justify the operation; rather, the patient will have to be referred to another hospital which is adequately equipped in this respect.

Up to this point we have discussed only the physician's liability arising from the so-called "wrongful act". This liability exists independently of any contractual relationships which may exist between physician and patient so that its principles apply in any case of medical treatment. In addition, however, there is also the physician's liability arising from a contract if a contract has in fact been established between him and the patient.

As a rule the contractual relationships between physician and patient are established by a medical contract which already exists merely due to the fact that the patient sees his physician and the physician starts an examination or treatment. This is the normal form of contract in the case of a free practitioner. This contract does not require any written document; as a rule it is concluded orally and even this not in the form of an expressed statement but merely through conclusive actions.

In the case of hospital treatment a distinction is made between three basic types of contracts:

First, we have the so-called hospital contract which is concluded between the hospital and the patient. It obligates the hospital to furnish all the services required for proper hospital treatment, including medical treatment and operations. Here the treating physician does not have any contractual relationship with the patient; he is merely the hospital's agent.

In the case of the so-called split hospital-physician's contract which is the most widespread type, the hospital is obligated to render all the services involved in the patient's care while the physician is obligated to furnish the specifically medical treatment such as diagnosis, operation, prescriptions, wound examination, etc. Consequently, contractual relationship exist on the same level with the hospital and with the physician. Here it is often difficult to draw the boundary line between the obligations of the hospital and those of the physician.

The third type is the total hospital contract with a physician's subcontract where the hospital is obligated to furnish all the patient care and medical services but where the patient, in addition, desires an especially close legal relationship with the physician employed by the hospital so that he concludes with him a physician's subcontract which obligates the hospital physician to perfrom special treatment and in turn entitles him to special compensation in addition to that given to the hospital.

Where the physician acts in the absence of a contract with his patient, for instance when a seriously injured person is unconscious so that a contract cannot be concluded, the physician's position will be that of the so-called agency of necessity. Since he is required even then to act in accordance with the patient's presumable intentions, which must be aimed at receiving proper treatment, special aspects will not normally arise from this situation.

Where a direct contractual relationship between physician and patient exists under the principles named above, the physician will be liable to the patient if he can be proved guilty of a positive infraction of the contract concluded - briefly called "positive violation of contract" or "positive violation of claim".

However, the physician's contractual obligations do not merely cover the purely medical treatment which must be up to the state of the art; rather, the physician is also required, and this on the basis of his contractual obligations, to adequately inform the patient of his plans and not to act without the patient's concent. If the physician violates these obligations in a wrongful, i. e. unlawful manner, he has committed a positive violation of contract which makes him liable for damages. This means that, practically, the same principles apply which have been described in detail when we discussed liability arising from an unlawful act, with the result that this liability arising from an unlawful act and the liability arising from breach of contract in most instances exist collaterally. The physician's contract which has been concluded also involves the obligation on the part of the physician to examine, inform, obtain the patient's consent etc. If he violates this obligation, grounds for damages require, as they do in the case of an unlawful act, that the physician was culpable for the violation. In addition the principles of liability - sustaining and liability-supporting causality, already described above, will also apply in this case.

Concerning Legal Responsibility in Neurosurgical Intensive Care Units

W. J. Bock, R. Lorenz, and B. Niedermeier

The question of the demarcation of responsibility between doctor and nursing personnel in the general sector of nursing can now be accepted as having been resolved in the following form:

Devolving on the doctor are all diagnostic and therapeutic decisions regarding the patient. Devolving on the nursing personnel, as the other hand, are the duties of nursing and tending to the patient.

In the decree of the Minister for Science and Research of the State of Nordrhein-Westfalen, dated 15.11.1973, the term "nursing personnel" is to be understood as comprising female nurses, pediatric nurses and male sick attendants. To these should be added the auxiliary female nurses and the auxiliary male nurses, who likewise must be recognized by the State.

If we take a look around in our supervision wards and intensive care units, however, we find in addition to the above a number of ancillary staff who are classified under the following designations: male and female auxiliary nurses, sick watching staff, Red Cross helpers, First Aid people, etc. i. e. persons who are not state-registered. Accordingly, what is protected is not the activity but the professional designation. These persons employed in a medical capacity attend to the nursing and care of the patients under the instructions of a doctor by virtue of the jurisdiction and of the medical professional code. In other words, there is theoretically a somewhat clear picture as regards the demarcation of the activities in a normal ward, the matter becomes problematical, however, within the context of intensive medicine. Here the demarcation between the duties of the doctor and those of the non-medical personnel is considerably more difficult. The central question is:

Is the nursing personnel allowed to give intramuscular injections, intravenous injections, infusions and transfusions as well as to take blood specimens? With respect to the legal position it must be stated in advance that there are neither laws, regulations or orders that forbid the nursing personnel to carry out these activities. Thus OPDERBECKE and WEISSAUER (10) express themselves in favour of delegating non-medical staff, within the context of intensive therapy, with the execution of diagnostic and therapeutic measures within certain limits, which, in their opinion, is in accordance with the requirements of modern medicine. The delegation of intramuscular and subcutaneous injections is not opposed in the literature as a whole. FREY (4) states in this connection that the nursing persons must have been instructed in the theory and practice during their training, that they may not give injections on their own initiative but only upon orders from the doctor. Also the puncturing of peripheral veins for the purpose of taking blood samples is regarded by all authors as well as embodied in court judgments that are accessible, as being capable of being delegated without scruple. With regard to the intravenous injections the position is otherwise, there being the possibility of the complication rate being substantially higher. OPDERBECKE and WEISSAUER (10), BRENNER (3) and LORENZ (8) agree to the giving of an intravenous injection as well as the administration of drugs via an indwelling catheter or in an infusion provided that the non-medical personnel has been instructed on the correct dosage, on the concentration, on the properties of the substance, on the rate of injection as well as on the incidence of complications. OPDERBECKE and WEISSBAUER (10) stress, however, that the direct venipuncture followed by an injection involves "some not inconsiderable danger factors", namely the paravenous injection possibly linked with pain, necrosis, vascular wall lesions, thrombosis or thrombophlebitis, which may lead to the loss of an extremity, for instance if an intra-arterial injection has been given by mistake. They therefore demand a particularly high standard of training, experience, and care in the nursing personnel. To be excepted from this arrangement, in their opinion, are patients with difficult vein conditions, as well as the administration of drugs that may cause necrosis or vascular wall lesions. The majority of authors separate the blood transfusion from the duties delegated in the above scope. OPDERBECKE and WEISSBAUER (10) regard the blood transfusion as a non-delegatory medical responsibility, since it corresponds to a transplantation of heterogeneous cells. This also includes the determination of the blood group, the Rh factor of donor and patient, the performance of serological specimen-taking and the matching of the transfusion to be given with the blood of the donor. The decree of the Minister for Science and Research of the State of Nordrhein-Westfalen, on the other hand, includes the transfusions among the medical duties that may be delegated. This opinion is also shared by BRENNER (3) and LORENZ (8).

BRENNER (3) only then draws a line for the delegation of duties to non-medical personnel if there are reasons present that render it necessary for the execution of such duties to be reserved to the doctor, for instance in the case of lack of training or in the event of there being risks in the measure to be carried out.

BRENNER (3) emphasizes that during the training period at the nursing colleges the technique of intravenous injections is not learned. There is quite another situation in Switzerland, France, and Great Britain, for example. He states, however, that the knowledge acquired during the training constitutes a basis for acquiring at a later date under medical instruction the knowledge required for carrying out the intravenous injections, transfusions and infusions. A similar demand is made in the edict of the Minister of the Interior of the State of Schleswig-Holstein, dated March 25th 1969. This qualification of a thorough training and a regular supervision are also regarded by SCHULZ as a pre-condition, which also finds expression in the judgment of the German Federal Court dating back to the year 1959. V. BRANDIS and PRIBILLA (2) stress, however, that in the delegation of medical duties to auxiliary medical personnel, the doctor has to assume the responsibility for his agents or assignees in every case. He states further that he may not rely blindly on the expertise and reliability of the person concerned, but may only employ him in conformity with the skills and experience acquired by him, as was also substantiated by SCHMELCHER, PONSOLD, FREY (4) and in judgments given by the German Federal Court.

In accordance with § 940 I of the Civil Code Book those jointly and severally liable towards the patient include in addition to the nurse possibly also the doctor in accordance with the provisions concerning unlawful acts, as MERGEN quotes in his book on the legal problems in medicine. Liability is construed as arising from the circumstances that the doctor has appointed the agents or assignees in accordance with § 831 of the Civil Code Book.

The seminar of the Federal Association of health insurance doctors dealing with the clarification of these problems therefore once again stressed on Jan. 16th 1974 that hypodermic, intramuscular and intra-venous injections as well as the application of infusions and trans-fusions are medical tasks that can be delegated, however. The persons to be considered for such duties should as a rule be such as have passed examinations in the paramedical professions. The pre-requisite for this is, however, that there is regular checking by the delegating doctor. Without the appropriate supervision by the latter these duties should not be carried out by the nursing staff. The responsibility must always lie with the delegating doctor except in the case of gross negligence by the auxiliary personnel.

Also the Federal Medical Council holds these duties to be medical measures, in connection with which it is emphasized that legal deci-sions are lacking and that we can only aid to assist in decisions. With respect to liability, reference is made to § 613, Sentence 1 of the Civil Code (GÜBBELS, 5). On the subject of liability BOCKELMANN (1) stresses that it is not the negligence in itself but the wilful act that constitutes negligence on the part of the doctor, related to the failure of the operation, which leads to the commission of bodily harm.

If one considers the conclusions that have been reached by the various authors, one finds no consensus of opinion, legal guidelines for as-sisting in decisions are hardly present in a clear form; amongst the medical guidelines there is a wide range of opinions which range from delegation without hesitation to complete rejection. The reason for this is seen by KUHLENDAHL (7) to be the significant contrast between legal and medical thinking that apparently consists in the fact that the lawyer judges from the extreme case to the mass of the normal cases, i. e. the everyday events in medical practice, whereas with the doctor it is just the opposite, judging from the more or less everyday standard case, and also exercising a theoretical and practi-cal approach to the extreme cases. Furthermore he states that it is precisely with respect to those advances in modern medicine that reach their culmination point within the context of so-called intensive med-icine, that the conceptions of the non-medical people have hitherto been apparently the least able to keep pace with the development.

In view of our own experience and the knowledge gained from the lit-erature and the legal judgments available to us we should like to ex-press in a summarized form the following recommendations:

1. Delegation to auxiliary medical personnel of hypodermic, intra-muscular, intravenous injections, of infusions and transfusions in the sphere of intensive medicine is possible.

2. The delegation of these measures may not be re-delegated to others.

3. The standard of training and the knowledge of persons who have passed their nursing examinations are prerequisites.

4. Over and above this knowledge there should be extension courses in the subject of infusions and transfusions etc.

5. On the occurrence of the slightest complication, an immediate interruption of the measure and the notification of the doctor is essential; under certain circumstances even before his arrival, re-
   animation measures should be initiated.

6. Within the context of the duty to exercise care, the responsibility
   of stating the indications and delegating the measures in question
   is incumbent on the doctor. For the accurate execution of such
   measures it is the person executing them that is responsible, however.

7. From medical side there is no difference between an indwelling
   cannula and one to be applied.

We trust that with these practice-oriented recommendations we have
made a contribution towards clarifying a set of problems with have
hitherto not been satisfactorily resolved from the legal viewpoint.

REFERENCES

1. BOCKELMANN, P.: Strafrecht des Arztes, S. 1 - 134. Stuttgart:
   Georg Thieme 1968.

2. Von BRANDIS, C., PRIBILLA, O.: Arzt und Kunstfehlervorwurf, S. 1 -
   131. München: Wilhelm Goldmann 1973.

3. BRENNER, G.: Darf das Krankenpflegepersonal Injektionen, Trans-
   fusionen, Infusionen und Blutentnahmen vornehmen? Medizinische
   Welt 23, 235 - 238 (1972).

4. FREY, R.: Intramuskuläre Injektionen durch examinierte Kranken-
   schwester? Dtsch. med. Wschr. 89, 1446 (1964).

5. GÖBBELS, H.: Ärztliche Haftung bei intravenösen Injektionen durch
   Hilfspersonal. Med. Welt 15, 311 (1964).

6. KRÄMER, M.: Injektionen durch Hilfspersonal? Anästhesist 23, 237
   (1974).

7. KUHLENDAHL, H.: Euthanasie-Sterbehilfe-Behandlungsabbruch. Neue
   Jur. Wschr. 27, 1419 - 1420 (1974).

8. LORENZ, R.: Intensivmedizin, S. 1 - 276. Stuttgart - Berlin - Köln-
   Mainz: W. Kohlhammer 1974.

9. MERGEN, A.: Die juristische Problematik in der Medizin, S. 1 - 278.
   München: Wilhelm Goldmann 1971.

10. OPDERBECKE, H. W., WEISSAUER, W.: Zur Abgrenzung der Aufgaben zwi-
    schen Arzt und nichtärztlichen Mitarbeitern in der Intensivthera-
    pie. Anästh. Inform. 14, 28 - 33 (1973).

Free Communications

Commission of Penal Offences and Cerebral Tumors

K. Hartmann

Not very long ago an actual case involving German domestic politics and the law drew the attention of large sections of the public to a possible connection between cerebral lesions and criminal actions.

Among our patients with intracranial space-occupying tumors there are some remarkable examples of this (1, 2, 3).

Three cases are reported on:

A 57-year-old very high-ranking police officer knocked down a gas street lamp while driving. Being under the influence of alcohol at the time, he was given a sentence of three weeks imprisonment in penal proceedings and, his licence was withdrawn, and in a disciplinary action had his salary reduced.

Two years later a left-sided sphenoidal bone tumor weighing 75 g was removed.

A study of the comprehensive files on the case threw up the question how such a high-ranking police official, who had hitherto been very conscious of duty, had taken his car and driven off after a police party, while under the influence of alcohol, notwithstanding the "drunkenness edict" of the Minister of the Interior, and this in spite of the fact that at his request the service car with driver was already en route to drive him home. There was no lack of attempts to explain this conduct which the official concerned put forward as reasons for the senselessness of his action, these culminating in the hypothesis that, taking all the attendant circumstances into account, a disturbance of consciousness had occurred due to the potentiation of the effects of alcohol and an enfeebled constitution.

In addition to uncharacteristic symptoms such as sleeplessness, irritability, tendency to tire more rapidly and exhaustion, he had occasionally observed momentary feelings of nausea and giddiness at the time in question - at least in the same year.

A good 6 months after he had committed the offence he received the first clinical treatment under the diagnosis of "cerebrovascular disturbances". During the further development of this disorder there were - initially at fairly long intervals - losses of consciousness, conditions which occurred suddenly but were only of short duration. These took place at his writing-desk and also during sleep. The police medical officer treated him for "cerebral-spastic insults of unclear aetiology".

A frequent repetition of the attacks attended by a loss of consciousness and tongue-biting, despite anticonvulsive drugs, rendered hospital treatment necessary once again, this time under the diagnosis of "senile epilepsy". The neurological examination which in agreement with the technical test results finally paved the way to the operation revealed clinically low grade, unilateral spastic symptoms on the right side with deficient synkinesis of the right arm and psychologically a weakening of memory, ability to concentrate, and power of recollection.

The official in question decided against a re-opening of the proceedings which in the opinion of our specialists would have had every prospect of success, since his impending promotion would not have come into effect as long as the proceedings were in progress.

As Chief Commissioner of the Police in a large city, he subsequently carried out his duties without complaint.

After having retired on reaching the age limit he now takes an active part as a long-standing member of a conservative party in the activities of his organization.

A 48-year old employee of the Federal Railways had committed a number of petty thefts and been dismissed without notice. Presenting the clinical picture of a FOSTER KENNEDY syndrome and considerable changes of character - according to the medical record data "not responsible for his actions", the patient was operated on a left frontal lesion half a year later. A huge cholesteatoma was removed that filled not only the whole left middle and in part also the anterior cranial fossa, but occupied large parts of the medial cranial fossa on the right side also. The left optic nerve had been transformed into an atrophic, brownish band. Two years before this he had already gradually lost the sight of his left eye.

A 44-year old engineer, confidential clerk with a well-known firm, had his driving licence withdrawn for having driven into a fence while under the influence of alcohol. 4 months later, again under the influence of alcohol, he had driven a company car, without a driving licence, down a slope during icy road conditions. Dismissed by his firm, he had to absolve a period of imprisonment after it had been attested in a neurological-psychiatric opinion that he was "compos mentis" (mentally sound).

A good year after this, only having just escaped being sent to a psychiatric institution, he came to us presenting with the clinical and angiographic picture of a frontal space-occupying process accompanied by anosmia and papilloedema on both sides and considerable changes in character. Within the context of a pronounced moria he made nothing but suggestive remarks, so that hardly a nurse dared to go to him. Later, when his attention was drawn to the things he said and did, he found it very embarrassing. The operation revealed a parasagittal meningioma which, about the size of a fist, occupied the whole right anterior cranial fossa and was firmly attached to the sinus and the falx cerebri, through which it had penetrated to the left side and had also formed there a tumor as big as a pigeon's egg. The meningioma together with the affected sinus and falx parts were removed. Backed by the specialist opinion of our clinic, the patient was exculpated and compensated in retrial proceedings.

20 years after the operation the now 65-year-old engineer is running his own firm with a staff of 60 persons. Apparently senseless thefts in the one case, an irresponsible indiscriminate behaviour in the other cases that involved persons who had hitherto been of irre-

proachable conduct, had led to drastic consequences in their social sphere and placed their financial existence in jeopardy. Granted, in two of the cases described there was the influence of alcohol per se, but also the changed tolerance to alcohol and drinking habits in terms of an increase in alcohol consumption have to be taken into account. Despite this, there remains the conspicuous fact that such offences were senseless and difficult to interpret (2).

In all these cases it was a question of extensive tumors of the anterior or middle cranial fossae, in part on both sides.

The misconduct which led to the commission of a penal offence can be classified chronologically in all cases as an early symptom.

This early symptom, as an expression of a lesion of the frontal or temporal brain areas, may manifest itself in a disturbance in the field of morals and ethics, in a lack of discrimination and reflection and in a change in character (1, 3).

The possibility of an intracranial tumor should receive appropriate attention in the judgment of penal offences.

REFERENCES

1. LESNIAK, R., SZYMUSIK, A., CHRZANOWSKI, R.: Multidirectional disorders of sexual drive in a case of brain tumor. Case report. Forensic Science 1, 333 - 338 (1972).

2. PETERS, K.: Fehlerquellen im Strafprozeß. Eine Untersuchung der Wiederaufnahmeverfahren in der Bundesrepublik Deutschland. Karlsruhe: C. F. Müller 1970, 1972.

3. SCHUSTER, P.: Psychische Störungen bei Hirntumoren, S. 368. Stuttgart: Ferdinand Enke 1902.

The Central Action of Free Serotonin on Blood Brain-Barrier and Regulation of Autonomic Functions

W. WINKELMÜLLER, E. MARKAKIS, G. HÜNEFELD, and H. W. KERSTING

Introduction

Serotonin is a naturally occuring monoamine stored in cell bodies of lower midbrain and upper pons. The serotoninergic neurons ascending involved with the regulation of temperature, sleep, psychomotor activity and sensory perception (1). An increased release of serotonin into the CSF is found under pathophysiological conditions in cases of brain injury, brain-tumors and cerebrovascular diseases (4, 5). The clinical significance of increased serotonin levels in CSF is not yet clear.

It was the aim of our study to examine - additionally to the well-known edema producing effect - the influence of serotonin on central autonomic functions.

Material and Methods

In 30 spontaneously breathing cats intracranial pressure, brain pulsations, arterial and central venous pressure, respiratory frequency and volume, mediastinal pressure, heart rate and electrocorticogram were recorded under light anestesia. Serotonin was injected into the lateral ventricle in the first group, into the subdural space in the second group and into the white matter of the left hemisphere in the third group.

Results

Following intraventricular and subdural application of serotonin significant changes in respiration were noticed in all animals. While respiratory frequency and mediastinal pressure amplitude increase, the respiratory volume - as indicated by the thermistor amplitude - is markedly reduced (Fig. 1).

These changes in respiration indicate a bronchospasm which is associated with an increase in central venous pressure. The cardiovascular reaction is characterized by a biphasic response. Following a shortlasting decrease in blood pressure and heart rate, both parameters tend to increase above the control level. The initial increase in intracranial pressure seems to be caused by a plethysmographic reaction during injection and by the rise in central venous pressure.

Statistical evaluation of the single groups shows significant changes following intraventricular and subdural serotonin injection (Fig. 2). The responses to intracerebral application during the 6 hours of observation time following the injection are minimal and statistically not significant. Based on these above results we conclude that the injected serotonin reaches the brain stem directly via CSF and stimulates neurons which respond to the excitation by a parasympathetic action. The diffusion of serotonin into the periventricular tissue produces a disturbance of blood brain barrier. The extent of the blood brain barrier damage, especially beneath the floor of fourth ventricle, could be demonstrated by means of Evans blue.

The respiratory and cardiovascular reactions are accompanied by micturition and defecation, tonic extension of the extremities and seizure discharges in the ECoG. Such phenomena are well known in the course of severe head injuries. The clinical observation of shifting of central autonomic homeostasis to the cholinergic side following brain injuries has led to the therapeutic application of anticholinergic substances (3).

In our experimental model the serotonin - induced parasympathicomimetic reaction can be antagonized by application of Orciprenalin, a β-sympathicomimetic drug (Fig. 3).

The pharmacological action of subdurally injected serotonin is likewise diminished by pretreating the animals with dexamethasone (Fig.4). The supposed effect of corticosteroids influencing serotonin metabolism is demonstrated by CURZON and GREEN (2) who found a significant decrease in the central amount of serotonin following injection of hydrocortisone.

Summary

Our experiments have shown that serotonin, which is released in high concentrations into the CSF in the presence of cerebral lesions, can damage the BBB, and cause autonomic and electroencephalographic changes. These informations allow us to spedify the functional neuronal alterations caused by biochemical irritation in the acute phase of cerebral lesions. Thus, dexamethasone and centrally acting anticholinergic drugs are of specific value in the treatment of brain edema and the cholinergic shift of central autonomic functions in cerebral lesions.

REFERENCES

1. BLOOM, F. E.: Serotonin neurons: localization and possible physiological role. Adv. Biochem. Psychopharmacol. 1, 27 - 47 (1969).

2. CURZON, G., GREEN, A. R.: Effect of hydrocortisone on rat brain 5-hydroxytryptamine. Life Sci. 7, 657 - 663 (1968).

3. HEPPNER, F., ARGYROPOULOS, G., LANNER, G.: Anticholinergische Behandlung des Schädelhirntraumas. Nachr. Unfallheilk. 76, 341 - 359 (1973).

4. MISRA, S. S., SINGH, K. S. P., GHARGAVA, K. P.: Estimation of 5-hydroxytryptamine (5 HT) level in cerebrospinal fluid of patients with intracranial or spinal lesions. J. Neurol. Neurosurg. Psychiat. 30, 163 - 165 (1967).

5. OSTERHOLM, J. L., BELL, J., MYER, R., PYENSON, J.: Experimental effects of free serotonin on the brain and its relation to brain injury. Part 1: The neurological consequences of intracerebral serotonin injections. Part 2: Trauma induced alterations in spinal fluid and brain. Part 3: Serotonin induced cerebral edema. J. Neurosurg. 31, 408 - 421 (1969).

6. REULEN, H. J., HADJIDIMOS, A., SCHÜRMANN, K.: The effect of dex-
   mathasone on water and electrolyte content and on rCBF in perifocal brain edema in man. Steroids and brain edema, S. 239 - 252.
   Berlin - Heidelberg - New York: Springer 1972.

7. SACHS, E., Jr.: Acetylcholine and serotonin in the spinal fluid.
   J. Neurosurg. 14, 22 - 27 (1957).

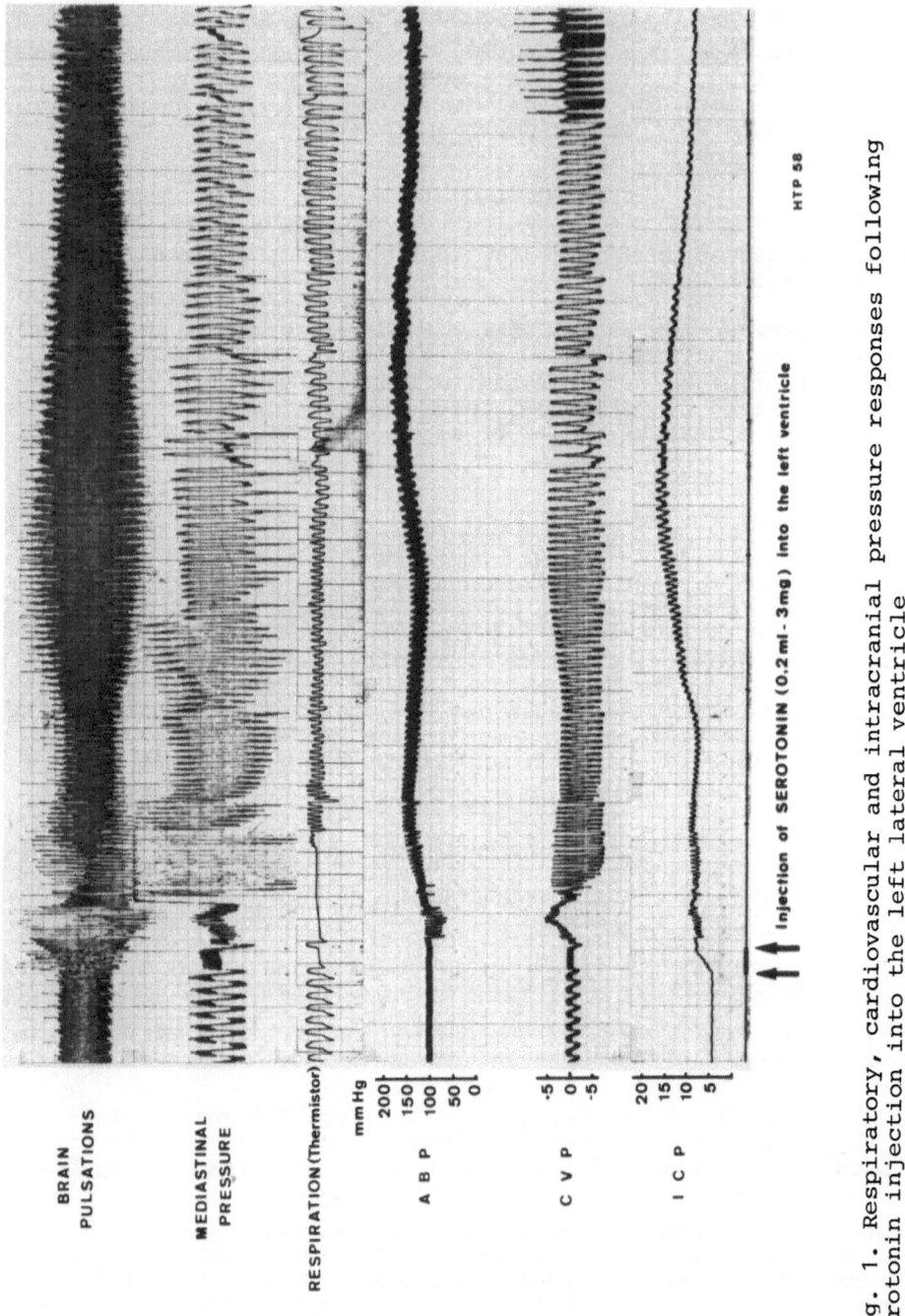

Fig. 1. Respiratory, cardiovascular and intracranial pressure responses following serotonin injection into the left lateral ventricle

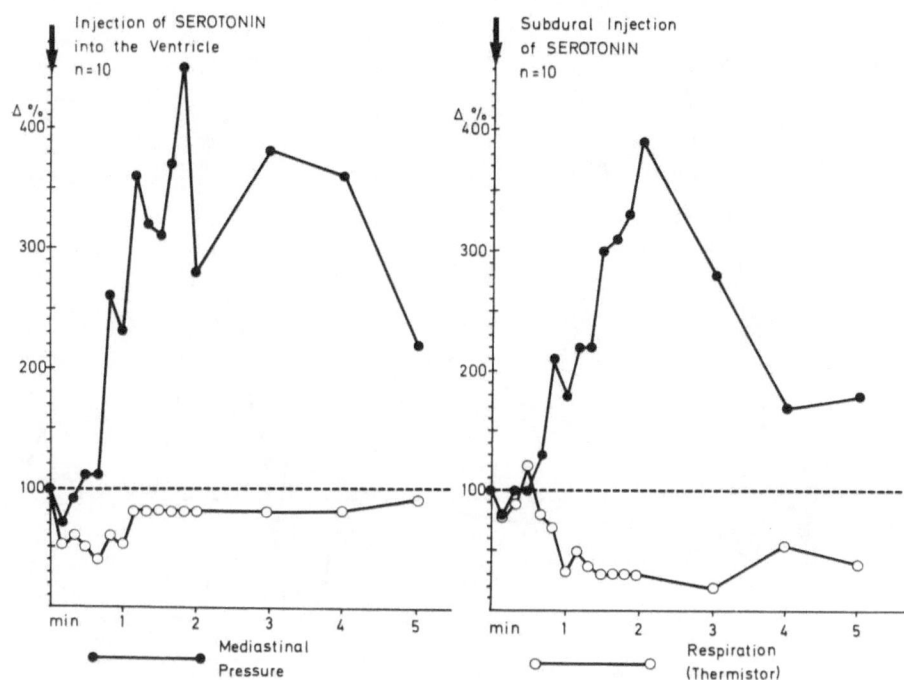

Fig. 2. Mean values (SD ± 2,4) of respiratory deviations (control = 100 %) following intraventricular and subdural serotonin application

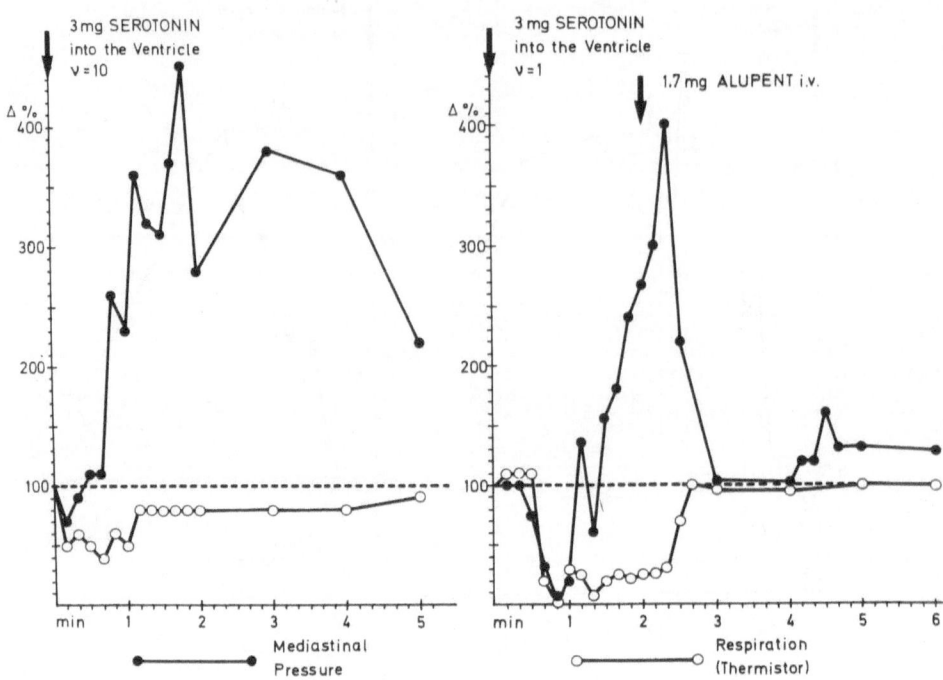

Fig. 3. Suppression of serotonin induced respiratory changes by i. v.
injection of orciprenalin Alupent[R])

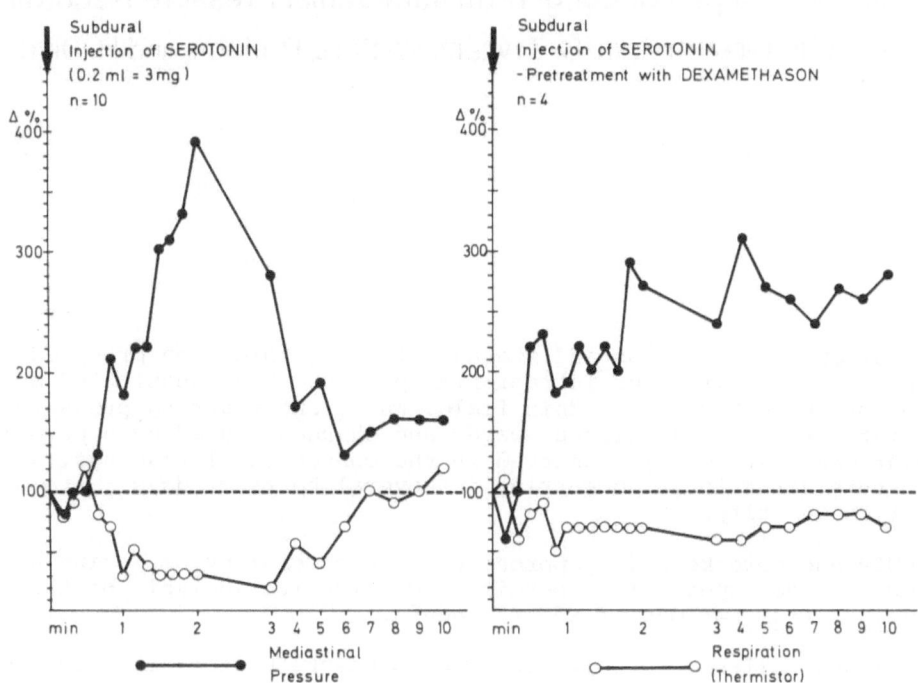

Fig. 4. Reduction of the maximal respiratory deviations in animals, pretreated with dexamethasone (0,22 mg/kg for 4 days)

Amplitude Analysis of Long-Term Intracranial Pressure Recordings*

M. BROCK, K. DIEFENTHÄLER, C. ZYWIETZ, W. PÖLL, P. MOCK, and H. DIETZ

Satisfactory evaluation and storage of the information provided by long term recordings of intracranial pressure has constituted a problem for those working in this field. While shortlasting pressure variations - such as plateau-waves and changes caused by hyperosmolar solutions - are easily observed in the conventional tracings, slower pressure variations - occurring in several hours or days - are difficult to quantify.

TROUPP and coworkers (1) approached this problem by employing a very slow recorder speed. This permits a qualitative analysis of the tracings from periods of several hours.

JANNY and collaborators (2) obtained pressure histograms with the aid of a computer, thus reaching a quantitative analysis of long-term pressure recordings. The same approach was adopted by KULLBERG (3), who developed a special equipment for the statistical analysis of intracranial pressure recordings.

Methods

We have developed an equipment similar to that described by KULLBERG (3) and which may be operated in connection with any conventional pressure recording device (Fig. 1). The pressure range being monitored in any given case can be subdivided in up to 10 input-proportional pressure classes of variable individual amplitude. Pressures are digitally stored at time-intervals of 0.1, 1.0 or 10.0 sec for pre-determined periods (minutes, hours or days). At the end of each recording period (e. g. 12 h), an alarm sound is emitted, data-storage is briefly discontinued, and the values for each class are recorded by the nurse on a special sheet of paper. These values are later transferred to punched cards by a technician and processed by a computer so as to producd the corresponding histograms (Fig. 2).

Results

Amplitude analysis of intracranial pressure has been performed without any complication in 10 patients who underwent routine continuous ICP-monitoring for several periods of time. Two kinds of problems have been met with:

1. The manual recording of the various class-values at the end of a pre-determined analysis period and their transfer to the punched cards are time and personel consuming operations, and constitute a source of error.

*Supported by a grant of the Deutsche Forschungsgemeinschaft.

2. Based on our present knowledge it is difficult to establish the
ideal period of analysis. Short periods of analysis - for example one
hour - increase unduly the bulk of recordings and to not provide sub-
stantial information additional to that obtained from direct visual
curve-analysis. Long periods of analysis - for example 24 hours -
appear to reduce somewhat the resolution-power of the method.

Comments

The problems posed by manual working-up of the information provided
by the analyzing equipment can be coped with by means of automatic
storage and re-setting, and by on-line transfer to a computer or to
a computer-compatible punched tape. Such an outfit is being presently devised.

As to the choice of the ideal periods of time for analysis, more
clinical experience is needed. We believe that the length of the
analysis periods will have to be established individually, according
to the clinical condition of the patient and to the therapeutic measures applied in each case.

Summary

Automatic or semi-automatic amplitude analysis of long-term ICP-recordings may contribute towards a more reliable evaluation of the
accumulated pressure data. A new and simple equipment for this purpose is described. Nevertheless, increasing experience with this
method of analysis will have to help in establishing the ideal length
of the periods of analysis in each individual case.

REFERENCES

1. TROUPP, H., KUURNE, T., KASTE, M., VAPALAHTI, M., VALTONEN, S.:
   Intraventricular pressure after severe brain injuries: prognostic
   value and correlation with blood pressure and jugular venous oxygen tension. In: Intracranial Pressure (eds. M. BROCK and H. DIETZ)
   pp. 222 - 226. Berlin - Heidelberg - New York: Springer 1972.

2. JANNY, P., JOUAN, P., JANNY, L., GOURGAND, M., GUEIT, U. M.: A
   statistical approach to long-term monitoring of intracranial pressure. In: Intracranial Pressure (eds. M. BROCK and H. DIETZ) pp.
   59 - 64. Berlin - Heidelberg - New York: Springer 1972.

3. KULLBERG, G.: A method for statistical analysis of intracranial
   pressure recordings. In: Intracranial Pressure (eds. M. BROCK and
   H. DIETZ) pp. 65 - 69. Berlin - Heidelberg - New York: Springer
   1972.

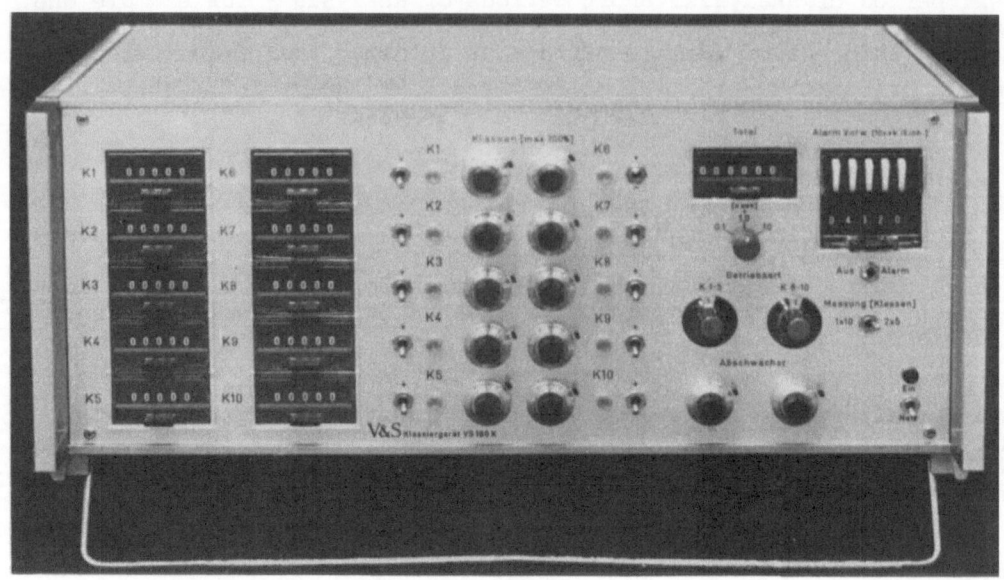

Fig. 1. Equipment for amplitude analysis of long-term continuous
ICP-recordings. The 10 "windows" on the left side correspond to the
10 pressure-classes

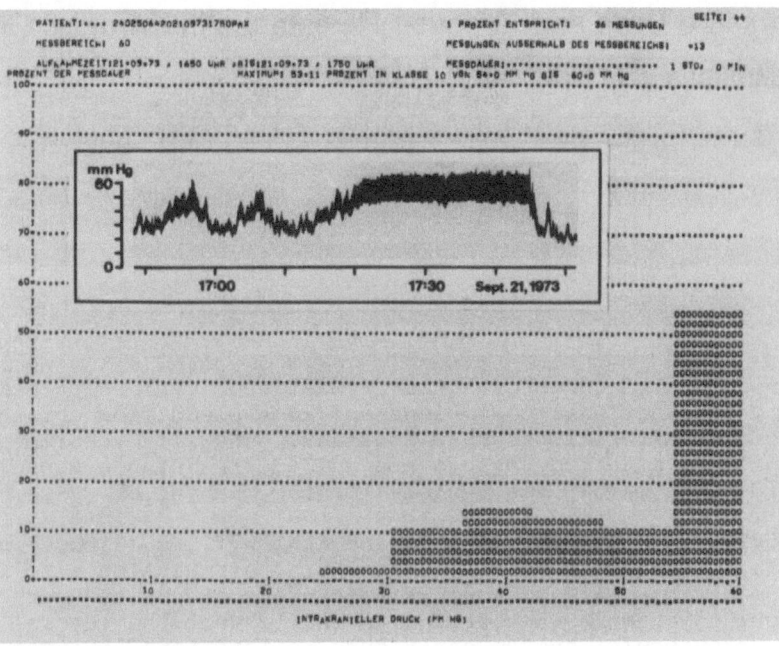

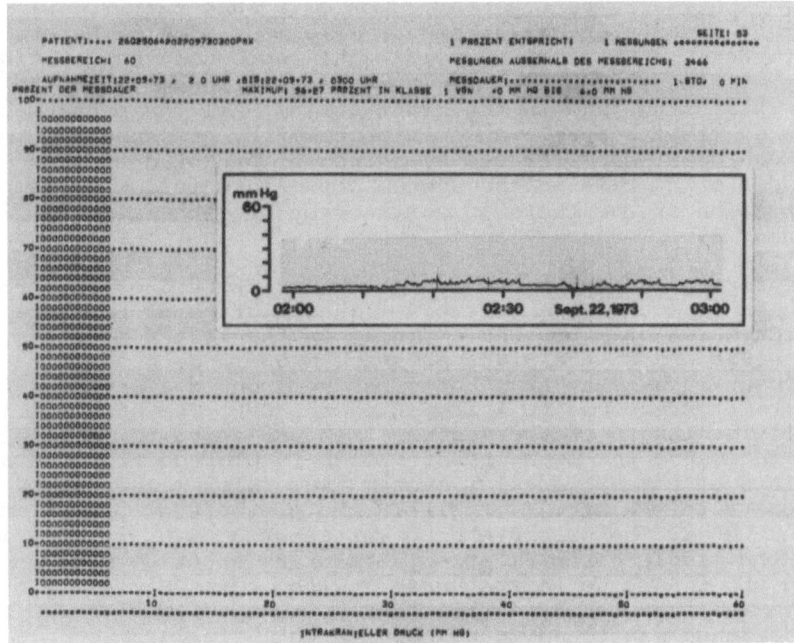

Fig. 2. One-hour pressure histograms in a case of posterior fossa tumor before (upper histogram) and after (lower histogram) open CSF drainage

Pressure Drop and Vascular Resistance in Cerebral Circulation*

J. Jansen and E. Kanzow

Variations of cerebrovascular resistance (CVR) adapt cerebral blood flow to functional conditions and keep blood flow during changes of systemic arterial pressure constant. Generally the immediately pre-capillary situated vessels are called "resistance vessels" and are held to be mainly responsible for the changes of CVR.

Studies of DIEÇKHOFF, JANSEN and KANZOW (1, 2, 3) have shown, that relatively large arteries in cerebral circulation also represent a considerable part of the CVR. Therefore it was the purpose of this paper to examine whether and to what extent the several parts of the cerebrovascular system contribute to functional changes of the flow resistance.

The experiments were performed on cats anaesthetized with chloralose-urethane. Pressure measurements were made with catheters and micro-catheters in the aortic arc, in the region of the carotid sinus, in the middle cerebral artery (origin and branches), in the superior sagittal sinus and in the right atrium. All the pressures were re-corded simultaneously and continuously by pressure transducers. The CVR changes were produced by infusions of Noradrenaline or Angio-tensin or by raising the systemic pressure following temporary con-striction of the thoracic aorta or by the inhalation of 10 % CO_2 in normal air.

The first figure (Fig. 1) shows the pressure drop in cerebral circu-lation in accordance to the well-known graph of pressure drop in the circulation of MALL. The ordinate on the left represents systemic pressure and on the right pressure drop in percent of the systemic pressure. The percentage of pressure drop in a section of the vascular system corresponds to its part of the CVR. The abscissa is about the relative length of the vessels from the aorta to the right atrium. At the curve the mean pressure drop is plotted from the aorta to those points of cerebrovascular system from which measurements were made. Even up to the circle of WILLIS the pressure drop was found to be about 25 %. The pressure drop was about 30 % up to the smaller branches of the middle cerebral artery measuring about 80 microns in diameter and about 40 % up to the vessels with about 40 microns outer diameter. From the superior sagittal sinus up to the right atrium the pressure difference was found to be about 6 %.

In the smallest pial vessels, pressure measurements were made either in the arterial or in the venous section. Therefore the investigation demonstrates: at least half the pressure drop, respectively correspon-ding to half of the CVR, is localized in relatively large vessels and less than half in the so-called precapillary resistance vessels.

---

*Supported by the Deutsche Forschungsgemeinschaft.

Fig. 2 shows the pressure drop distribution during increased CVR due to noradrenaline-infusion. The relative pressure drop from the aorta to the circle of WILLIS decreases by only about 2,7 % and from the superior sagittal sinus to the right atrium by about 3,2 %.

Nearly the same was found during angiotensin-infusion: The relative pressure drop from the aorta to the circle of WILLIS decreases by only about 3 % and from superior sagittal sinus to the right atrium by about 4,3 %.

In the same manner the CVR rises proportional to increased aortic pressure during mechanical compression of the thoracic aorta. In contrast to the pharmacological raising of CVR in these experiments the relative pressure drop up to the circle of WILLIS is completely recovered after a short time.

The effect of a decreased CVR during hypercapnia on pressure drop distribution is shown in Fig. 3. Pressure drop increases up to the circle of WILLIS by about 3,6 % and from the superior sagittal sinus to the right atrium about 2,8 %. The shifting of the relative pressure drop is very small considering that hypercapnia provokes an increase of cerebral blood flow (CBF) by about 50 - 100 % corresponding to a decrease of CVR to about one half.

A more important shifting of the pressure drop in the greater arteries should be expected if the small, so called resistance vessels, alone change the CVR. The distribution of the pressure drop remains unchanged during variations in CVR. Therefore these findings demonstrate that the greater vessels in the cerebral circulation are an essential part of CVR not only anatomically but also functionally and that they participate in regulating the CBF.

REFERENCES

1. DIECKHOFF, D., KANZOW, E.: Über die Lokalisation des Strömungs-
   widerstandes im Hirnkreislauf. Pflügers Arch. 310, 75 - 85 (1969).

2. JANSEN, J., BERNDT, U., KANZOW, E.: Anpassungsmechanismen der
   Widerstandsverteilung im Hirnkreislauf. Folia Angiologica 21, 353 -
   355 (1973).

3. KANZOW, E., JANSEN, J., DIECKHOFF, D.: Druckabfall und Strömungs-
   widerstand in den Arterien des Gehirn- und Extremitätenkreislaufes.
   In: Vascular Smooth Muscle (Hrsg. E. BETZ), S. 80 - 83. Berlin -
   Heidelberg - New York: Springer 1972.

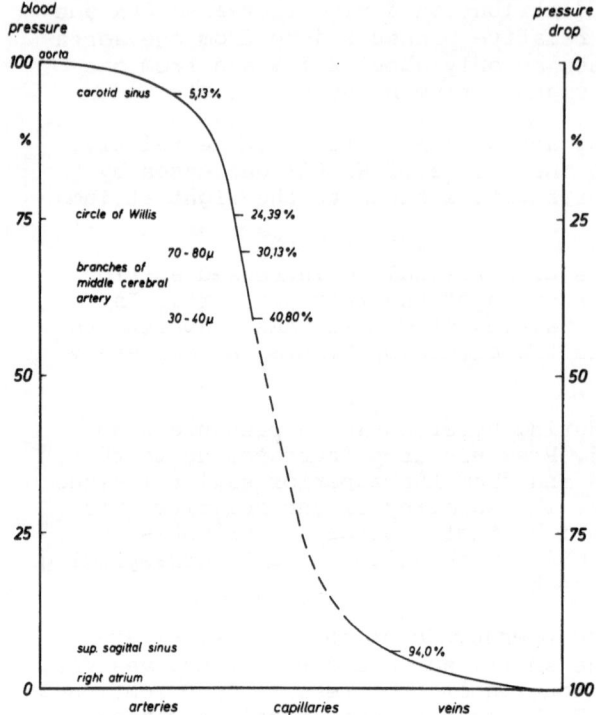

Fig. 1. Pressure drop and distribution of vascular resistance in
cerebral circulation

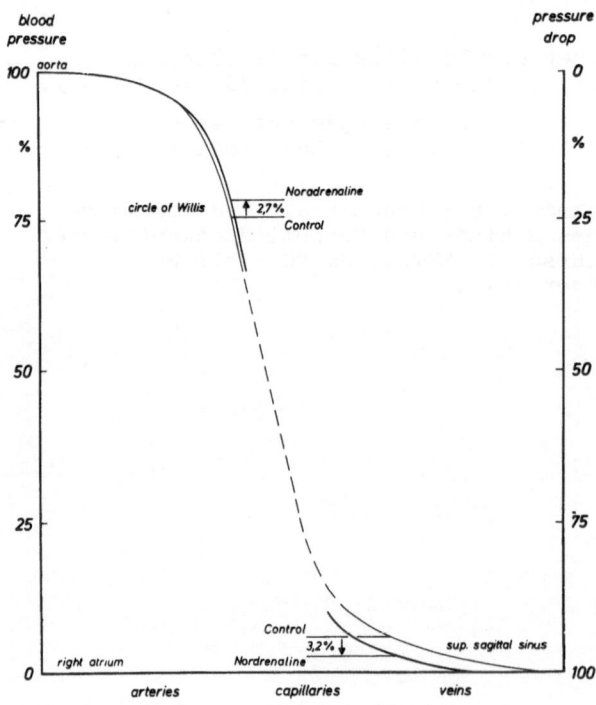

Fig. 2. Pressure drop and
distribution of vascular
resistance in cerebral
circulation during nor-
adrenaline

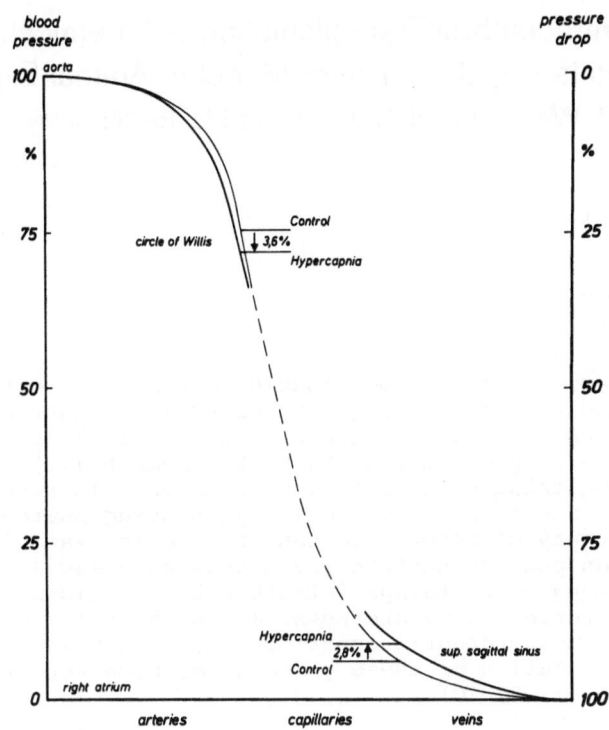

Fig. 3. Pressure drop and distribution of vascular resistance in cerebral circulation during hypercapnia

Intracerebral Transplantation of Chemically Induced Gliomas in Rats – A Brain Tumor Model in Animal Experiment

H. Waldbaur, H. Schmidt, and U. Engelmann

Various brain tumor models have been used to test diagnostic isotopes and cytostatic drugs. Numerous investigations (e. g. 6, 7, 8) have been carried out with a transplantable ependymoma in the mouse which was originally induced by ZIMMERMANN (12) through the intracerebral implantation of methylcholanthrene. In recent years DRUCKREY (2, 3, 4) succeeded in selectively inducing neuroepithelial tumors in rats by way of resorptive cancerogenesis. Rat gliomas induced by his methods possess certain advantages as a model over mouse ependymomas. Among other things intrathecal injections and infusions into the carotid artery are possible in the rat - a fact that is important for chemotherapeutic experiments for example (11). However, the transplantation of these gliomas has been reported only in a few instances (1, 5, 9, 10).

For a period of almost 9 months, we gave 15 BD-II rats a weekly intravenous injection of 5 mg/kg methylnitrosourea. In 12 animals tumor growth was observed betwwen the 243rd and 378th day after initiation of the experimental series. Glioblastomas of the brain were found in 11 rats (in 8 rats solitary and in 3 multiple tumors) and a glioblastoma of the spinal cord in the 12th rat. The brain tumors were located chiefly in the cerebral hemispheres. One rat with a cerebral glioblastoma was found to have a fibrosarcoma of the base of the skull as well.

Three glioblastomas were transplanted to animals of the same strain.

The *tumor of rat No. 4* was carried by serial intracerebral transfer for 9 consecutive generations. We implanted solid tumor specimens with a trocar in the right parietal region. The reddish and spongy transplantation tumors infiltrated the surrounding tissue of the lateral ventricles and revealed a tendency to invade the ventricular system. Histologically they showed the characteristics of multiform glioblastomas and were sometimes combined with oligodendroglioma and astrocytoma structures. There were no significant changes compared with the histology of the methylnitrosourea-induced primary tumor.

The *tumor of rat No. 6* was transferred subcutaneously in the first generation and by intracerebral transplantation in all following generations. All intracerebrally transplanted tumors again had the histological characteristics of glioblastomas. With respect to the macroscopic picture and the infiltrating growth they were similar to the transplantation tumors of glioblastoma 4.

The transplantation of the *tumor of rat No. 9* was performed in the same way as that of glioblastoma 6: one subcutaneous transplantation followed by intracerebral passages. Here a transformation into fibroblastic spindle cell or polymorphous sarcomas was observed. The grey and relatively firm transplantation tumors grew mainly in the area of the implantation wound, some also in extracerebral and extracranial sites without invasion of the ventricular system.

Summarizing, our experiments showed that it is possible to preserve the initial histological structure of gliomas in rats for several generations by exclusive intracerebral transplantations. After intracerebral transplantation secondary to one subcutaneous passage, gliomatous or sarcomatous tumors can develop, depending on which fragments of the subcutaneously transplanted tumor are transferred.

Recently we have worked with the glioblastoma 6 which is now in the 15th generation. For the last passages the take rate was 100 % at a median survival time of 17 days. Considering this take rate, we feel that this tumor is a good model for chemotherapeutic experiments in particular. It may, however, also be a suitable model for biochemical and immunological studies.

REFERENCES

1. BENDA, P., SOMEDA, K., MESSER, J., SWEET, W. H.: Morphological and immunochemical studies of rat glial tumors and clonal strains propagated in culture. J. Neurosurg. 34, 310 - 323 (1971).

2. DRUCKREY, H., JVANKOVIC, S., PREUSSMANN, R.: Selektive Erzeugung maligner Tumoren im Gehirn und Rückenmark von Ratten durch N-methyl-N-nitrosoharnstoff. Z. Krebsforsch. 66, 389 - 408 (1965).

3. DRUCKREY, H., SCHAGEN, B., JVANKOVIC, S.: Erzeugung neurogener Malignome durch einmalige Gabe von Äthyl-nitrosoharnstoff (ÄHN) an neugeborene und junge BD IX-Ratten. Z. Krebsforsch. 74, 141 - 161 (1970).

4. JVANKOVIC, S., DRUCKREY, H.: Transplacentare Erzeugung maligner Tumoren des Nervensystems. I. Äthyl-nitrosoharnstoff an BD IX-Ratten. Z. Krebsforsch. 71, 320 - 360 (1968).

5. LEE, J. C.: Direct transplantation of intracranial tumors. Anat. Rec. 160, 481 (1968).

6. LONG, R. G., McAFEE, J. G., WINKELMAN, J.: Evaluation of radioactive compounds for the external detection of cerebral tumors. Cancer Res. 23, 98 - 108 (1963).

7. SHAPIRO, W. R., AUSMAN, J. I., RALL, D. P.: Studies on the chemotherapy of experimental brain tumors: Evaluation of 1,3 - bis (2-chloroethyl)-1-nitrosourea, cyclophosphamide, mithramycin, and methotrexate. Cancer Res. 30, 2401 - 2413 (1970).

8. SHAPIRO, W. R.: Studies on the chemotherapy of experimental brain tumors: Evaluation of 1-(2-chloroethyl)-3-cyclohexyl-1-nitrosourea, vincristine, and 5-fluorouracil. J. Natl. Cancer Inst. 46, 359 - 368 (1971).

9. THUST, R., WARZOK, R.: Comparative studies on the in vitro and in vivo morphology of clones of experimental CNS tumors in the rat. Acta Neuropath. 20, 248 - 257 (1972).

10. WECHSLER, W., RAMADAN, M. A., GIESELER, A.: Isogenic transplantation of ethylnitrosourea induced tumors of the central and peripheral nervous system in two different inbred rat strains. Naturwissenschaften 59, 474 (1972).

11. WILSON, C. B., BATES, E. A.: Transplantable brain tumors. In: The Experimental Biology of Brain Tumors, pp. 19 - 56 (eds.

W. M. KIRSCH, E. GROSSI-PAOLETTI, P. PAOLETTI). Springfield/Ill.: C. C. Thomas 1972.

12. ZIMMERMANN, H. M., ARNOLD, H.: Experimental brain tumors. I. Tumors produced with methylcholanthrene. Cancer Res. 1, 919 - 924 (1941).

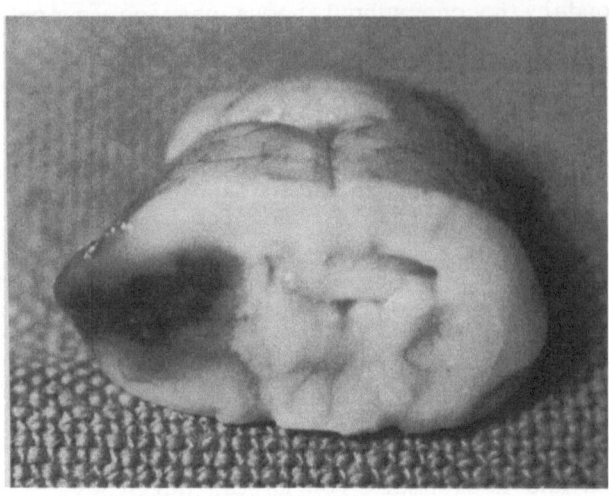

Fig. 1. Rat No. 6. Brain tumor with hemorrhages and necrotic portions induced by chronic administration of methylnitrosourea (glioblastoma)

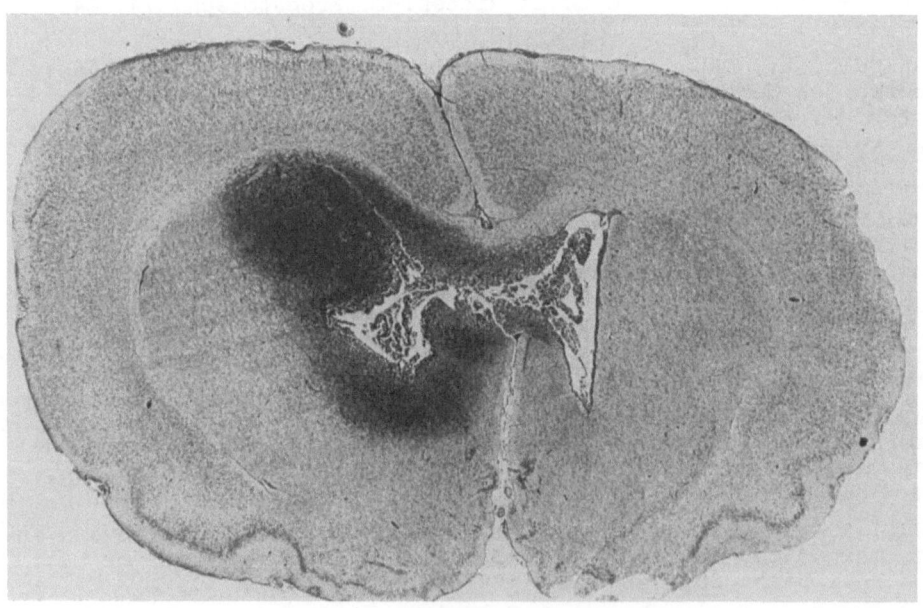

Fig. 2. Rat No. 117. Glioblastoma 6 transplanted intracerebrally. Infiltrating growth near the right lateral ventricle and growth within both lateral ventricles

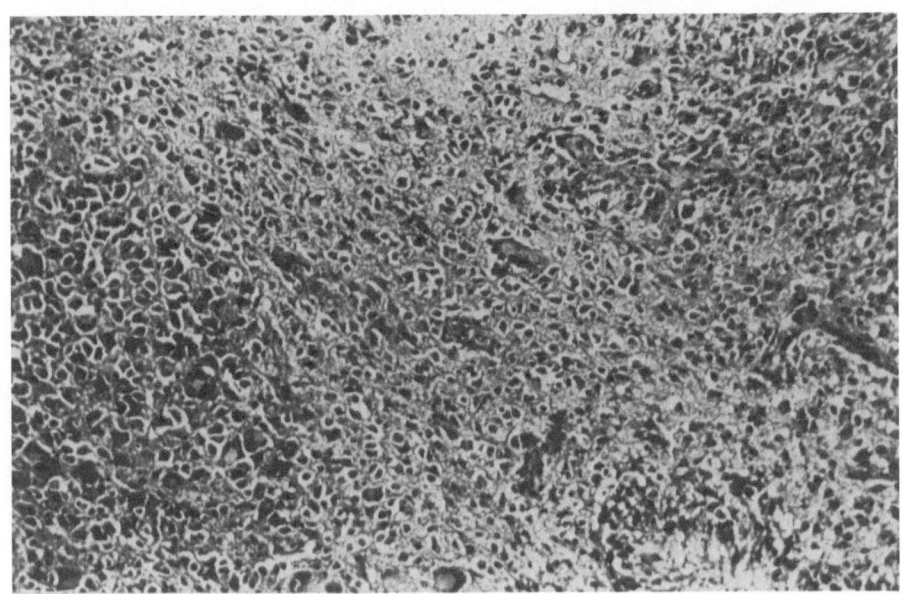

Fig. 3. Rat No. 4. Glioblastoma induced by methylnitrosourea. Stained with cresyl-violet

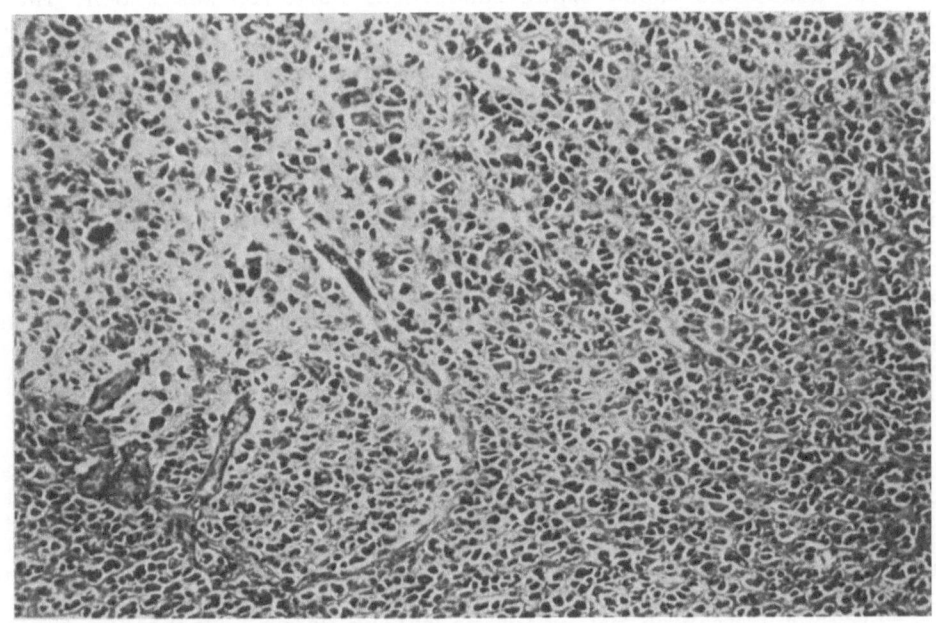

Fig. 4. Rat No. 109. Glioblastoma 4 transplanted intracerebrally (second passage). The tumor has retained its gliomatous structures. Stained with cresyl-violet

Causes of Stenoses and Embolic Occlusions in Microsurgical Anastomosis (Experimental Study)

R. Meyermann and G. Kletter

In the last decades vascular surgery has gained considerable importance. Such interventions are not limited to the removal of lesions which narrow the lumen, but an increasing number of angioplastic and bypass operations are being performed. Reports on histological studies following such operations have been presented now and then (1, 3). The results do not differ essentially from those of other healing processes of injured vascular walls (5). However, we believe that in the case of microsurgical procedures in vessels with a diameter of 0.5 - 1 mm, systematic studies are indispensible, as tissue reactions decisively influence the sufficiency of the anastomosis.

In 30 rats the common carotid artery was severed on both sides and end-to-end anastomoses were performed by means of microsurgical techniques (6). The diameter of the vessels ranged from 0.7 - 1.0 mm. Two animals were sacrificed immediately after the operation, and then two at a time at intervals of 24 hours so that after 14 days 60 anastomoses were available whose exact functional duration was known. The vessels taken out were neither fixed by perfusion nor washed out in order to avoid artificial removal of loosely adhering coagulum. The material was fixed in buffered formalin (pH 7.4), embedded in paraffin and cut into serial sections. Hemotoxylin-eosin (H.-E.), azan and elastica - van Gieson stains were prepared from these sections.

During the first days after the operation, thrombus formation was the dominating feature. This is known to be caused by damage to the endothelium, which results in the release of tissue thrombocinase and thus in the formation of lateral thrombi (4). Since the damage of the endothelium at the puncture point of the needle is unavoidable, one can understand that the formation of thrombi occurs regularly at this point after the operation (Fig. 1 a - c). The mushroomlike thrombus emerges out of the puncture channel and spreads over the adjoining uninjured endothelium (Fig. 1 c). These thrombi may spread relatively far, since channel lacerations of all layers of the wall occur in the neighbourhood of the puncture (Fig. 1 b).

It is striking that the area of the anastomosis itself is completely free of thrombi (Fig. 1 a). This is doubtless due to the fact that the cut ends of the vessel are turned inside out when the suture is performed so that intima covers intima and no part of the injured intima comes into contact with blood, once the circulation is allowed to continue. When the cut ends of the vessel are turned outside in, the thrombus formation may reach an extent which jeopardizes the result of the operation (Fig. 2 a - b).

Up to the 4th day after the operation, the stratified thrombus plainly grew in size (Fig. 1 d), later on the thrombi become smaller or at least retain the same size. Unlike other lateral thrombi, also examined on the 7th day after the operation, no clear proliferation of vessels into the thrombus can be found (Fig. 2 c). This is probably due to the fact that the walls of vessels with such a small diameter are supplied mainly by diffusion from the lumen and this is rendered difficult by the superimposed thrombi.

The same fact is probably also the cause why signs of cellular destruction can be found in all layers of the wall of the cut ends of the vessel between the stitches as early as 24 hours after the operation. Only isolated cellular nuclei are still demonstrable (Fig. 3 a). The same finding can be obtained in all anastomoses up to the 7th day after the operation. After that additional indications of the destruction of elastic fibres appear (Fig. 3 b).

11 to 14 days after the operation of the rats, the total operation area is completely replaced by cicatricial tissue. In particular when the stitches reach too far, sections of vascular walls are found within the cicatricial tissue which have not yet been absorbed (Fig. 4 b). However, the cut ends of the vessels are always completely separated and held together only by scar tissue (Fig. 4 a - b). The interior of the vascular lumen is lined by a tissue substitute consisting of several layers of cells, which additionally narrow the lumen. This hyperplasia of the intima was also described by BAXTER and his co-workers in the case of damage to vessels with a diameter about 1 mm (2).

In summary, anastomosis operations have a natural lower limit in the size of the vessel diameter, due to unavoidable thrombus formation and cicatrization as well as by physical and physiological conditions. On the other hand, the existing risk of an insufficient anastomosis operation may be lowered considerably by certain technical conditions, as has been demonstrated by this investigation .

REFERENCES

1. ACLAND, R.: Signs of patency in small vessel anastomosis. Surg. 72, 744 - 748 (1972).

2. BAXTER, Th. J., O'BRIEN, B. McC., HENDERSON, P. N., BENNETT, R. C.: The histopathology of small vessels following microvascular repair. Brit. J. Surg. 59, 617 - 622 (1972).

3. BARKER, W. F., CANNON, J. A.: Anatomical result of endarterectomy Surg. Forum 6, 266 - 284 (1955).

4. BÜCHNER, F.: Allgemeine Pathologie, S. 227 - 237. München - Berlin: Urban und Schwarzenberg 1962.

5. TEXON, M., IMPARATO, A. M., LORD, J. J., HEIPERN, M.: Experimental production of arterial lesion. Arch. intern. Med. 110, 50 - 58 (1962).

6. YASARGIL, M. G.: Microsurgery applied to Neurosurgery. Stuttgart: Georg Thieme 1969.

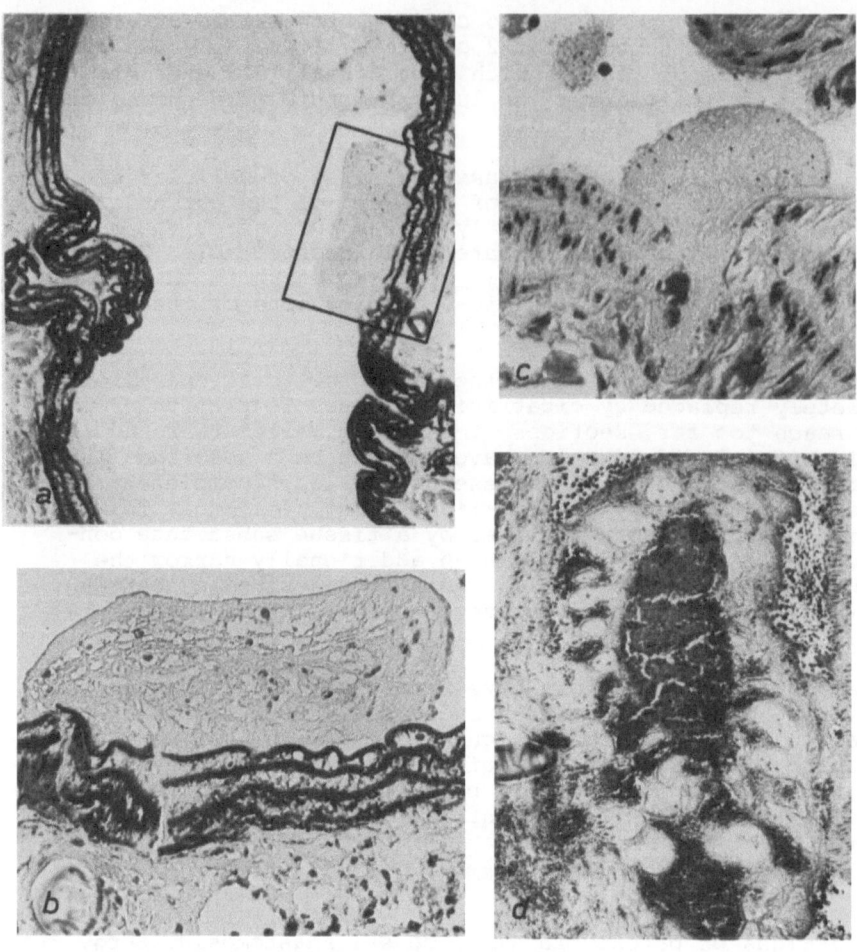

Fig. 1.
a) End-to-end anastomosis, 2nd day after the operation, thrombus only over the puncture channel, not over the anastomosed ends of the vessel, E.-v.G. X 40
b) Higher magnification of Fig. 1 a to demonstrate the damaged wall of the vessel, E.-v.G. X 100
c) 1/2 hour after the operation, mushroomlike thrombus in the puncture channel, H.-E. X 100
d) 4th day after the operation, enlargement of thrombus, typical structure of a stratified lateral thrombus, H.-E. X 40

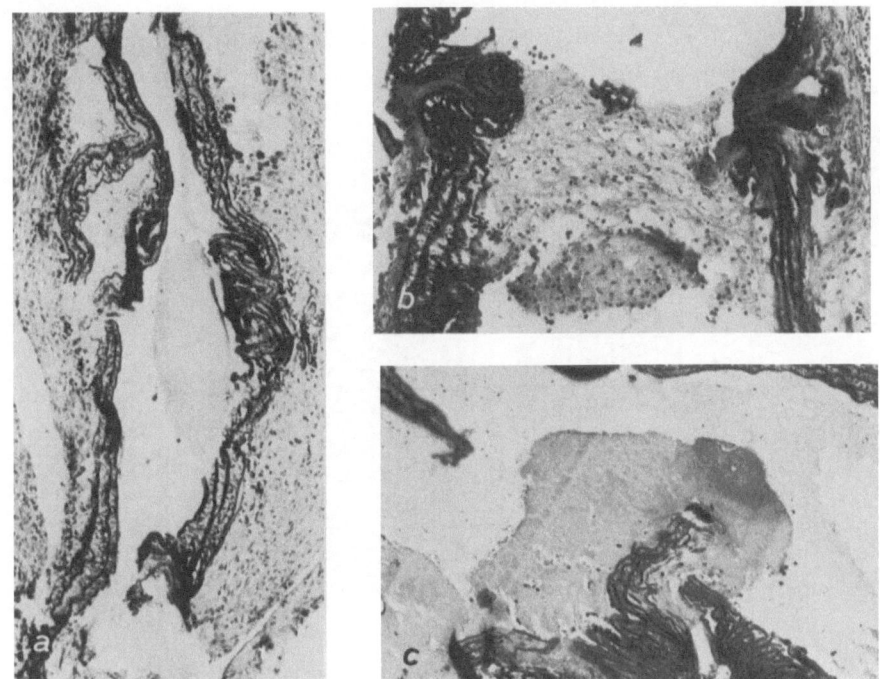

Fig. 2.
a) Anastomosis, 4th day after the operation, cut ends of the vessel
turned into the lumen bearing a large thrombus, E.-v.G. X 40
b) 2nd day after the operation, obliteration of the vessel by thrombus,
caused by cut ends of the vessel turned into the lumen, E.-v.G. X 50
c) 7th day after the operation, thrombus without vascular proliferation,
H.-E. X 40

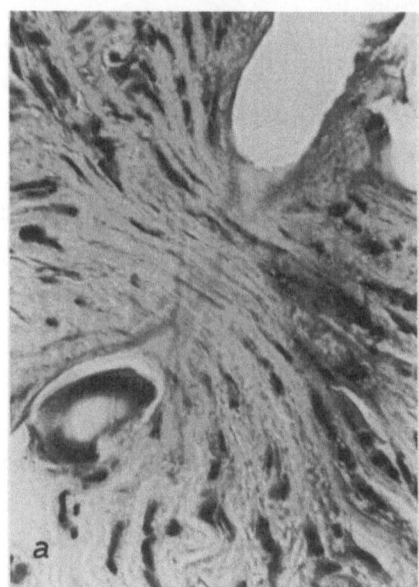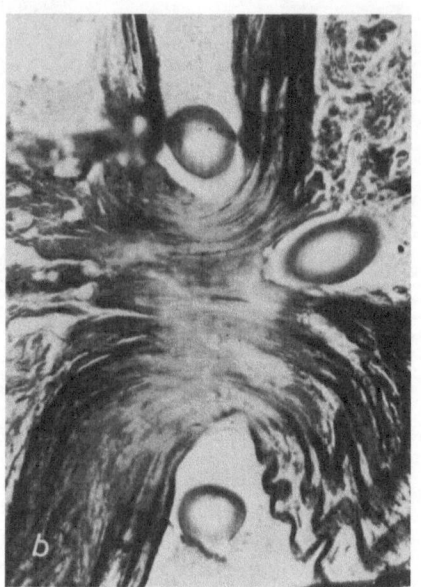

Fig. 3
a) Anastomosis 24 hours after the operation, cellular destruction,
H.-E. X 160
b) 10th day after the operation, destruction of the elastica, E.-v.G.
X 100

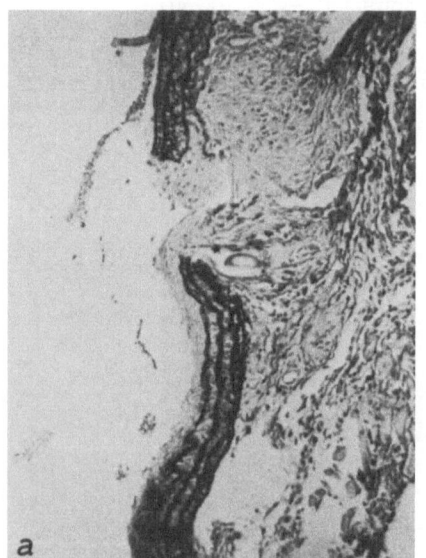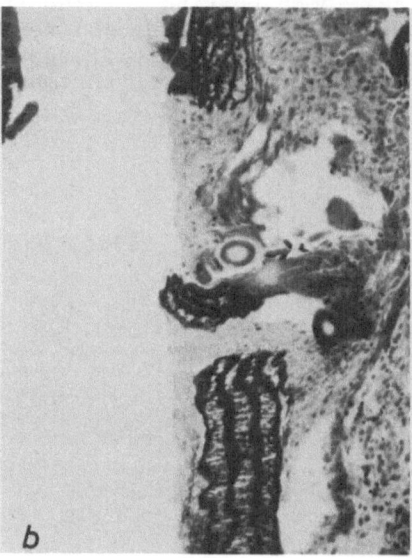

Fig. 4
a) 14th day after the operation, scarred anastomosis with separation
of the cut ends of the vessel, hyperplasia of intima, E.-v.G. X 40
b) 14th day after the operation, scarred anastomosis like Fig. 4 a,
including non-absorbed parts of the cut ends of the vessel, hyperplasia of intima, E.-v.G. X 50

Hormone Concentrations in Patients with Pituitary Tumors in the Postoperative Period with Regard to Hormone Replacement Therapy

K. v. WILD, F.-D. HOFFMANN, M. NEUBAUER, P.-H. ALTHOFF, and J. HAPP

Investigations about the endocrine activity of the anterior pituitary lobe in the acute postoperative period after removal of pituitary tumors are rare as compared to those in general surgery (1, 7, 12, 19, 37). In patients with pituitary tumors there are great variations in the preoperative hormonal state as well as in the extent of tissue destruction by neurosurgical procedures (18, 20, 35). Inevitably there must be great differences in the need for hormone replacement therapy during the acute operative period. Therefore it cannot be satisfying to use a fixed scheme (3, 10, 21, 25) that would be valid in all cases especially in regard to the side effects of the hormones used (5, 32). This is why we started our investigations by studying the pattern of some clinically important hormones (23, 33) during the immediate postoperative period in our neurosurgical patients (16).

In the last two years we measured the plasma concentrations of cortisol, LH, FSH and growth hormone (GH) by radioimmunological methods in 29 patients with pituitary adenomas and in 4 patients with craniopharyngiomas. Thyroid function was estimated by determining the total thyroxine and TBG index. At the onset of this study ACTH and TSH radioimmunoassays were not yet available in our laboratory. Blood samples were taken as follows: directly before and after operation (13, 15, 17, 25, 29); then at six hour intervals starting at 6 p. m. until the morning of the 3rd day; finally on the 7th and 14th postoperative day. If possible hormones were not administered unless necessary due to the clinical situation. Recently in 3 patients with craniotomies dexamethasone was given to avoid edema of the brain (5, 7, 28). Our operative control groups consisted of 8 males and females: 5 patients with brain tumors, 2 patients with lumbar disc prolapses, and 1 patient with neurolysis of the ulnar nerve.

The mean values of cortisol, LH, FSH and GH are shown in Fig. 1. For comparable results concerning LH and FSH only males and concerning GH only patients with endocrine inactive pituitary tumors were considered. The preoperative mean levels of the hormones investigated were in the normal range. Directly postoperatively there was a distinct increase in cortisol concentrations followed by a slight decline on the same day. Thereafter the mean cortisol level remained above the preoperative concentration until the 14th postoperative day. The LH concentrations were constantly in the lower normal range (3, 14, 22) whereas FSH gradually fell to the lower normal range limit. The pattern of GH was not characteristic in patients with endocrine inactive pituitary tumors (8, 31, 42).

In 5 patients suffering from acromegaly (Fig. 2) the concentrations of GH were elevated and showed a variable postoperative course (21, 37). Only in two patients was there an immediate postoperative decrease of GH (19).

The levels of thyroxine are not presented. They were in the normal range pre- and postoperatively without a decrease during the period studied (8, 37).

Of particular interest with respect to postoperative hormone replacement therapy was the pattern of cortisol (6, 41) during the postoperative period. A comparison of the results from the patients suffering from pituitary tumors with those of the control groups (Fig. 3) revealed a distinctly higher increase of plasma cortisol after all brain operations. Furthermore the mean cortisol levels remained above the normal range with a disturbed circadian rhythm (24) during the whole observation period. These observations were reported as well by BOUZARTH et al. (7) in 1972. Following extracranial operations, however, cortisol levels and circadian rhythm had been normalized by the second postoperative day (7, 8, 11, 26, 27, 42). The 3 patients treated with dexamethasone (1 pituitary adenoma operated by transfrontal approach and 2 intracranial meningiomas) showed the expected suppression of plasma cortisol (4, 5, 6, 7). Nevertheless an increased cortisol concentration during the first 48 hours due to the operative stress was observed as reported by other authors (4, 41, 42). Particularly interesting was the plasma cortisol pattern in a patient with severe insufficiency of the anterior pituitary lobe due to a tumor (9). It showed a similar even though delayed course as seen in our dexamethasone group. Due to this observation we would like to conclude that even in this patient with severe disturbance of pituitary function there was still active pituitary tissue present after the operation (37, 40).

Considering the cortisol concentrations following pituitary operations with regard to the operative approach, a more distinct cortisol peak directly postoperatively is evident in the transfrontal procedure group (Fig. 4). This is possibly caused by an irritation of the hypothalamic centers (7). On the other hand cortisol levels in patients with intrasellar pituitary tumors compared to those with large suprasellar extension (Fig. 5) showed no significant differences in contrast to the findings of OSTERMANN et al. (24).

Finally we have compared the cortisol levels of patients with and without preoperative adrenal insufficiency (Fig. 6). With the exception of the initial postoperative peak, plasma cortisol was slightly lower during the first three days, though still in the normal range.

Conclusions

1. Preoperatively a severe pituitary insufficiency was rare (9, 19).

2. In most of the patients with pituitary tumors, a rapid decrease of hormone levels due to the operative procedure, as would be expected, was absent.

3. In all these patients a distinct but variable increase of plasma cortisol occurred immediately after operation. This increase was less in patients undergoing the transsphenoidal approach.

4. The cortisol levels remained above the preoperative values until the 14th postoperative day. These results are the same as in patients with other kinds of brain procedures.

5. In patients with secondary pituitary insufficiency, cortisol levels well above the preoperative concentrations were observed even though the curve was flatter.

Table 1

No. of cases	Various types of neurosurgical therapy		
33 Pituitary tumors	16 Transfrontal approach	15 Transsphenoidal approach	2 Per cutaneous implantation of seeds
4 Craniopharyngiomas	3	1	
22 Non secretory adenomas	12	10	
7 Secretory adenomas	1	4	2

No. of cases	Craniotomy for brain tumor	Extracranial surgery
8 Controls		3 Extracranial surgery
4 Meningiomas	2 Transfrontal	
	2 Parietal	
1 Cerebello-pontine-angle exploration	1 Posterior fossa	
2 Lumbar discs		2 Interlaminectomy
1 Periph. ulnar		1 Neurolysis
1 Ulnar nerve		

6. In the light of these findings, we now use the following regimen of hormone replacement therapy during the operative period:

In patients with transsphenoidal procedures and preoperative adrenal insufficiency we continue the hormone replacement therapy. In the course of dexamethasone treatment (28) when craniotomies were performed, additional mineralocorticosteroids are necessary if disturbances of the electrolyte balance, or serious hypotension occur. Final hormone replacement therapy is established about 2 months after the operation depending on the results of hypophyseal function tests (30, 33, 34, 36, 38, 39, 43).

REFERENCES

1. ALTHOFF, P. H., HAPP, J., GRABS, V., SCHNEIDER, B., BEYER, J., SCHÖFFLING, K.: The early rise of growth hormone in acromegalic patients following intravenous glucagon-sign of secondary hypothalamic acromegaly. Acta endocr. (Kbh.) Supp. 184, 7 (1974).

2. AONO, T., KURACHI, K., MIZUTANI, S., HAMANAKA, Y., ZOZUMI, T., NAKASIMA, A., KOSHIYAMA, K., MATSUMOTO, K.: Influence of major surgical stress on plasma levels of testosterone luteinizing hormone and follicle stimulating hormone in male patients. J. Clin. Endocrinol. Metab. 35, 535 - 542 (1972).

3. ARSENI, C., MARETSIS, M.: Craniopharyngioma. Neurochirurgica 1, 25 - 32 (1972).

4. ASFELDT, V. H., ELB, S.: Hypothalamo-pituitary-adrenal response during major surgical stress. Acta endocr. (Kbh.) 59, 67 - 75 (1968).

5. BEKS, W. F., DOORENBOS, H., WALSTRA, G. J. M.: Clinical experiences with steroids in neurosurgical patients. In: Steroids and brain edema (eds. H. J. REULEN, K. SCHÜRMANN), pp. 233 - 238. Berlin - Heidelberg - New York: Springer 1972.

6. BINNS, T. B.: Diskussionsbeitrag. In: ACTH - eine Standortbestimmung für die Praxis (Hrsg. R. SCHUPPLI), S. 40. Bern - Stuttgart - Wien: Huber 1973.

7. BOUZARTH, W. F., SHENKLIN, H. A., GUTTERMAN, P.: Adrenal cortical response to neurosurgical problems, noting the effects of exogenous steroids. In: Steroids and brain edema (eds. J. J. REULEN, K. SCHÜRMANN), P. 183 - 193. Berlin - Heidelberg - New York: Springer 1972.

8. CARTERS, A. C., ODELL, W. D., THOMPSON, J. C.: Anterior pituitary function during surgical stress and convalescence. Radioimmunoassay measurement of blood TSH, LH, FSH and Growth Hormone. J. Clin. Endocr. 29, 63 - 71 (1969).

9. COPE, C. L., PEARSON, J.: Zitiert bei WINKELMANN et al. (1973).

10. ELKINGTON, S. G., BUCKELL, M., JENKINS, J. S.: Endocrine function following treatment of pituitary adenoma. Acta endocr. (Kbh.) 55, 146 - 152 (1967).

11. FAIMAN, C., WINTER, J. S. D.: Diurnal cycles in plasma FSH, testosterone and cortisol in men. J. Clin. Endocr. 33, 186 - 191 (1971).

12. FEUERLE, G., REISERT, P. M., EMRICH, D., KÖNIG, A., BUCHE, K.-A.: Untersuchungen zur klinischen und endokrinologischen Diagnostik von hypophysären und suprasellären Tumoren. Dtsch. med. Wschr. 95, 1051 - 1058 (1970).

13. GUIOT, G., THIBAUT, B.: L'exsirpation des adenomes hypophysaires par voi trans-sphénoidale. Neurochir. 1, 133 - 150 (1959).

14. HAPP, J., BEYER, J., SZAMAK, F., NEUBAUER, M., DEMISCH, K., SCHÖFFLING, K.: LH, FSH testosterone and estrogens in serum of healthy men after prolonged infusion of synthetic LH-RH. Acta endocr. (Kbh.) Suppl. 184, 20 (1974).

15. HARDY, J., WIGSMER, S. M.: Trans-sphenoidal surgery of pituitary fossa tumors with televised radioflourscopic control. J. Neurosurg. 23, 612 - 619 (1965).

16. HOFFMANN, F.-D.: Inaug. Diss. Frankfurt/Main (in Vorbereitung).

17. KLAR, E.: Bericht über 456 Hypophysenausschaltungen (472 Eingriffe) mittels Elektrokoagulation bzw. Radio-Gold-Implantation auf percutanem, paranasalem Wege. Langenbecks Arch. klin. Chir. 294, 497 - 510 (1960).

18. KRACHT, J., HACHMEISTER, U.: Hormonbildungsstätten im Hypophysenvorderlappen des Menschen. In: Oestrogene, Hypophysentumoren (Hrsg. J. KRACHT), p. 200 - 205. Berlin - Heidelberg - New York: Springer 1969.

19. KNAPPE, G., MENNING, H., ROHDE, W.: Evaluation of hypophyseal function in acromegaly before and after removal of pituitary adenoma by the transethmoidal-transsphenoidal approach. Acta endocr. (Kbh.), Suppl. 177, 264 (1973).

20. LABHART, A.: Die Adenohypophyse. In: Klinik der inneren Sekretion. 2. Aufl. (Hrsg. A. LABHART), S. 70 - 129. Berlin - Heidelberg - New York: Springer 1971.

21. LAZARUS, L., BLAESEL, K. F., CONNELLEY, T. J., YOUNG, J. D.: Serum-growth-hormone in acromegaly. Lancet 90 - 91 (1966).

22. MONDEN, Y., KOSHIYAMA, K., TANAKA, H., MIZUTANI, S., AONO, T., HAMANAKA, Y., UOZUMI, T., MATSUMOTO, K.: Influence of major surgical Stress on plasma testosterone, plasma LH and urinary steroids. Acta endocr. 69, 542 - 552 (1972).

23. NEY, R. L., ORTH, D. N., LIDDLE, G. W.: Evaluation of pituitary-adrenal function in man. In: The investigation of hypothalamic-pituitary-adrenal function (eds. V. H. T. JAMES, J. LANDON), pp. 285 - 294. Cambridge: University-Press 1968.

24. OSTERMANN, P. O., LINDBERG, P. O., WIDE, L.: The Level and circadian rhythm of plasma free 11-hydroxycorticoids in patients with localized intracranial processes, especially in the sellar region. Acta Neurol. Scandinav. 49, 115 - 132 (1973).

25. RAY, B. S.: Intracranial hypophysektomy. J. Neurosurg. 28, 180 - 186 (1968).

26. RETIENE, K.: Die circadiane Rhythmik endokriner Funktionen und ihre Bedeutung für die klinische Medizin. Habilitationsschrift in Frankfurt/Main (1969).

27. RETIENE, G., FROHNS, T., SCHULZ, F.: Experimentelle Untersuchungen zur Chronopharmakologie von Corticosteroiden. Verh. Dtsch. Ges. Inn. Med. 73, 990 (1967).

28. REULEN, H. J., HADJIDIMOS, A., HASE, U.: Steroids in the treatment of brain edema. In: Advances in neurosurgery 1 (eds. K. SCHÜRMANN, M. BROCK, H. J. REULEN, D. VOTH), pp. 92 - 105. Berlin - Heidelberg - New York: Springer 1973.

29. RUF, H.: Über die transfrontale Freilegung der Sellaregion. Dtsch. med. Wschr. 95, 2233 - 2236 (1970).

30. RUF, H., von WILD, K., NEUBAUER, M.: Follow-up studies on 33 craniopharyngiomas and 95 cases of chromophobe and acidophil pituitary adenomas after treatment by transfrontal operation. In: Modern aspects of neurosurgery, Vol. IV (eds. H. KUHLENDAHL, M. BROCK, D. Le VAY, T. J. WESTON), pp. 152 - 161. Amsterdam: Excerpta Medica 1973.

31. SCHALCH, D. S.: The influence of physical stress and exercise on growth hormone and insulin secretion in man. J. Lab. & Clin. Med. 69, 256 - 269 (1967).

32. SCHÄFER, E. L., BUCHHOLZ, R.: Nebenwirkungen und Gefahren der Hormontherapie. Stuttgart: Georg Thieme 1974.

33. SCRIBA, P. C.: Postoperative Diagnostik und Substitionstherapie bei Hypophysentumoren. In: Oestrogene Hypophysentumoren (Hrsg. J. KRACHT), S. 274 - 288. Berlin - Heidelberg - New York: Springer 1969.

34. SCRIBA, P. C.: Endocrinology of the hypothalamus and pituitary gland. In: Modern aspects of neurosurgery, Vol. IV (eds. H. KUHLENDAHL, M. BROCK, D. Le VAY, T. J. WESTON), pp, 83 - 89. Amsterdam: Excerpta Medica 1973.

35. SCRIBA, P. C., Von WERDER, K., SCHWARZ, K.: Hypothalamus und Hypophyse. In: Klinische Pathophysiologie, 2. Aufl. (Hrsg. W. SIEGENTHALER), S. 266. Stuttgart: Georg Thieme 1973.

36. SOLBACH, H. G., BETHGE, H., ZIMMERMANN, H.: Funktionsdiagnostik der Hypophysentumoren. In: Oestrogene Hypophysentumoren (Hrsg. J. KRACHT), S. 236 - 255. Berlin - Heidelberg - New York: Springer 1969.

37. WEISBECKER, L., SCHEMMEL, K., KINET, M., STÖWSAND, D., LEYBOLD, K., LAHRTZ, H. G., MOKMOL, V., ZEPF, S.: Untersuchungen zum hormonalen Status nach Hypophysektomie. Verh. Dtsch. Ges. Inn. Med. 78, 1525 - 1529 (1972).

38. Von WILD, K.: Notfallausweis für Hypophysenoperierte Patienten. Neurochirurgica 5, 177 - 178 (1972).

39. Von WILD, K.: Zur Diagnose der Hypophysentumoren. Nervenarzt 43, 587 - 589 (1972).

40. Von WILD, K., RÜTTGER, P., KRÜCKE, W.: Recurrent adenoma of the adenohypophysis in connection with polyadenomatosis of endocrine glands, pheochromocytoma and alopecia totalis. In: Modern aspects of neurosurgery, Vol. IV (eds. H. KUHLENDAHL, M. BROCK, D. Le VAY, T. J. WESTON), pp. 175 - 179. Amsterdam: Excerpta Medica 1973.

41. WINKELMANN, W., BETHGE, H., HACKENBERG, K., SOLBACH, H. G.: Cortisol und Cortikosteronsekretion bei Hypophysentumoren. In: Oestrogene Hypophysentumoren (Hrsg. J. KRACHT), S. 309 - 311. Berlin - Heidelberg - New York: Springer 1969.

42. YALOW, R. S., VARSANO-AHARON, N., ECHEMENDIA, E., BERSON, A.: HGH and ACTH secretory responses to stress. Horm. Metab. Res. 1, 3 - 8 (1969).

43. ZIMMERMANN, H., SOLBACH, H. G., WIEGELMANN, W.: Pre- and postoperative hormone substitution in pituitary tumors. In: Modern aspects of neurosurgery, Vol. IV (eds. H. KUHLENDAHL, M. BROCK, D. Le VAY, T. J. WESTON), pp. 191 - 196. Amsterdam: Excerpta Medica 1973.

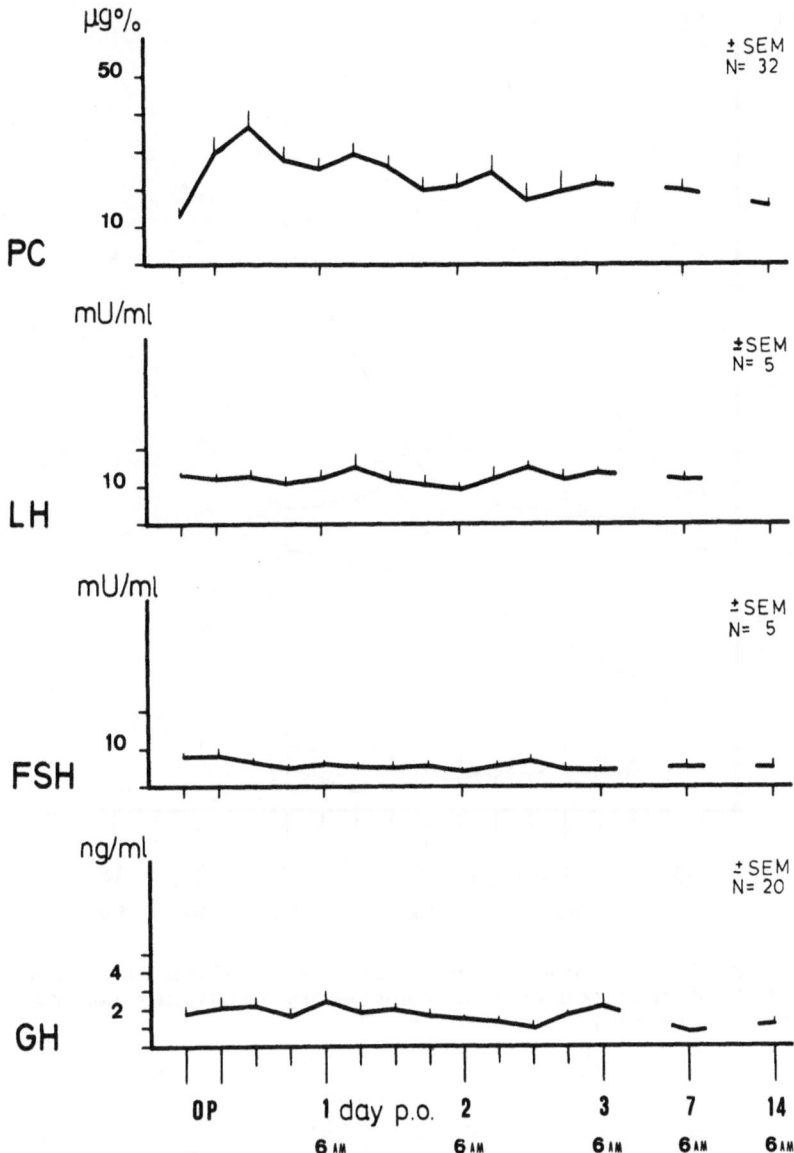

Fig. 1. Plasma cortisol, LH, FSH and growth hormone levels after removal of pituitary tumors

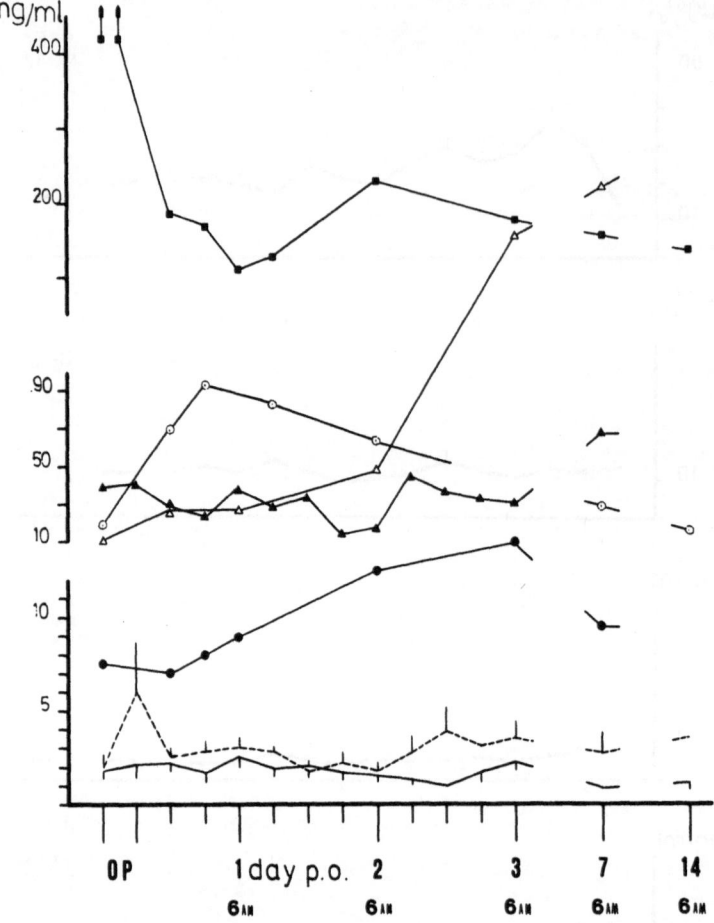

Fig. 2. Growth hormone levels in acromegalics after operative treatment in comparison with non secretory pituitary tumors (———) and controls (-----)

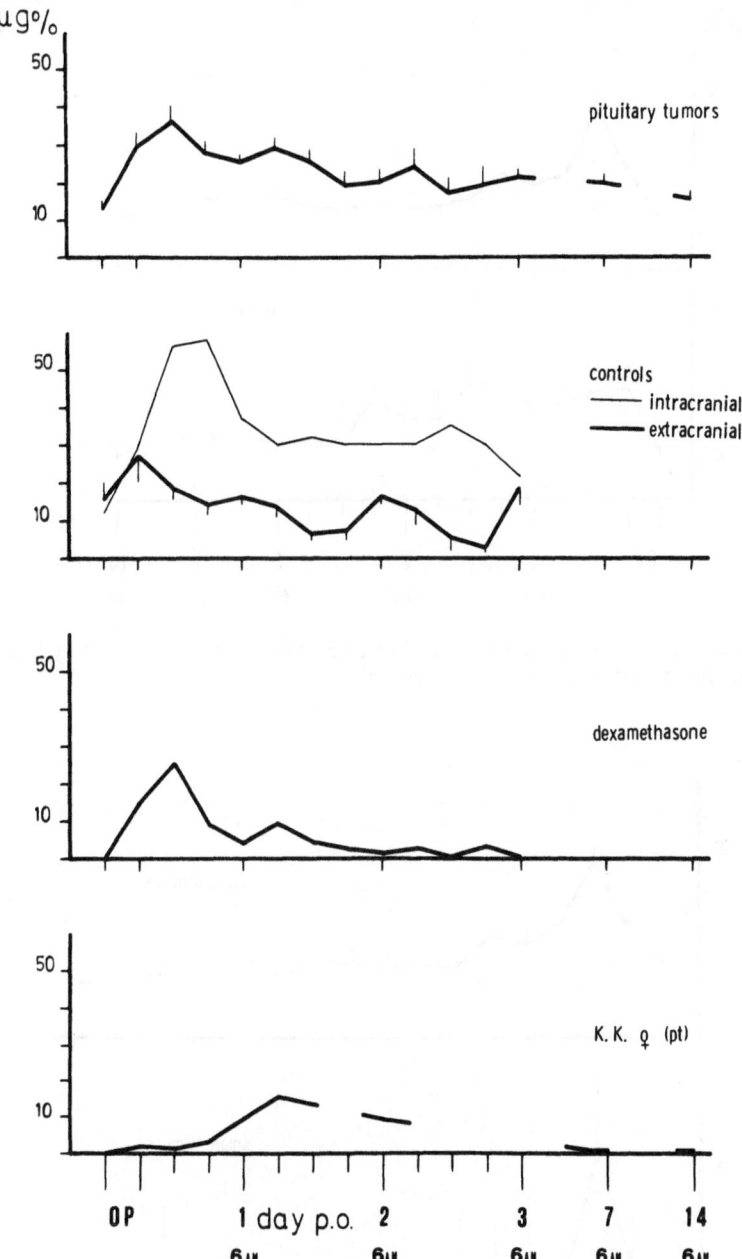

Fig. 3. Plasma cortisol levels after surgical treatment

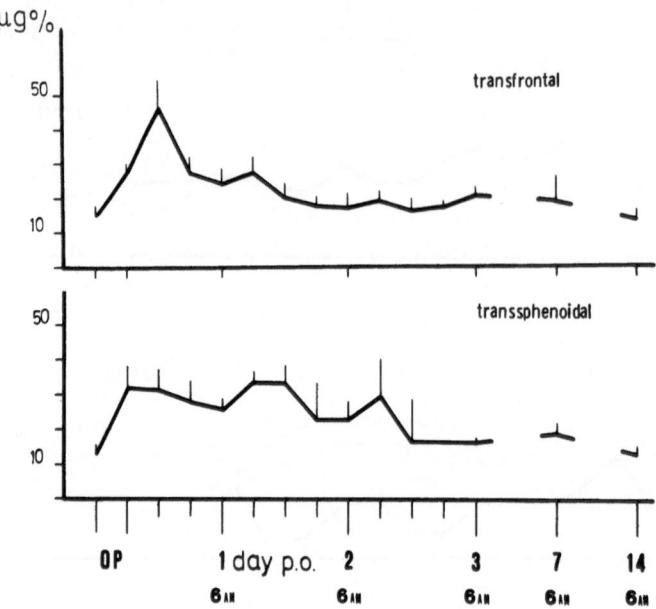

Fig. 4. Plasma cortisol levels after removal of pituitary tumors in respect to surgical approach

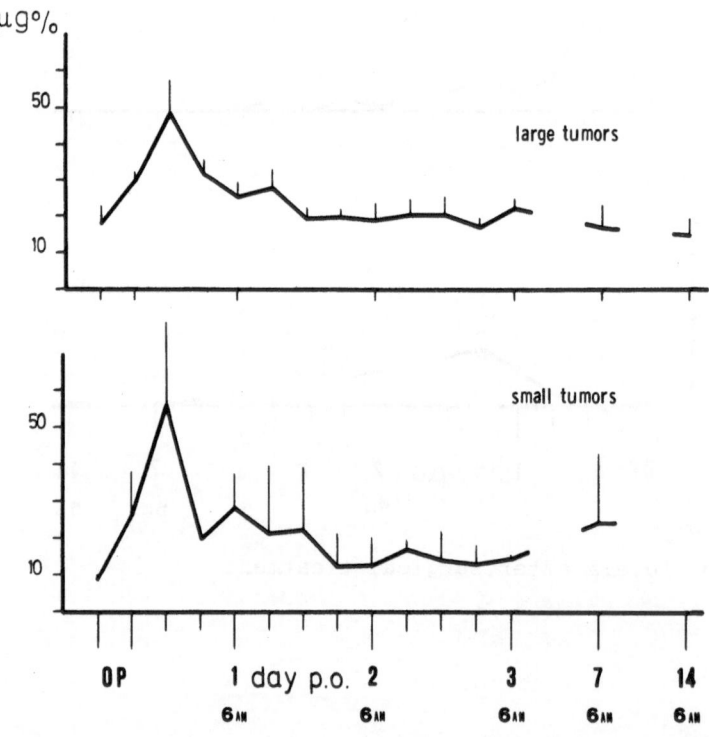

Fig. 5. Plasma cortisol levels after surgical treatment in respect to size of pituitary tumor

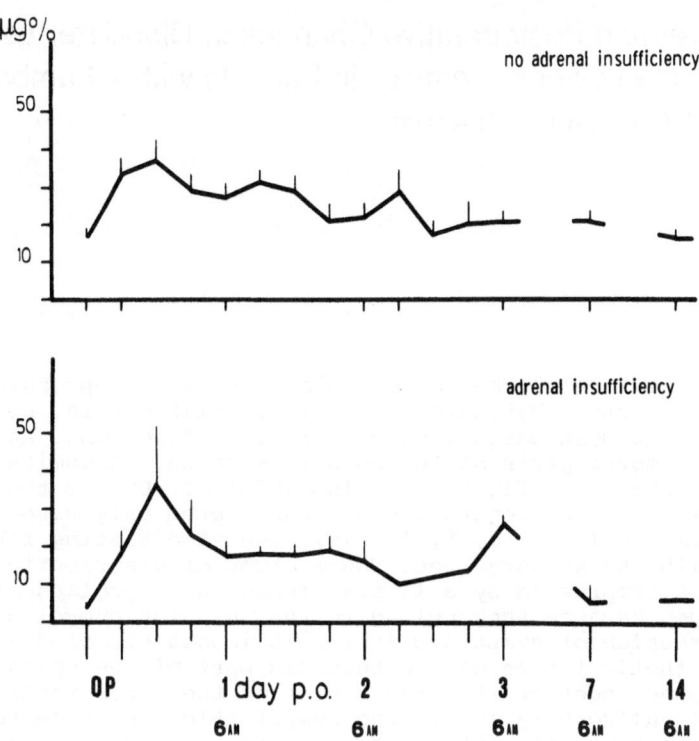

Fig. 6. Plasma cortisol level after surgical treatment in respect to hormonal state

Pre- and Postoperative Changes in Blood Perfusion of the Muscle of the Lower Extremities in Patients with a Lumbar Disc Prolapse

W. Elies and H. Seboldt

The lateral lumbar disc prolapse causes compression of the spinal
nerve root. Patients show severe sciatic pain, neurological signs
and in most cases vasovegetative dysfunctions. Apart from the sensory
and motor parts of the spinal nerve the concomitant vegetative parts
of the nerve fibres are also affected. Due to the topographic relations of the vegetative nervous system only vasodilating structures are
damaged (3, 4, 5, 8, 10, 14). The vasodilating fibres go together
with the sensory ones. Their order of distribution is segmental. They
are compressed by a lateral lumbar disc prolapse and are easily damaged because they belong to the thinnest unmyelinated nerves. Compression of sympathic fibres is impossible caudal to L 2. The sympathetic fibres of the thoracic part of the spinal cord leave the
spine together with the fibres of the nerve roots as far down as L 2.
Distal to this level, the sympathetic fibres leave their ganglia
lateral to the intervertebral foramina as rami communicantes grisei
and enter the spinal nerves. As about 90 % of the lumbar disc prolapse syndromes occur at the levels of L 4 / L 5 and L 5 / S 1 (6, 11),
vasodilation is altered although sympathetic innervation is not affected. The segmentally intensified tonus of the sympathetic system
manifests itself by vasoconstriction with a subsequent decrease in the
temperature of the extremity (8). Patients often complain about a
sensation of coldness in the aching leg which is reinforced when the
leg is cooled. This fact shows that the alteration of the parasym-
pathetic-sympathetic balance is of clinical relevance. This symptom
is mentioned in literature several times (7, 8, 9, 12, 13, 15). In
1958 REISCHAUER mentioned sciatic disturbance of the blood flow in
the legs. KOLLAR published results of pre- and postoperative examinations of vegetative dysregulations in patients with a lumbar disc prolapse in 1973 for the first time. Both authors used oscillography and
measurement of skin temperature in order to objectify vegetative dysfunctions. But until now no data about the real changes in blood perfusion are available.

Material and Methods

In 28 patients with a lateral lumbar disc prolapse, blood perfusion
of the lower legs was measured. Clinical diagnosis was verified by
myelography in all cases. Blood flow was measured in both calves and
feet at rest and after an arterial occlusion of three minutes. We did
this in the preoperative phase and usually on the 15th postoperative
day by means of a two-channel venous occlusion plethysmograph[1] which
works on a pneumatic principle. Our normal values of plethysmography
are listed in Table 1. The reactive hyperemia after three minutes of

---

[1] Infraton Vasoskript VVP 33 nach Prof. Barbey; Fa. Boucke, D - 74
Tübingen, Germany

arterial occlusion is a good hemodynamic parameter and an exactly comparable and reproducible equivalent for physical strain.

Table 1. Normal values of venous-occlusion plethysmography; value in ml/min/100 ml of tissue

	Blood flow at rest	Reactive hyperemia after three minutes of arterial occlusion
Calf	1 - 4	more than 15
Foot	1 - 5	more than 5,5

Results

Clinical data of the examined patients correspond to those given in literature [(2, 7, 11), Table 2]. The average age was 44 + 12 years. The percentage of male cases was higher than that of female cases. Lumbar disc prolapses situated at the level of L 4 / L 5 were more frequent than those at L 5 / S 1.

Table 2. Clinical data of the patients

Number of patients	28
male	17
female	11
Length of history (months)	40 + 37
Level of the disc prolapse	
L 4 / L 5	18
L 5 / S 1	10

Patients were grouped according to their preoperative neurological state (Table 3). Most of them had severe sciatic pains combined with neurological signs. Few showed pain only and it was only in one case that we found segmental paresis of the calf muscles. Therapeutic procedure consisted of the removal of the disc prolapse after enlargement of the interlaminar space or by hemilaminectomy. Results were checked after a fortnight. 23 patients recovered totally or at least subtotally. Only five patients said their symptoms had decreased slightly. Before the operation all patients reported that they felt sensations of coldness in the painful leg which increased after cooling. Some reported this symptom spontaneously, others only after we had asked them.

Table 3. Preoperative state in patients with lumbar disc prolapse

Severe sciatic pain only	8 patients
Severe sciatic pain combined with neurological signs	19 patients
Segmental paresis of the shank muscles	1 patient

Preoperative blood flow of both calves at rest was not pathologically
reduced. The blood flow of the calf on the side corresponding to the
prolapse (3,2 ± 1,5 ml/min/100 ml of muscle tissue) was 25 % less
than the flow on the other side (4,0 ± 1,6). This difference was not
significant, but became clearer after arterial occlusion. We found a
highly significant decrease (- 25 %) of blood perfusion in the calf
homolateral to the disc prolapse (Table 4). The values (13,4 ± 4,7)
were equal to those found in mild arterial occlusion diseases (10 -
15; according to BOLLINGER). The results measured in the foot were
similar to those of the calf. In comparison with our normal values
we had a reduction of about 30 %. During the postoperative phase
blood perfusion was normal and showed no differences between the two
sides. After arterial occlusion the blood flow in the extremity homolateral to the disc prolapse became normal (more than 15). It rose by
about 25 % up to 16,4 ± 4,7 and was equal to the other side. During
the postoperative phase patients hardly complained about sensations
of coldness in the leg. In five cases only we still found some symptoms. Significant relationships between blood flow and the neurological state could not be established. We should like to point out that
the normal blood flow values measured in our patients were relatively
low.

Table 4. Blood perfusion of the calves at rest (A) and after three
minutes of arterial occlusion (B)
+ = values of significant difference

| | Calf to the disc prolapse | | Foot to the disc prolapse | |
	homolateral	contralateral	homolateral	contralateral
Pre-operative				
A	3,2 ± 1,5	4,0 ± 1,6	1,0 ± 0,7	1,2 ± 1,0
B	13,4 ± 4,7[+]	16,5 ± 3,9[+]	6,7 ± 2,3[+]	8,3 ± 2,4[+]
	n = 28	n = 28	n = 27	n = 27
Post-operative				
A	3,2 ± 1,5	3,4 ± 1,8	0,9 ± 0,5	1,0 ± 0,9
B	16,7 ± 4,7[+]	16,4 ± 5,0	7,8 ± 1,3	8,0 ± 2,3
	n = 17	n = 17	n = 16	n = 16

Discussion

In the past oscillography and measurements of skin temperature were
used to objectify sciatic disturbances of blood flow in the legs.
Those methods give only weak data when the hemodynamic characteristics
of the vascular system are considered. To characterize the vascular
system hemodynamically, we measured the arterial blood perfusion of
the lower extremities. The values found after arterial occlusion are
well reproducible and comparable. They can be regarded as an expression of physical strain. During the preoperative phase, blood flow
is not reduced in both calves. After three minutes of arterial occlusion we found a significant decrease in blood perfusion of the homo-

lateral calf. With 13,4 ml/min/100 ml of muscle tissue, it corresponds
to values found in mild arterial occlusion diseases (1). But they were
different from genuine arterial occlusion disease by a normal course
of time of the reactive hyperemia. The curve of the blood flow showed
a normal steep initial rise with a subsequent normal course. Therefore we assume that the reason for the disturbances of blood flow of
the calf in patients with a lumbar disc prolapse is the irritation of
vasodilating fibres. Together with other authors we are of the opinion
that the pressure of the protruding disc prolapse damages the vasodilating fibres which are situated in close vicinity to the sensory
parts of the spinal nerve while the sympathetic fibres are not impaired that the degree of vasodilation is more prominent than we could
find in our measurements. We measured the blood flow of the whole calf
which is innervated by several lumbar nerve roots. Since only one
nerve root is damaged in most cases, we measured normotonic as well
as dystonic areas of the muscles. After operative decompression, the
vasodilating fibres recovered quickly. This can be shown by normal
blood flow values and the absence of sensations of coldness in the
legs. The quick recovery of the vasodilating fibres is of remarkable
contrast to the longstanding segmental dysfunctions of sensibility.
The normal values of blood perfusion tend towards the lower end of
the distribution curve. Our explanation for this is little or no
training of calf muscles, due to sciatic pains.

Summary

In 28 patients with lateral lumbar disc prolapse the blood flow of
the lower extremities was measured pre- and postoperatively by using
a venous-occlusion plethysmograph. The blood perfusion three minutes
after arterial occlusion, a comparable and reproducible parameter of
physical strain, was significantly reduced in the calf and foot homolateral to the disc prolapse during the preoperative phase. The difference to the genuine arterial occlusion disease was the normal run
of the curve of the blood flow. Postoperatively the blood flow was
normal. Preoperative blood flow disturbances are due to a vasoneuro-
pathia, caused by a compression of the vasodilating fibres in the
spinal nerve roots.

REFERENCES

1. BOLLINGER, A.: Durchblutungsmessungen in der klinischen Angiolo-
   gie. Bern - Stuttgart: Huber-Verlag 1969.

2. BRADFORD, F., SPURLING, R. G.: The intervertebral disc. 2nd edition. Springfield/Ill.: C. Thomas 1945.

3. BRODAL, A.: Neurological Anatomy in Relation to Clinical Medicine,
   p. 612. London - Toronto - New York: Oxford University Press 1969.

4. CLARA, M.: Das Nervensystem des Menschen. 3. Aufl. S. 252. Leipzig: J. A. Barth 1959.

5. FOERSTER, O.: Über die Vasodilatatoren in den peripheren Nerven
   und hinteren Rückenmarkswurzeln beim Menschen. Dtsch. Z. Nerven-
   hlk. 107, 41 - 56 (1929).

6. GURDJIAN, E. St., THOMAS, L. M.: Operative Neurosurgery. 3rd edition. Baltimore: Williams and Wilkins 1970.

7. JUNGHANNS, H.: Die gesunde und die kranke Wirbelsäule in Röntgen-
   bild und Klinik. Stuttgart: Georg Thieme 1968.

8. KOLLAR, W. A. F.: Untersuchungen zur Frage der postischialgischen Durchblutungsstörung; prä- und postoperative Befunde nach Laminotomien. Neurochirurgia 16, 9 - 23 (1973).

9. LJUBINSCHEW, S. A., KENTS, V. V.: Zur Differentialdiagnostik von Gefäßstörungen bei Lumbosacral-Radikulitiden und Endarteriitis obliterans. Zh. Nevropat. Psikhiat. (Moskva) 5, 647 - 651 (1968).

10. MUMENTHALER, M., SCHLIACK, H.: Läsionen peripherer Nerven, S. 75. Stuttgart: Georg Thieme 1973.

11. OLDENKOTT, P.: Zur medizinischen und medizinisch-sozialen Problematik beim lumbalen Bandscheibenvorfall. Tübingen, Habil. (1971).

12. REISCHAUER, F.: Über die postischialgische Durchblutungsstörung des Beines. Med. Klin. 14, 579 - 584 (1958).

13. SCHRADER, A. E.: Die Bedeutung des Bandscheibenschadens für die Manifestation von arteriellen Durchblutungsstörungen. Dtsch. Z. Nervenhk. 160, 400 - 412 (1949).

14. WALDEYER, A.: Anatomie des Menschen. Bd. I, S. 81. Berlin: De Gruyter 1957.

15. WLASOW, N. A.: Vegetative changes in lumbar osteochondrosis. Zh. Nevropat. Psikhiat. (Moskva) 5, 665 - 669 (1968).

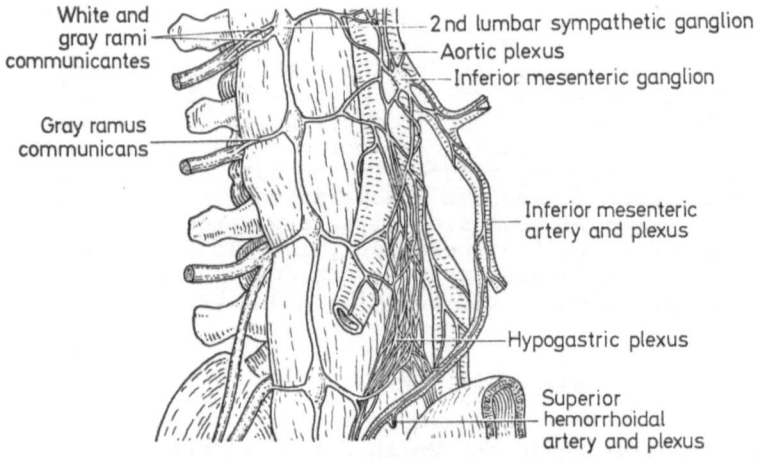

Fig. 1. Autonomic nerves and ganglia in the pelvis

Problems of Hospitalism in Neurosurgical Intensive Care

H. SOLLMANN, F. K. BÖCKEM, and K. SCHMIDT

During the last years an increasing number of endemic infections of
seriously ill patients in Intensive Care Units have been observed all
over the world. The infectious agents have been almost exclusively
gram-negative germs, resistent to all or almost all the antibiotics
available.

The patients this paper refers to, were mainly comatous and in a state
of protracted shock, they were intubated for a long period of time or
under artificial respiration. The causes for the increasing rate of
infection are multiple: Increasing number of very young and very old
people, contamination of technical material used, immunosuppressive
therapy, increasing resistence to antibiotics, increasing chance of
survival of the seriously-ill. Endemic infections often appear as relatively harmless but persistent cystopyelitis. In the seriously-ill,
however, they appear as acute or subchronic, and finally, lethal
pneumonias. The pneumonias caused by Klebsiella are characterized by
their rapid course, lobe filling secretions, and death within 24
hours after the onset of the clinical signs. In addition,
lethal meningitis due to Klebsiella, presumably hematogenous, is observed occasionally. We have seen 3 cases of this kind in our clinic.

Our investigations are based on the bacteriological examinations and
the antibiograms of pathogenic germs from October 1971 to June 1974.
All pathogenic germs were registered, their sensitivity to the antibiotics was tested and listed. In every patient a tracheal swab and
an urine sample was examined twice weekly for bacteria.

The number of Intensive Care Unit patients is specified in relation
to the patients who died and to the ICU patients with pneumonia. For
patients who died of pneumonia, the autopsy protocol certified the
cause of death as pneumonia and in the pre and postmortal swabs
Klebsiella were found (Fig. 1).

A more precise analysis of the death cases in the ICU and of the
deaths by pneumonia in relation to the percentage of Klebsiella-
strains in all pathogenic germs and urinary cultures (October 1971
to June 1974) shows that the peak of mortality is followed by a peak
of mortality due to pneumonia. Also mortality and percentage of
Klebsiella in all pathogenic germs can be correlated (Fig. 2).

The organisation of the ICU has an important influence on the mortality: Highest mortality occurs with a high number of patients
confined to a single room. On the other hand, isolation of patients
and personnel (one nurse and one patient per room) and rigorous
sanitizing measures showed striking positive results. Furthermore,
it is intersting to note that during the time of prophylactic application of antibiotics the gram-negative strains dominated the gram-

positive. During the same time the sensitivity of these germs to antibiotics decreased down to almost zero. When used specifically, the gram-positive germs rose. When antibiotic therapy was stopped, the amount of gram-negative bacteria diminished in regard to the gram-positive strains. During this time the sensitivity to antibiotics increased (Fig. 3) (Table 1).

In addition the reciprocity of Klebsiella and Staphylococcus aureus is interesting. We have to assume that the gram-negative germs are suppressed when gram-positive strains are numerous (Fig. 4).

The percentage of sensitivity in all antibiograms from October 1971 to June 1974 for gentamycin, cephalosporines, carbenicillin, and tetracyclines (the percentage of all other antibiotics being tested was below this level) shows that the sensitivity largely depends on the application of these antibiotics. The sensitivity of all strains present was most responsive to gentamycin. At any rate during the constant application of this antibiotic the sensitivity sank from 32 % in 1971 to 18 % in 1974. From October 1971 to June 1974 the combination of gentamycin with cephalosporines was chiefly given prophylactically. During this period, the sensitivity to cephalosporines decreased from 24 % to 9 %. Only when removed from the therapeutic schedule, did the sensitivity increase. Similar observations were made with carbenicillin', which was employed 1973 and 1974 specifically: the sensitivity decreased from 14 % to 7 %. Tetracyclines were given rarely. Their sensitivity increased from 4 % in 1971 to 16 % in 1974 (Fig. 5), (Table 2).

When reviewing the different therapeutic schedules applied, we have noticed that concentration of several seriously ill patients in one room and the presence of only one nurse for several patients is most favourable for cross-infections. In spite of the temporary closing of this one-room Intensive Care Unit, followed by disinfection and re-opening, the suppression of antibiotic prophylaxis and strict antiseptic measures (concerning doctors and medical personnel) remained without the success expected. Only complete isolation of every ICU-patient in a single room equipped with one person per patient during 24 hours (3 shifts) improved the results.

A further reduction of infections is possible by strict hygienic measures leading to a progressive decrease of the pathogenic germs to a level without danger, i. e. below the infectious level. The constant disinfection of rooms and floors before admitting a new patient, the disinfection of beds in the "shelter" using an aldehyde-alcohol-combination (Buraton^R, Incidin^R) has proved very effective. These measures are supported by the largest possible use of one-way materials. Wearing protective clothing is indispensable for an ICU. The whole medical staff (doctors and nurses) have to be trained regularly. Regular bacteriological controls have to be performed automatically.

In conclusion, the most important rules in a hopeful struggle against endemic hospitalism by Klebsiella-infection are the following:

1. Isolation of ICU-patients in single room is indispensable.

2. The ICU-patients have to be supervised during 24 hours by one person per room.

3. No prophylactic use of antibiotics is permitted, but only specific employment according to the antibiogram.

Table 1. Percentage of the most frequent gram-positive and gram-negative germs from October 1971 to June 1974 and the percentage of all strains during the whole period 1971 – 1974

Percentage of strains %	Klebs.	E. coli	Pyocy.	Proteus.	Staph. aureus	Enterok.	Staph. epid.	Strepto pyogenes
1971	18,3	-	15,8	18,3	15,8	10,5	2,6	2,6
1972	33,24	14,42	20,16	11,06	3,98	10,3	1,02	3,12
1973	21,74	19,14	6,15	8,81	27,81	10,9	2,65	2,92
1974	3,06	25,78	3,46	5,92	37,92	10,28	3,38	10,18
1971 – 1974	19,66	18,81	10,20	9,3	23,33	10,65	2,41	5,12

Table 2. Percentage of sensitivity of the different groups of antibiotic figuring in the antibiograms during different years and the percentage during the whole period 1971 – 1974

Sensitivity %	1971	1972	1973	1974	1971 – 1974
Gentamycin	32,3	20,58	16,31	18,0	21,8
Carbenicillin	11,8	12,66	13,2	7,12	11,23
Cephalospor.	23,5	9,22	11,96	12,32	14,26
Furadantin	13,2	14,5	10,11	8,64	11,61
Tetracyclin	4,4	11,0	9,81	16,02	10,03
Chloramphenicol	5,9	8,58	11,61	12,43	9,6
Ampicillin	-	6,1	10,72	12,0	7,2
Oxacillin	2,9	0,5	4,42	9,52	4,2
Nalidixins.	-	10,4	2,38	-	3,2
Polym./Colistin	-	2,6	6,2	2,0	2,7

4. Permanent reduction of germs by disinfection of rooms, floors apparatus and beds (shelter), disinfection of hands, employment of protective clothes and one-way material is absolutely essential.

5. Training of medical staff.

6. Regular bacteriological controls of patients and of contact surfaces.

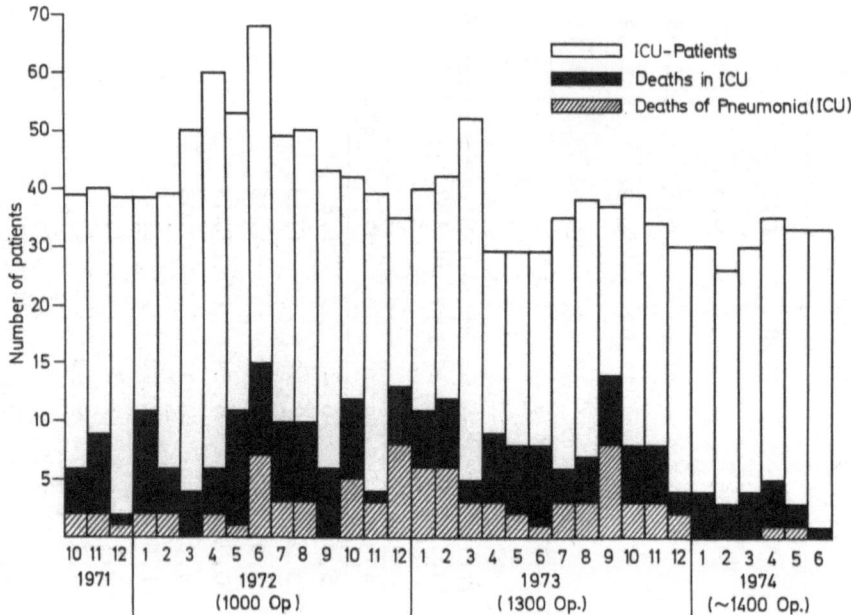

Fig. 1. Monthly number of Intensive Care patients in relation to the lethal cases and to the Intensive Care patients who died of pneumonia from October 1971 to July 1974

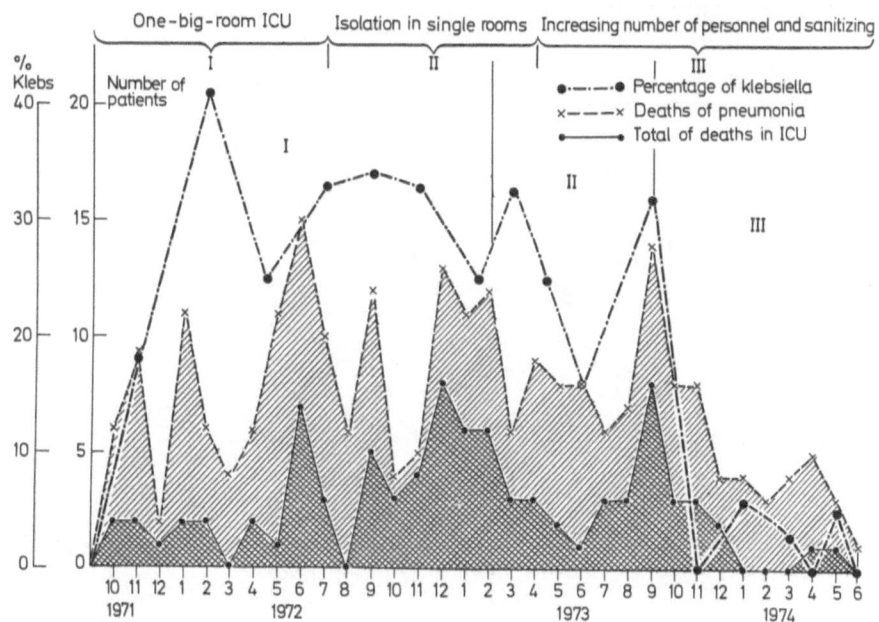

Fig. 2. The total of all Intensive Care patients and of the patients
who died of pneumonia from October 1971 to June 1974 is compared with
the percentage of Klebsiella in all pathogenic germs counted in tracheal swabs and urine cultures during the same time. One can recognize the three periods as related to one room-big surface Intensive
Care Unit, isolation in single rooms and increasing number of personnel in addition to sanitizing procedures

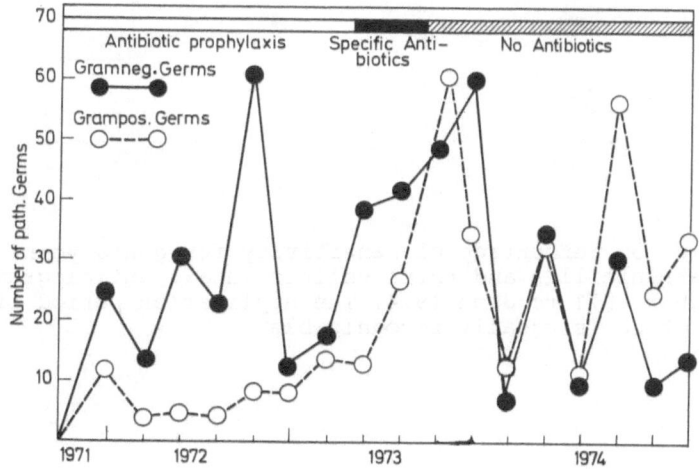

Fig. 3. Relation of gramnegative to grampositive pathogenic germs
during the period October 1971 to June 1974 in relation to the application of antibiotics

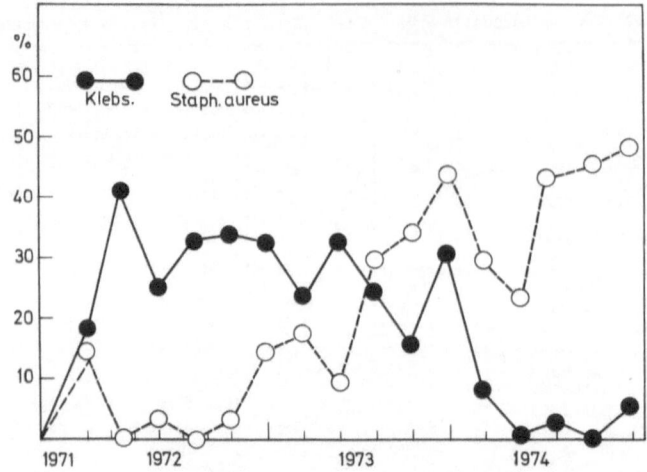

Fig. 4. Percentage of Klebsiella and Staphylococcus aureus in all pathogenic germs recorded from 1971 to 1974

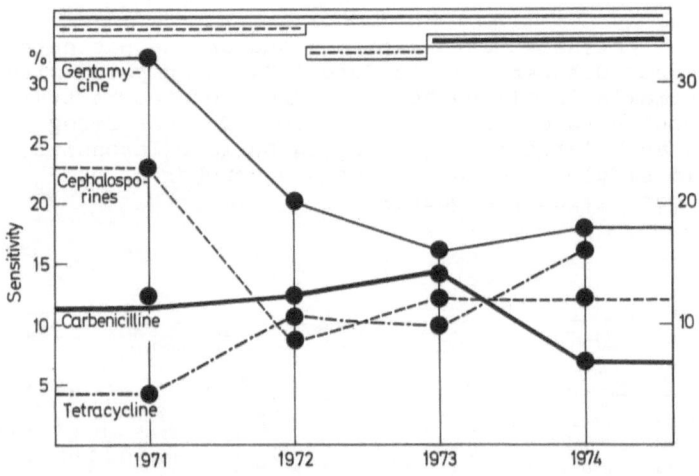

Fig. 5. Percentage of sensitivity for gentamycin, cephalosporines, carbenicillin and tetracyclines in all antibiograms made from October 1971 to June 1974. The application period of these four antibiotics is equally recognizable

The Influence of Antibiotics on the Development, Clinic and Treatment of Brain Abscess

A. KARIMI-NEJAD

Clinical analyses of 170 cases of brain abscess, 10 of which were early, 98 by extension, 47 metastatic and 15 cryptogenetic abscesses show a certain regularity in the development and course of abscesses.

Clinic and Course

In 160 cases of haematogenous and brain abscess by direct extension, 3 stages were to be seen in retrospect as mentioned by WEBER (12) according to the corresponding pathological-anatomic changes; i. e. the acute beginning of the disease with meningitic symptoms resulting from a local cerebral infection with perifocal edema. This was followed by a latent stage due to the gradual disappearance of the perifocal edema or the walling-off and encapsulation of the process respectively.

This latent stage was eventually followed by symptoms of intracranial pressure or by the abscess rupturing into the ventricle system, which led in general to fatal pyocephalus internus.

It was only in about 8 % of the cases that the acute beginning of a local cerebral infection with meningitic and local symptoms such as pareses or severe local pain could be verified. In more than 70 % of the cases these abscesses did not receive clinical treatment until local symptoms and symptoms of increasing intracranial pressure had begun to show. It was only in 5 patients (3 %) that fatal ventricle rupture with diffuse meningoencephalitis occurred without any previous symptoms.

The clinical symptomatology and the course of 10 cases of early incipient brain abscess followed from their pathogenesis which was markedly different from that of haematogenous abscesses and abscesses due to direct extension (10, 11, 9, 3, 7). The early brain abscess presupposes an open brain injury. If this leads to an open brain wound, however slight, an early brain abscess may develop. A focus of encephalomalacia and, eventually, a wound cavity may develop in the injured region of the brain. Insufficient wound toilet leads to a retention of the secretion. In case of infection, the secretion is converted into pus and the wound cavity into an abscess. Unlike traumatic brain abscesses, due to direct extension, early brain abscesses developed only at the cerebral convexity, if an obstructed bone gap caused retention of the secretion. Consequently, the previously mentioned phases that allow definition and walling-off of the process in cases of haematogenous abscesses and abscesses by extension are missing in cases of early, incipient brain abscesses. That is why clinical signs and symptomatology in about 80 % of the cases were characterized by an acute beginning with symptoms of a persistent diffuse cerebral infection with increasing intracranial pressure. In 3 patients with Clostridium brain abscess, spontaneous intracranial collection of gas was observed. One patient having an open brain wound caused by the heel of a shoe, received primary treatment on the open skull wound and survived the infection. The other 2 patients, whose skull injuries had been considered of "no great importance" and had been closed primarily, died with symptoms of acute therapy-resistant cerebral edema (7, 5).

Clinical diagnosis of an early brain abscess and - above all - its distinction from a mere meningoencephalitis after an open brain injury often prove to be difficult, since an early, incipient abscess seldom occurs without accompanying meningoencephalitis. As further local symptoms show, it is only by revising the wound that an incipient abscess can be eliminated.

Localisation of an Abscess

Localisation and mortality of the 170 cases of brain abscess in our clinic are given in Table 1. Apart from the well-known preferred temporal, infratentorial and frontal localisations of abscesses by extension resulting from otitis and sinusitis, a relatively frequent localisation of haematogenous abscesses in the parieto-occipital region is striking.

Frequency of Papilledema

In about half of the cases papilledema was observed as a symptom of increasing intracranial pressure. Table 2 shows the frequency of papilledemas and their effect on the course. Irrespective of the kind of abscess they suffered from, patients with papilledema generally had a less favourable prognosis than those without papilledema. It is especially striking that, unlike in other intracranial space-narrowing processes, papilledema was found relatively more frequently in cases of infratentorial abscess. This may also be one of the reasons for the well-known diagnostic difficulties in cases of infratentorial abscess.

On the whole, *the change of cell count in CSF* never gave similar results and was, thus, of no particular help as to the diagnosis of brain abscess. Fig. 1 shows that in about 10 - 15 % of the examined cases the cell count was normal. We found, however, pleocytosis of varying intensity depending on the intensity of the meningitic symptoms. It was only in patients with meningitic symptoms that we found more than 500 cells/mm^3. CSF examinations in 3 cases of *incipient* brain abscess with acute beginning revealed a severe pleocytosis of up to 15.000 cells/mm^3. It is striking that in cases of infratentorial abscess, the cell count in the CSF is also more often normal or just insignificantly increased than is the case in supratentorial abscesses. There was, however, no definite difference between haematogenous abscesses and abscesses by extension as to an increase in cell count in CSF.

Unlike meningitic symptoms, an increased cell count in CSF does not show a definite dependence on the type of organism of the abscess.

The number of bacteria occurring simultaneously in 140 cases of abscess that were examined is shown in Fig. 2. Unlike in infections of other parts of the body and tracheo-bronchial infections of neuro-

Table 1. Localisation of 170 brain abscesses and their mortality

Type of abscess	frontal		temp.-pariet.		occipital		fossa posterior		multip.		total	
	No.of cases	Mort. %	No.of cases	Mort. %	No.of cases	Mort. %	No.of cases	Mort. %	No.of cases	Mort. %	No.of cases	Mort. %
Early	2	50	7	43	-	-	-	-	1	100	10	50
By ex-tension ten-sion traumatic	15	20	6	33	2	50	1	0	2	50	26	27
non-traum.	20	26	30	33	3	33	16	56	3	100	72	39
Total	35	23	36	33	5	40	17	53	5	80	98	36
Metastatic	19	37	20	35	6	17	1	100	1	10	47	36
Cryptogenetic	9	67	3	67	1	100	1	0	1	100	15	60
Total	65	34	66	36	12	25	19	53	8	88	170	39
Abscess by extension	37	24	43	33	5	40	17	53	6	83	108	37
Haematogenous	28	46	23	39	7	14	2	50	2	100	62	42

Table 2. Frequency of papilledema in cases of brain abscess and its effect on course of disease

		With papilledema		without papilledema	
		No. of cases	Mortality	No. of cases	Mortality
Early brain abscesses	10	3 (30)	33 %	7 (70)	57 %
Abscess by extension — traumatic	26	9 (35)	22 %	17 (65)	29 %
non-traum.	72	34 (47)	44 %	38 (53)	34 %
total	98	43 (44)	40 %	55 (56)	33 %
Metastatic	47	23 (49)	35 %	24 (51)	33 %
Cryptogenetic	15	6 (40)	83 %	9 (60)	44 %
Total	170	75 (44)	43 %	95 (56)	36 %
Infratentorial	19	6 (32)	83 %	13 (68)	68 %
Supratentorial	151	69 (46)	39 %	82 (54)	35 %

The figures in brackets show percentage of present and absent papilledema respectively surgical patients (6), the majority of cases showed only one type of organism in the abscess contents. As usual, it is the gram-positive cocci that are prevailing. Even in recent years, there has been no evidence of a relative increase of gram-negative bacteria, so that there was no need for a special drawing-up.

It was the type of infection that was decisive for the reaction of the surrounding cerebral tissue, i. e., the perifocal edema caused in the first phase of abscess development. The severest reaction to therapy-resistent acute brain edema was observed in 3 patients with gas-gangrene infections. In line with the experimental observations of FALCONER et al. (1, 2), we found no evidence that the type of bacterium might influence the encapsulation of the abscess.

Walling-off of the process and encapsulation of the abscess were, however, decisive for the course. Table 3 shows that the mortality in cases of encapsulated abscess was only 18 %, whereas it was as high as 61 % in non-encapsulated abscesses. Cases of encapsulated but multi-chambered abscess show a mortality of 47 %. The frequency of encapsulation was nearly similar to haematogenous and abscesses due to extension.

Preceding antibiotic treatment was of greatest importance for both the walling-off of local encephalitis and the process of encapsulation. Fig. 3 shows that, in this way, genuine encapsulation was a-chieved in 50 % of the cases. We should, however, mention that as a rule local antibiotic treatment was only given if previous puncture had shown encapsulation of the abscess.

If sterility of the abscess contents was achieved by intensive pa-renteral and local antibiotic treatment before removing the capsule, the mortality could be reduced to 27 %. If, at the time of operation, the abscess contents were not yet sterile, the mortality was as high as 46 % (cf. Table 4). In the last two years, the beginning of a local cerebral infection in 2 patients with purulent sinusitis was so dramatic that clinical treatment had to be initiated in the early phase of abscess development. A maximum of antibiotic therapy was carried through at this stage. Angiography showed that, as a symptom of the local cerebral infection with perifocal edema, both patients suffered from a massive frontal displacement of A. cerebri anterior. Repeated needling through a burr-hole did not produce any pus. Gradual and finally complete disappearance of the narrowing and displacement was achieved under angiographic control. Both patients recovered completely without showing any subsequent symptoms. Because of the early antibiotic treatment both patients escaped an abscess formation of the local encephalitis or the cerebral "phlegmons" respectively. HEINEMANN et al. (4) report on similar cases.

Therapy of Brain Abscess

These favourable therapeutic results without surgical treatment are, nevertheless, to be considered as exceptional. Table 5 shows the results of treatment of 170 cases of brain abscess as well as the catamneses of surviving patients as far as obtainable. According to observations by SCHIEFER (8), the mortality was lowest, i. e. 17 %, under combined surgical treatment with primary needling through a burr-hole and removal of the capsule later on. Subsequent symptoms, especially neurological sequelae were, however, more marked with 13 and 23 %, which was obviously due to the major surgical intervention.

Table 3. Dependence of course of disease on capsular development

Brain abscesses	Encapsulated		Not encapsulated		Chambered		Undefined		Total	
	No.of cases	Mort. %	No.of cases	Mort. %	No.of cases	Mort. %	No.of cases	Mort. %	No.	Mort. %
Early	4	0	5	80	1	100	-	-	10	50
Abscess by extension traumatic	11	18	7	43	4	50	4	0	26	27
non-traum.	28	14	24	69	9	33	11	27	72	39
total	39	15	31	68	13	38	15	20	98	36
Metastatic	20	20	20	40	1	100	6	67	47	36
Cryptogenetic	4	50	8	75	2	50	1	0	15	60
Total	67	18	64	61	17	47	22	32	170	39
Abscess by extension	43	14	36	69	14	43	15	20	108	37
Haematogenous	24	25	28	50	3	67	7	57	62	42

Table 4. Interdependence of course of disease and sterility of abscess contents before operation (159 cases)

	No Antibiotics		Antibiotics parenteral		Antibiotics parenteral & local		Total	
	No. of cases	Mortality	No. of cases	Mortality	No. of cases	Mortality	No. of cases	Mortality
Contents *not* sterile	8	89 %	49	46 %	19	30 %	76	46 %
Contents sterile	0	0	49	30 %	34	22 %	83	27 %
Total	8	89 %	98	39 %	53	25 %	159	36 %

Table 5. Result of treatment in 170 cases of brain abscess

	No surgical treatment	burr-hole	immediate total extirp.	burr-hole & caps. extirp.
No. of cases	11	54	40	65
Mortality	82 %	54 %	42 %	17 %

Sequelae in surviving patients with known catamnesis

	No surgical treatment	burr-hole	immediate total extirp.	burr-hole & caps. extirp.
No. of cases	0	13	17	52
Recurrence	?	0 %	5 %	4 %
Neurol. sequelae	?	0 %	15 %	13 %
Seizures	?	14 %	25 %	23 %
General trouble	?	21 %	25 %	21 %
No symptoms	?	79 %	26 %	35 %

If preceding needling did not result in genuine encapsulation, following surgical treatment to remove the capsule generally led to a higher percentage of sequelae. It is, however, not possible to give a more detailed account in the present paper. If sterility of the abscess contents is achieved under combined antibiotic treatment with preceding needling of the abscess through a burr-hole, removal of the capsule later on does not seem to be necessary, if angiographic control shows no more space narrowing and displacement. Only in cases of existing space narrowing, even if only local, caused by the formation of a thick and voluminous capsule, removal of the capsule is indicated under all circumstances.

The different pathological-anatomical changes and their corresponding clinical course mentioned in the beginning, require a different treatment of early brain abscesses. Because of the missing walling-off of the process by encapsulation and despite the abundance of antibiotics, early brain abscesses still require the open method of treatment recommended by TÖNNIS (11) with opening of the abscess and subsequent drainage.

Summary

Clinical analysis of 170 cases of brain abscess, 10 of which were early, 98 by extension and 62 haematogenous abscesses, provides important leads for diagnosis and treatment of abscesses. According to pathological-anatomical changes, the beginning of the process in cases of incipient brain abscess was acute and dramatic with symptoms of diffuse cerebral infection. Haematogenous abscesses and abscesses by extension, however, often did not receive clinical treatment until symptoms of increasing intracranial pressure showed. It rarely happened that the acute beginning of these abscesses was so dramatic that treatment was initiated very early. Under early, intensive antibiotic treatment during the initial phases, 2 cases showed complete disappearance of the local cerebral infection without formation of an abscess and encapsulation of the "phlegmons" under angiographic control.

In the light of these findings and catamneses, provided by 170 cases of intracranial abscess, aspects of surgical treatment are being discussed.

REFERENCES

FALCONER, M., McFARLAN, A. M., RUSSELL, D. S.: Experimental brain abscesses in the rabbit. Journ. Neurol. and Psychiat. 4, 273 (1941).

FALCONER, M.: Experimental brain abscesses in the rabbit. Brit. J. Surg. 30, 245 - 260 (1943).

IRSIGLER, F. J.: The Neurosurgical Approach to intracranial Infections. Berlin - Göttingen - Heidelberg: Springer 1961.

HEINEMANN, H. S., BRAUDE, A. I., OSTERHOLM, J. L.: Intracranial Suppurative Disease. JAMA 218, 1542 - 1547 (1971).

HEINEN, M.: Gasbrandabscess des Gehirns nach "Bagatellverletzung" des Kopfes. Z. Rechtsmedizin 73, 245 - 253 (1973).

KARIMI-NEJAD, A.: Zur Verhütung und Behandlung der entzündlichen Lungenkomplikationen im akuten und subakuten Stadium einer Hinrschädigung. Acta Neurochirurgica 30, 167 - 202 (1974).

KARIMI-NEJAD, A., KRENKEL, W.: Clostridium Brain Abscess after a Scalp Wound. German Medical Monthly 10, 399 - 403 (1966).

SCHIEFER, W.: Die operative Behandlung des Hirnabszesses. Zbl. Neurochir. 18, 332 - 348 (1958).

SPATZ, H.: Gehirnpathologie im Kriege. Von den Gehirnwunden. Zbl. Neurochir. 6, 162 - 212 (1941).

TÖNNIS, W.: Schußverletzung des Gehirnes. Zbl. Neurochir. 6, 113 - 162 (1941).

TÖNNIS, W.: Operative Versorgung der Hirnschüsse. Acta Chirurg. Scandinavica 90, 275 - 294 (1945).

WEBER, G.: Der Hirnabszess. Stuttgart: Georg Thieme 1957.

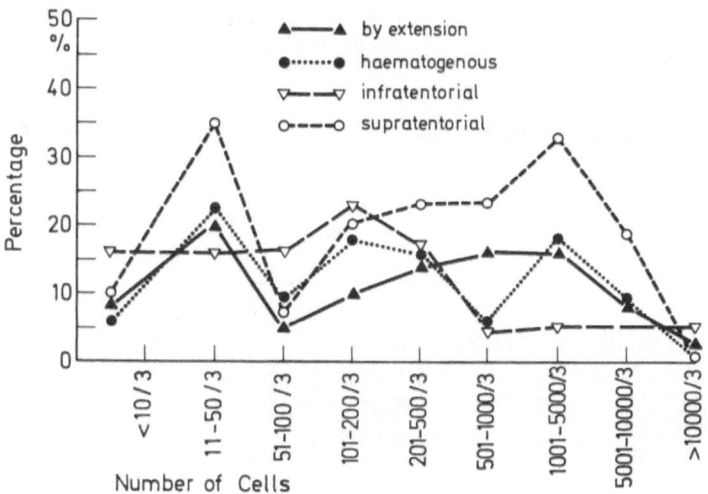

Fig. 1. Number of cells in CSF in 154 cases of brain abscess

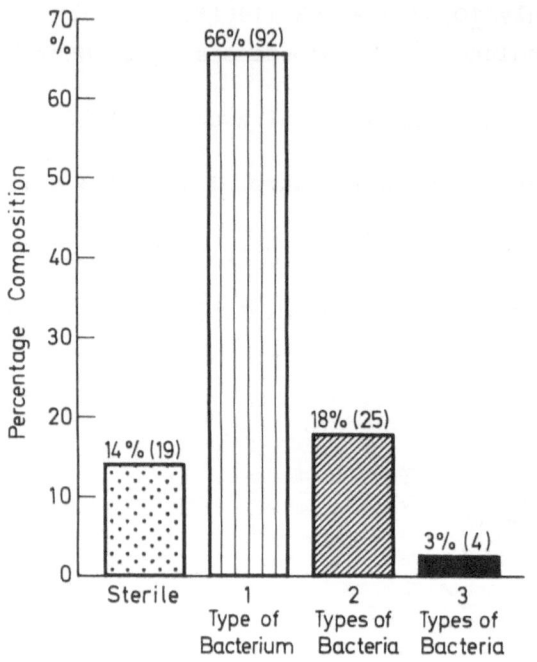

Fig. 2. Number of bacteria
occurring simultaneously in
one brain abscess in 140
examined patients

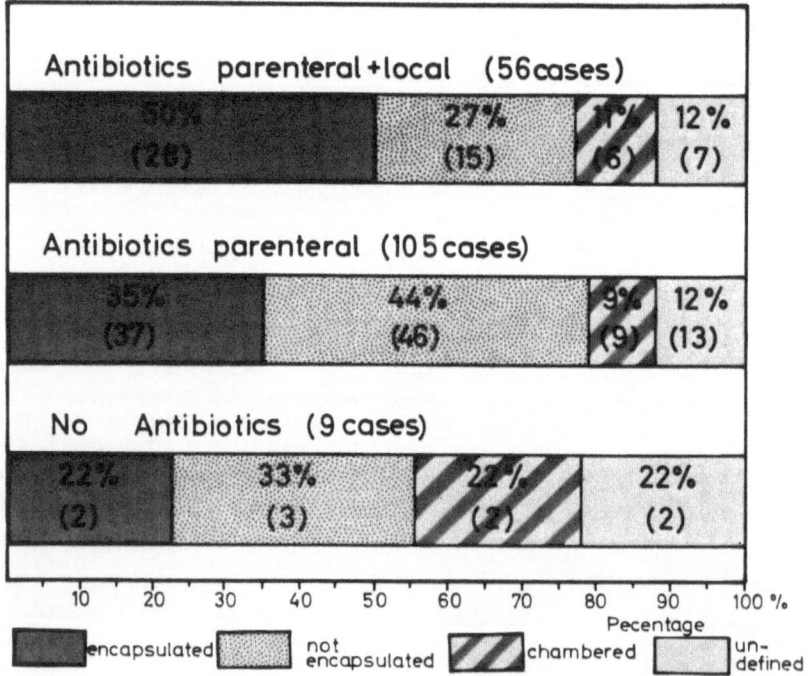

Fig. 3. Influence of antibiotics on capsular development of brain abscesses

A Simplified Procedure and a New Equipment for Stereotaxic Brain Operations

K. Schmidt

Stereotaxic surgery has become more expensive and complicated especially due to the use of extensive computer calculations.

The author has used the installation of X-rays and a new stereotaxic equipment to obtain the greatest possible simplification, low cost, improved handling and wider and more versatile applications in various operative neurosurgical procedures.

First, the possibility was devised of making antero-posterior and lateral pneumoencephalographic X-ray pictures of the skull in a simple way in the radiological department both with the patient sitting up and lying down, under the control of an image intensifier, with a focus-film distance of 4 m and a distortion of 5 % (Focus-film distance to image plane-film distance 0 : 1). Lateral tomography is possible.

In the operating theater, the X-ray equipment is installed for ap and lateral radiological control, with the stereotaxic equipment fitted to the patient, for exposures at a 4 m focus-film distance with a 5 & distortion also. The constant distortion of 5 % simplifies the single but essential conversion from the model brain to the X-ray picture and back to the patient's brain, and the transfer of the target from the pneumoencephalogram to the surgical field with the attached mounting ring, by congruent superposition of the X-ray films without measurement and calculation.

The new stereotaxic equipment consists essentially of a mounting ring fixed to the skull. Attached to it are a coordinate system and a sagittal segmental arch, which, in turn, carries the lateral segmental arch with the equipment guide.

The equipment permits the direct adjustment of the three coordinates without a phantom and without calculation. The coordinates can also be altered at will during operations with several targets. The segmental arches in 2 planes allow a free choice of sagittal and lateral angles of incidence, since by adjustment of the depth gauge to 0, the instrument tip (exploring tip, drill tip, implantation cannula tip etc.) always remains in the target, even if the angle of incidence changes.

The carrier permits the use of various instruments such as the drill, conduction probes, stimulation and coagulation probes for elimination operations within the brain, 10 mm ball trephine for transmaxillary hypophysectomy, implantation devices for transnasal radionuclide implantation into the hypophysic etc.

359

The function and use of the method were illustrated with slides (open transmaxillary hypophysectomy and transnasal implantation) and a film of an operation (intention tremor).

Is the Automatic Midline Determination with the Midliner Really an Improvement in Ultrasound Diagnosis? - A Comparative Investigation of 1889 Cases

M. Klinger, G. Graef, Th. Grumme, K.-H. Hartmann,
H. Hopman, E. Kazner, W. Meese, and B. Vogel

Introduction

At the annual meeting of the German Neurosurgical society in Mainz
last year, HOPMAN, KAZNER and VOGEL (12) reported on first results
of the automatic midline determination. In order to establish the
diagnostic value of this method of examination, there was a need for
a large series of investigations. A co-operative study by several
neurosurgical clinics promised to be the best way of reaching this
goal in a relatively short time.

The automatic midline determination with the midliner was developed
in order to achieve a standardization of the ultrasound examination
and to eliminate the factor "experience" which plays an important
role in A-scan echoencephalography, so that non-medical personnel
could quickly learn to handle the equipment (1, 3).

Results and Discussion

In answer to the above-mentioned question, the results of the co-operative study are presented. Altogether 1889 patients of the Neurosurgical University Clinics in Berlin, Erlangen and Munich underwent the
midliner investigation. Table 1 presents a survey of the diagnoses of
these patients: there were 591 brain tumors, 312 head injuries, nearly 200 cases of cerebrovascular disease and 414 patients with various
intracranial diseases. Only 374 subjects were unremarkable at clinical
and echoencephalographic examination and these serve as the control
group. Since the accuracy of the diagnosis is particularly important
in these patients, all findings were compared to an A-scan echoencephalogram carried out by an experienced physician. In order to prevent
operator bias, most of the midliner measurements were carried out by
untrained students.

Table 2 shows the results of the comparison between these midliner
histograms and the A-scan echogram performed by a trained physician.
In 1889 cases the histograms were found to be unshifted 1111 times.
In 1100 cases this was confirmed so that the accuracy for the normal
midline echo was 99 %.

Of the 434 cases of midliner displacement, 401 (92 %) were confirmed
and thus correct and 33 (8 %) were incorrect. Drawing the group of
unsatisfactory cases into consideration, which comprised no less than
18 %, the overall accuracy of the midline computer measurements was
only 80 %. The high percentage of unsatisfactory histograms in the
Berlin series is due to their particular age distribution.

Table 1. Midliner measurements of 1889 patients

DIAGNOSIS	BERLIN	ERLANGEN	MÜNCHEN	Total
Brain tumors	127	183	281	591
Head injuries	115	73	124	312
Cerebrovascular lesions	43	37	118	198
Intracranial disease of other etiology	95	20	299	414
Normal	249	117	8	374
Total	629	430	830	1889

Table 2. Results of automatic midline determination in 1889 patients

Histogram	Number of cases				Comparison with A-scan echo-encephalography	
	Berlin	Erlangen	München	Total	correct	incorrect
No shift	322	277	512	1111	1100 (99%)	11 (1%)
Shift	118	102	214	434	401 (92%)	33 (8%)
Unsatisfactory	189 (30%)	51 (12%)	104 (13%)	344 (18%)		
Total	629	430	830	1889	1501 (80%)	44 (2%)

Table 3 gives a survey of the 388 unsatisfactory and incorrect measurements. In a total of 44 patients, the results of the two methods of examination (midliner and A-scan) did not agree. The midliner showed a displacement which could not be verified in 33 cases, in other words, a false positive result. Considerably more dangerous is a false negative finding in which the midline appears to be normal in the histogram while the cerebral midline is actually displaced. This occurred 11 times, so that the percentage of such errors in the entire group of 1889 patients was 0.6 %; relating these cases to the number of shifts, the error quota was found to be 2,7 %. Technical difficulties were met in 207 cases: most of these had histograms containing many scattered values without an unequivocal midline echo column.

Table 3. Causes of unsatisfactory and incorrect histograms in 388 cases

	BERLIN	ERLANGEN	MÜNCHEN	Total
False positive („shifted" in midliner although midline unshifted)	15	8	10	33
False negative („unshifted" in midliner although midline shifted)	4	3	4	11
Technically inadequate (widely scattered measurements, no unequivocal midline echo)	145	14	48	207
No record obtainable (thickness of skull, age)	44	18	37	137
Echo from one side only (Trauma or swelling of opposite side)		19	19	
Total	208	62	118	**388**

Whenever the consistency of the skull bone is altered, e. g. increased thickness of the bony skull or pneumatisation of the bone, the midliner is unable to record a value because the ultrasound beam is absorbed too strongly. As Table 4 shows, this is particularly true for patients over the age of 60, which tend to cause difficulties for A-scan echo-encephalography as well. According to the manufacturer, the high rate of non-recordable cases in infants is due to the setting of the apparatus for the diameter of the skull, which is limited to 130 to 180 mm.

A large proportion of the unsatisfactory measurements was due to the failure to record an echo from one side or not at all. Since a sub-galeal hematoma generally prevents the detection of an unequivocal M-echo, a considerable number of patients with head injuries could not be examined. For this reason, the agreement between histogram and A-scan echoencephalogram in Table 5 was rather poor in this group: the accuracy of the midliner in cases of head injuries was only 68 %. Because of the large number of unsatisfactory midliner measurements, only 79 of 102 midline shifts could be detected using the midliner (77 %).

Although the midliner reading-out was thought to be entirely objective and independent of the experience of the examiner, this assumption is contradicted by Table 6. This table shows two succeeding series of 150 cases, each performed by the same untrained student. The total error rate sank from 29 % in the first series of 150 cases to 8 % in the succeeding group - the difference is no doubt due to experience with the midliner technique.

Table 4. Midliner measurements in 249 normal controls of various age groups (Neurosurgical University Clinic Berlin)

Age group	Number of cases	Unshifted	Shifted	Unsatisfactory	Midliner-Display correct	Midliner-Display incorrect
Children under 1 year	55	14	1	40 (72%)	14	1
Children up to 16 years	74	49	0	25 (34%)	49	-
Adults 16-60 years	61	57	1	3 (5%)	57	1
Adults over 60 years	59	38	0	21 (36%)	38	-
Total	249	158	2	89 (36%)	158	2

Table 5. Comparison of midline determination by midliner and A-scan echo-encephalograph in 196 patients with intracranial lesions (Neurosurgical University Clinic Erlangen)

	No of Cases	Midliner Unshifted	Midliner Shifted	Midliner Unsatisfactory	A-scan Unshifted	A-scan Shifted	Agreement
Tumors	132	49	57	26	62	70	98 = 74,2%
Head injuries	41	13	15	13	17	24	28 = 68,3%
Cerebrovascular lesions	23	13	7	3	15	8	20 = 87%

Summary

In summary, the accuracy of the midliner is high as soon as a normal histogram can acutally be obtained - 1100 of the 1111 measurements were found to be correct, an accuracy of 99 %. However, no less than 18 % or almost 1/5 of the measurements were unsatisfactory. Although the midliner may be regarded as a first step to automatic midline determination, it can never replace A-scan echoencephalography. In some unclear cases, the use of the midliner in addition to A-scan

Table 6. Causes of incorrect and unsatisfactory histograms in 2 subsequent series (Neurosurgical University Clinic Erlangen)

	I. Series 150 Cases	II. Series 150 Cases
Echo from one side only (Trauma or swelling of the opposite side)	13	3
No record (Skull thickness, age)	11	5
Technically inadequate (Widely scattered measurements, no unequivocal midline echo)	10	2
False positive („shifted" in midliner although midline unshifted)	6	1
False negative („unshifted" in midliner although midline shifted)	3	1
Total error rate:	43=28,6 %	12 = 8 %

echoencephalography may provide further information so that its use as a *second apparatus* in a neurological or neurosurgical clinic is feasible. With an overall accuracy of only 80 %, it is of limited use for practicing neurologists and emergency departments of small hospitals. As experience in all three clinics in this study has indicated, the computerized determination of the midline echo is not reliable enough to recommend it for routine use in cases of head injuries.

REFERENCES

1. GALICICH, J. H., WILLIAMS, J. B.: A computerized echoencephalograph. J. Neurosurg. 35, 453 - 460 (1971).

2. HOPMAN, E., KAZNER, E., VOGEL, B.: Comparative Study of Computerized and A-Mode Midline Echo-encephalography. In: Advances in Neurosurgery 1 (eds. K. SCHÜRMANN, M. BROCK, H.-J. REULEN, D. VOTH) pp. 299 - 302. Berlin - Heidelberg - New York: Springer 1973.

3. WHITE, D. N.: Midline Echo-encephalography with the Automatic Midline Computer. Comput. Biol. Med. 2, 273 - 284 (1972).

Results of Two-Dimensional Ultrasonic Examination in Supratentorial Space-Occupying Lesions

Th. Grumme

Introduction

Direct evidence of a supratentorial tumor with the A-scan echo-encephalograph is successful in 25,6 % of cases (6), the temporal glioblastoma giving the best results, namely in 70 % of all cases with a
tumor echo. The chronic subdural hematoma can be detected in 80 % (4)
or 83 % (3) by a hematoma-echo. A special echo complex of a hematoma
can be shown in 35 % (4) of the non-traumatic cases.

ADAPON et al. (1966) and LOMBROSO et al. (1970) reported on examinations with the parallel B-scan in 60 and 97 cases respectively with
supratentorial lesions (1, 5). LOMBROSO et al. (1970) showed the tumors of the midline and of the base of skull best, that is in 86 %.
The percentage of direct tumor echos for all tumors together is 34 %.
In temporal tumors the astrocytomas yield the best results. Frontal
and occipital tumors could hardly ever be shown directly. A hematoma
echo could be found in about 30 % in chronic subdural hematomas. Corresponding results with the compound scan in a greater number of supratentorial space-occupying lesions could not be found.

Material and Method

From 1971 until now, 225 supratentorial space-occupying lesions were
examined in children and adults by two-dimensional echoencephalography.
The type of two-dimensional scan performed was the compound scan using
the apparatus of the KRETZ-Company. The probe was 15 mm in diameter,
1 MHz in adults, 2 MHz in children. The horizontal examination is related to the line: external auditory meatus - lateral angle of the
eye, the vertical examination to a line standing at right angles to it
through the external auditory meatus. Horizontally, the parallel
planes generally lie 2 - 5 cm above the above mentioned line, vertically from 3 cm ahead of to 3 cm behind the ear. Each patient was
examined horizontally in different planes; in cases of suspected
space-occupying lesions of the midline and parietal region an investigation in a vertical plane was also performed. The B-scan findings
were always compared to the results of the A-scan and to neuroradiological, histological, and if possible to postmortal examinations as
well as to the site of operation. In about half of the cases, the
neuroradiological examinations had already bèen performed in other
departments before the B-scan examination.

Results

1. Brain Tumors

The position of a supratentorial tumor can be investigated by the kind of the midline-shift: in frontal tumors we find evidence that the midline shift increases towards the front of the skull, although the echo is not shifted greatly.

In temporal tumors a nearly parallel shift of the midline occurs over a larger distance while tumors in the occipital region lead to an increase of the midline shift towards the back. Unfortunately, the examinations performed so far indicate that a diagnosis of the tumor's position by the kind of midline shift is possible in only 25 %. The reason for this can be found in the unfavourable sounding-conditions of the midlines, because these are not hit by the ultrasound beam at an angle of 90° although they are only moderately shifted in a frontal tumor.

The results of direct tumor evidence are shown in summary in Table 1. In 52 % of all cases direct evidence of the tumor could be demonstrated. It is remarkable that the group of the gliomas could be detected most frequently with 69 %. Metastases had the poorest results; they could only be located in the temporal region if they were rather large, or presented hemorrhage and cysts. Adenomas of the pituitary body with an extensive suprasellar expansion could be shown in nearly every case. The rather low share of meningiomas is easily accounted for by the frequent parietal or parasagittal site of these tumors. Among the tumors shown in the picture as "others" are summarized 3 arachnoid cysts, 2 colloidal cysts, 2 ependymomas, 1 papilloma of the choriod plexus, 1 cholesteatoma, 1 pinealoma, and 1 sarcoma.

Table 1. Type of tumor and incidence of direct tumor evidence. The number in the parentheses relate to children

Kind of tumor	Number of cases	Tumor echo Number	%
Glioblastoma	52 (1)	26 (1)	50
Astrocytoma	17 (1) ⎫	11 ⎫	
Oligodendroglioma	16 (1) ⎬ 39	11 ⎬ 27 (3)	69
Spongioblastoma	6 (2) ⎭	5 ⎭	
Meningioma	32	14	44
Pituitary adenoma	14	7	50
Craniopharyngioma	4	3	
Metastasis	21	6	28
Others	11 (2)	8 (1)	
	173	91	52

Fig. 1 shows the incidence of direct tumor proof in relation to the localization. It is apparent that the fronto-temporal tumors as well as the midline tumors can be shown best, because the sounding-conditions are best in these regions. The tumors of the midline are best qualified for visualization in several planes as a "three-dimensional" picture, as shown in 2 examples of an adenoma of the pituitary body, one in the horizontal, the other side in the vertical picture (Figs. 2 and 3). Even with an appropriate technique, parietal tumors are difficult to demonstrate, while tumors located in the occipital region alone can not be shown at all. In 65 % of all recurrences, direct tumor proof was positive. A histological diagnosis could not be provided. This is shown in Figs. 4 and 5. The plotting of a cyst in a tumor only turned out in rare cases. According to our experience the size of a tumor found in the two-dimensional pictures, states nothing about the real extent, which is found by neuroradiological methods or by operation.

Two brain abscesses were examined by the two-dimensional method. The walls of a frontal abscess could clearly be shown in one case.

2. Hematomas

The results in cases with hematomas are shown in Table 2.

Table 2. Incidence of the direct hematoma evidence. Numbers in parentheses relate to children

	Number of cases	Hematoma echo number	%
Intracerebral hematomas	15 (1)	7	46
Extracerebral hematomas	36 (10)	10 (4)	27

Intracerebral hematomas of non-traumatic origin (Fig. 6) could be shown directly in 46 %. 5 out of 7 hematoma echoes were located in the temporal region. Here, the B-scan was clearly more effective than the A-scan, which only showed 3 out of the 7 hematomas detected by the B-scan. The results with the extracerebral hematoma, especially the chronic subdural hematoma, were disappointing. The good spatial evidence with the vertical technique (Fig. 7) only turned out in 27 %. In these cases, the A-scan was more effective than the B-scan. The reason probably lies in the unfavourable sounding conditions of the parietal region for the B-scan, whereas by special tilting of the probe in the A-scan, the parietal region can easily be reached by the ultrasound beam.

Concluding Remarks

1. The B-scan provides an advantage in the diagnosis of supratentorial space-occupying lesions over the A-scan. Brain tumors and intracerebral hematomas can be shown better and more often in this way. The tumors could be demonstrated twice as often as with the A-scan. On the other hand, the results in chronic subdural hematomas are clearly poorer than with the A-scan.

2. In general, the compound scan shows better results than the parallel- and sector-scan.

3. The B-scan in its present form offers no possibility for further development. The future lies in computerized transverse axial tomography.

Summary

Two-dimensional echoencephalography investigations in 225 supratentorial space-occupying lesions with the compound scan. Direct proof of brain tumors in 52 %, of intracerebral hematomas in 46 %, and of chronic subdural hematomas in 27 %. Frontotemporal tumors and midline-tumors can be shown best.

REFERENCES

1. ADAPON, B. D., CHASE, N. E., KIRCHEFF, I. I., HATTISTA, A. F.: B-Scan encephalography. Acta radiol. (Stockh.) 5, 730 - 739 (1966).

2. GRUMME, Th.: Der Wert der Echo-Enzephalographie bei Schädel-Hirn-Verletzten. Zeitschr. ärtzl. Fortbildung 59, Heft 7 (1970).

3. GRUMME, Th.: Die zweidimensionale Echoenzephalographie (B-Scan). Deut. Med. Wochschr. 98, 1234 - 1238 (1973).

4. KAZNER, E.: Erfahrungen mit der Echo-Enzephalographie bei raumfordernden intrakraniellen Blutungen. Ultrasonographie medica, S. 197 - 207. Wien: Wiener Med. Akademie 1969.

5. LOMBROSO, C. T., ERBA, G., YOGO, T., LOGOWITZ, N., HILAIRE, J. St.: Two-dimensional sonar scanning for detection of intracranial lesions. Arch. Neurol. (Chic.) 23, 518 - 527 (1970).

6. SCHIEFER, W., KAZNER, E.: Klinische Echoencephalographie. Berlin - Heidelberg - New York: Springer 1967.

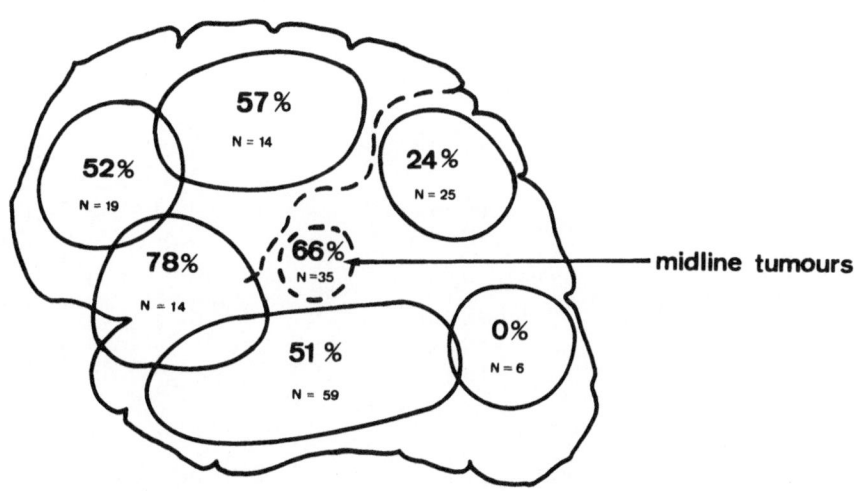

Fig. 1. Relation between site and direct evidence of the tumor. n = number of cases

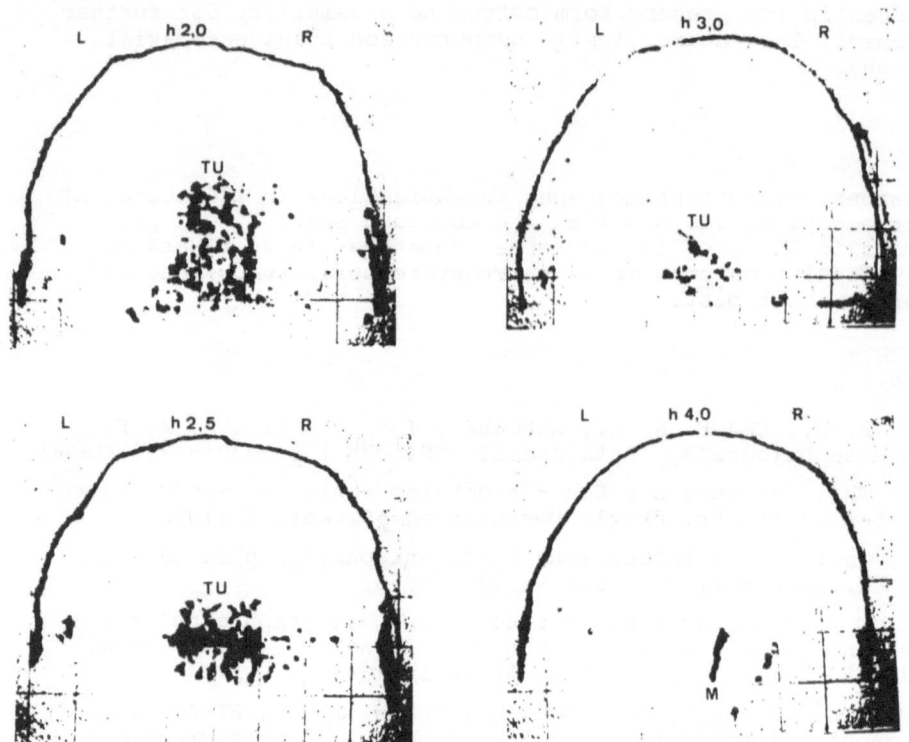

Fig. 2. Chromophobe pituitary adenoma with suprasellar extension in 4 horizontal planes. h = horizontal scan; 2,0 = above the horizontal plane; L = Left; R = Right; TU = tumor; M = midline

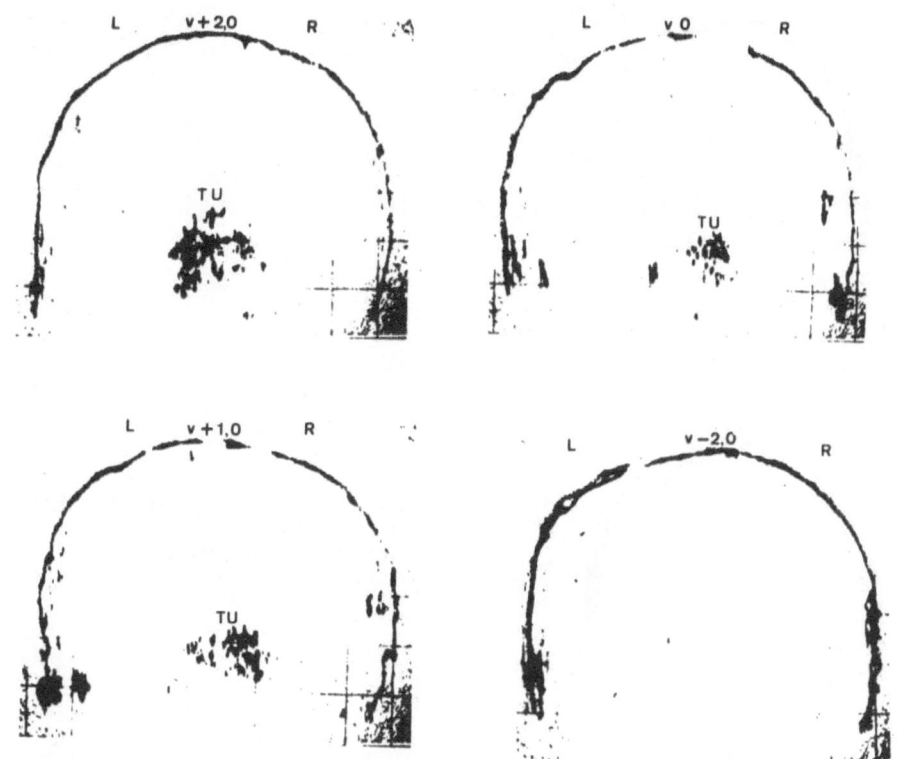

Fig. 3. Chromophobe pituitary adenoma with suprasellar extension in 4 vertical planes. v = vertical scan; + = scan infront of; - = scan behind the vertical plane

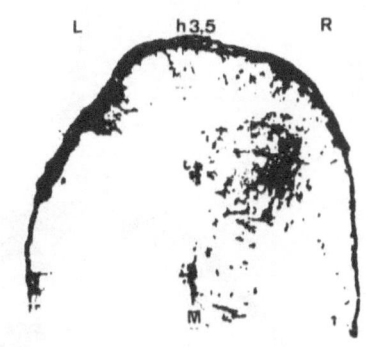

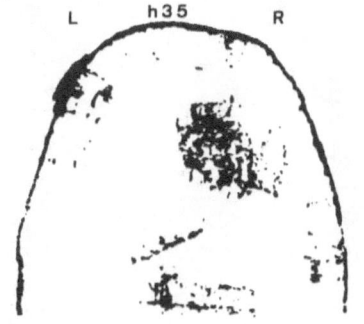

Fig. 4. Upper Picture: temporal glioblastoma, middle picture: meningioma of the sphenoid bone, lower picture: temporal metastasis with perifocal edema

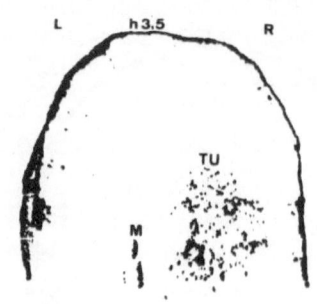

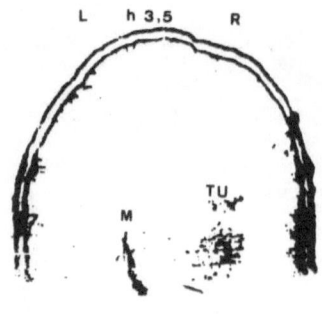

Fig. 5. Upper picture: frontal glioblastoma, lower picture: frontal meningioma

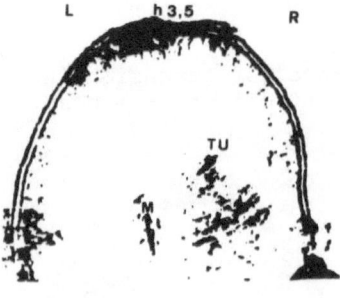

Fig. 6. Frontal intracerebral hematoma (H)

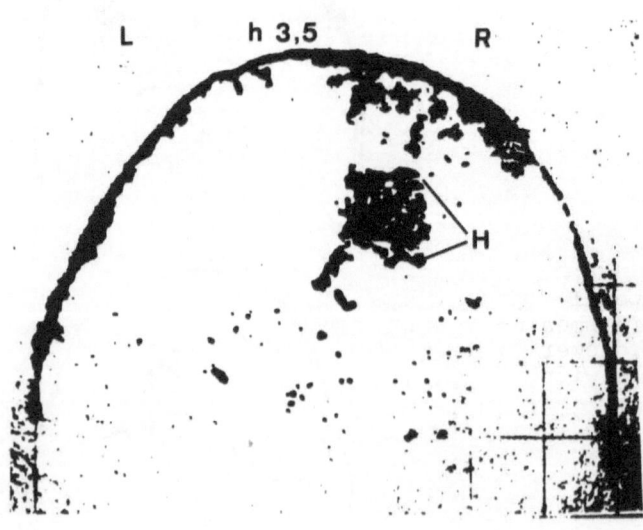

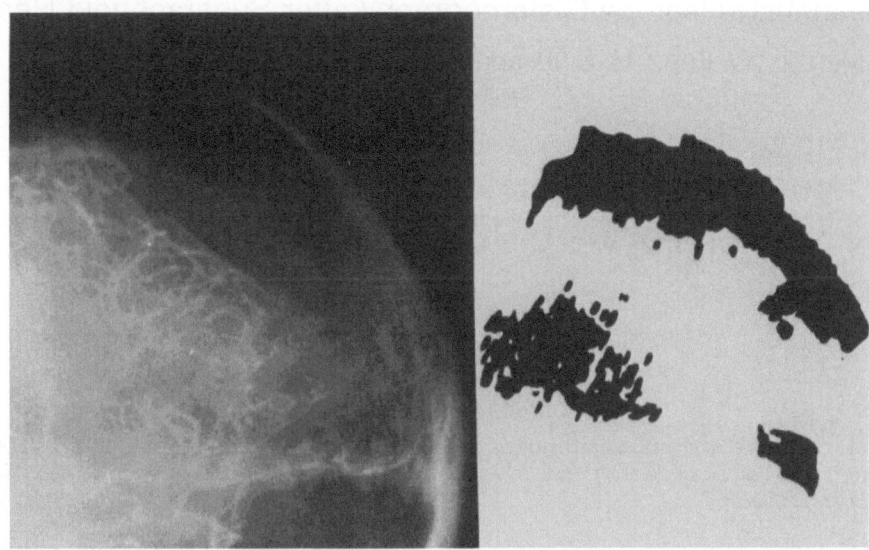

Fig. 7. Chronic subdural hematoma: section of a picture of a vertical scan in comparison to the angiogram

The Diagnostic and Prognostic Significance of Qualitative and Quantitative Isotope Cisternography after Subarachnoid Hemorrhage

J. MENZEL, G. ERBS, H. SINN, and P. GEORGI

The concept of subarachnoid hermorrhage is not to be understood in the nosological sense of the term or as a disease sui generis but as a syndrome (5).

The pathophysiological mechanism which leads to a communicating hydrocephalus either acutely or latently after a subarachnoid hemorrhage regardless of its etiology is always the same.

The acute form accompanied by increased intracranial pressure is due to a complete blockage of the cerebrospinal fluid (CSF) circulation in the basal cisterns caused by corpuscular blood elements (2, 7, 8). If this blockage is caused by a closure of the subarachnoid space due to reactive changes in the leptomeninges a chronic communicating hydrocephalus can develop (4, 1, 3).

Fig. 1. shows the pathological mechanism representative of both forms of disturbed CSF-circulation and its morphological consequences. The chronic form in its final phase is of great clinical interest because of the three symptoms: dementia, gait ataxia and incontinence. All of these symptoms may however be encountered in different degrees of severity and in isolation from the others.

In order to follow up changes in CSF-circulation after subarachnoid hemorrhage 129 patients were examined on the basis of isotope cisternographic studies over a period of 1 1/2 years. Spontaneous subarachnoid hemorrhage was encountered in 66 cases while 63 patients showed a traumatic subarachnoid hemorrhage.

After suboccipital puncture all patients received ^{111}In-HSA in a dose of 350 to 500 microcuries. Scintiphotos in at least two planes were taken 1 - 2, 24 and 48 hours after injection.

Three forms of CSF-circulation were evaluated:

1. The dynamics of normal CSF-circulation (Fig. 2 and Fig. 3).

2. Ventricular reflux, sufficient clearance within 24 to 48 hours and differing activity over the surface (Fig. 4).

3. Ventricular reflux, delayed clearance or stasis and no activity over the surface (Fig. 5).

Rare disturbances of CSF-circulation were summarized. Table 1 shows CSF-circulation in operated aneurysms. Normal CSF-dynamics were en-

Table 1. Operated aneurysms

LOCALISATION	NO OF CASES	NORMAL CSF-CIRCULATION	DISTURBED CSF-CIRCULATION
ANT. COMM. ART.	18	11	7
MID. CER. ART.	13	10	3
POST. COMM. ART.	8	4	4
INT. CAROT. ART.	6	5	1
ANT. CER. ART.	3	2	1
TOTAL	48	32 (66,7%)	16 (33,3%)

countered in 32 of 48 patients while 16 showed pathological CSF-dynamics. A similar proportion of operated supra- and infratentorial angiomas is indicated by Table 2.

Table 2. Operated angiomas

LOCALISATION	NO OF CASES	NORMAL CSF-CIRCULATION	DISTURBED CSF-CIRCULATION
SUPRATENTORIAL	15	11	4
INFRATENTORIAL	3	2	1
TOTAL	18	13 (72,2%)	5 (27,8%)

Fig. 6 presents a relationship between the incidence of disturbed CSF-dynamics and time since the spontaneous subarachnoid hemorrhage. The peak of pathological patterns between the 10th and the 15th day after hemorrhage is significant. The forms of disturbed CSF-circulation and the resulting therapeutic consequences are illustrated in Table 3. 5 patients who satisfied the criteria of the first group received ventriculo-atrial shunts. In one patient a severe psycho-syndrome had already existed over several years so that surgical treatment did not seem indicated any more. In one case quantitative measurements indicated a sufficient clearance so that a shunt was refrained from for the time being.

Table 3. Patterns of disturbed CSF-circulation after spontaneous SAH

CSF - DYNAMICS	NO OF CASES	SHUNT-INDICATION
VENTRICULAR REFLUX DELAYED CLEARANCE OR STASIS NO ACTIVITY OVER THE SURFACE	7	+
VENTRICULAR REFLUX SUFFICIENT CLEARANCE ACTIVITY OVER THE SURFACE	11	-
OTHER	3	-

To sum up: Out of 66 patients with spontaneous subarachnoid hemorrhage 21 or 31,5 % had disturbed CSF-circulation. 5 received ventriculo-atrial shunts, that is 7,5 % of the total sample or 23,8 % of those in whom a pathological CSF-circulation was encountered.

In a second group 63 patients with traumatic subarachnoid hemorrhage were examined (Table 4), only 20 of which had undisturbed CSF-dynamics. In 68,5 % pathological patterns were evaluated. Fig. 7 presents the incidence of pathological CSF-dynamics in relationship to time after the trauma. In contrast to the curve obtained in the cases of spontaneous subarachnoid hemorrhage here, the broader peak lies higher and declines in the long-term post-examination phase only down to 55,0 %.

Table 5 illustrates the patterns of disturbed CSF-circulation with the operative consequences. In group 1 three of the patients received ventriculo-atrial shunts. As the psychological examination in one case was inconspicuous except for a poor memory, a shunt was refrained from.

To sum up: Of 63 patients with traumatic subarachnoid hemorrhage 43 or 68,5 % showed a pathological CSF-circulation. Three of them received ventriculo-atrial shunts, that is 4,8 % of the total sample or 7,0 % of those with a pathological CSF-circulation.

Table 4. Traumatic SAH

	NO OF CASES	NORMAL CSF-CIRCULATION	DISTURBED CSF-CIRCULATION
CEREBRAL CONTUSION	38	12	26
CEREBRAL CONTUSION WITH HEMATOMA	25	8	17
TOTAL	63	20 (31,5%)	43 (68,5%)

Table 5. Patterns of disturbed CSF-circulation after traumatic SAH

CSF - DYNAMICS	NO OF CASES	SHUNT-INDICATION
VENTRICULAR REFLUX DELAYED CLEARANCE OR STASIS NO ACTIVITY OVER THE SURFACE	4	+
VENTRICULAR REFLUX SUFFICIENT CLEARANCE ACTIVITY OVER THE SURFACE	11	-
OTHER	3	-

5 received ventriculo-atrial shunts, that is 7,5 % of the total sample or 23,8 % of those in whom a pathological CSF-circulation was encountered.

In a second group 63 patients with traumatic subarachnoid hemorrhage were examined (Table 4), only 20 of which had undisturbed CSF-dynamics. In 68,5 % pathological patterns were evaluated. Fig. 7 presents the incidence of pathological CSF-dynamics in relationship to time after

the trauma. In contrast to the curve obtained in the cases of spontaneous subarachnoid hemorrhage here the broader peak lies higher
and declines in the long-term post-examination phase only down to 55,0 %.
Table 5 illustrates the patterns of disturbed CSF-circulation with
the operative consequences. In group 1 three of the patients received
ventriculo-atrial shunts. As the psychological examination in one
case was inconspicuous except for a poor memory, a shunt was refrained
from.

To sum up: Of 63 patients with traumatic subarachnoid hemorrhage 43
or 68,5 % showed a pathological CSF-circulation. Three of them received ventriculo-atrial shunts, that is 4,8 % of the total sample or
7,0 % of those with a pathological CSF-circulation.

In order to evaluate CSF-dynamics quantitatively, additional measurements of the serum activity were performed 2,24 and 48 hours after
injection. Fig. 8 shows characteristic values in the case of a normal
(upper curve) and a pathological (lower curve) qualitative cisternogram. The curve between both of the above represents a scintigram
with ventricular reflux and just adequate clearance. An indication
for operation can only be observed in the course of the lower curve.

Finally we propose qualitative and quantitative isotope cisternography as the most significant single examination for registering
disturbed CSF-circulation after subarachnoid hemorrhage. It is ad-
visible however, to take into account the clinical picture before
indicating a ventriculo-atrial shunt.

Summary

After a subarachnoid hemorrhage 10 - 43 % of the patients develop the
acute or chronic form of a communicating hydrocephalus. Only 40 - 60 %
of these however, require a shunt. In the present study 129 patients
were examined using isotope cisternography after subarachnoid hemorrhage due to aneurysms, angiomas and trauma. The different patterns
of disturbed CSF-circulation and -reabsorption are presented. The
parameters after which a permanent shunt was necessary are discussed.

REFERENCES

1. ADAMS, R. D., FISCHER, C. M., HAKIM, S., OJEMANN, R. D., SWEET,
   H. H.: Symptomatic occult hydrocephalus with "normal" cerebrospinal fluid pressure. A treatable syndrom. New Eng. J. Med. 273,
   117 - 126 (1965).

2. BAGLEY, C.: Blood in the cerebrospinal fluid. Resultant functional
   and organic alterations in the central nervous system. B. Clinical
   data. Arch. Surg. (Chicago) 17, 39 - 81 (1928).

3. BANNISTER, R., GILFORD, E., KOCEN, R.: Isotope encephalography in
   the diagnosis of dementia due to communicating hydrocephalus.
   Lancet 2, 1014 - 1018 (1967).

4. HAKIM, S., ADAMS, R. D.: The special clinical problem of symptomatic hydrocephalus with normal cerebrospinal fluid pressure. J.
   Neurol. Sci. 2, 307 - 327 (1965).

5. HEIDRICH, R.: Die subarachnoideale Blutung. Leipzig: VEG Georg
   Thieme 1970.

6. HEINZ, E. R., DAVIS, D. O., KARP, H. R.: Abnormal isotope cisternography in symptomatic occult hydrocephalus. Radiology 95, 109 -
120 (1970).

7. KUSSKE, J. A., TURNER, P. T., OJEMANN, G. A., HARRIS, A. B.: Ven-
triculostomy for the treatment of acute hydrocephalus following
subarachnoid hemorrhage. J. Neurosurg. 38, 591 - 595 (1973).

8. PERTUISET, B., HOUTTEVILLE, J. P., GEORGE, B., MARGENT, P.:
Dilatation ventriculaire précoce et hydrocéphalies consécutives
à la rupture d'aneurysmes artériels sus-tentoriels. Neurochirurgia
4, 113 - 126 (1972).

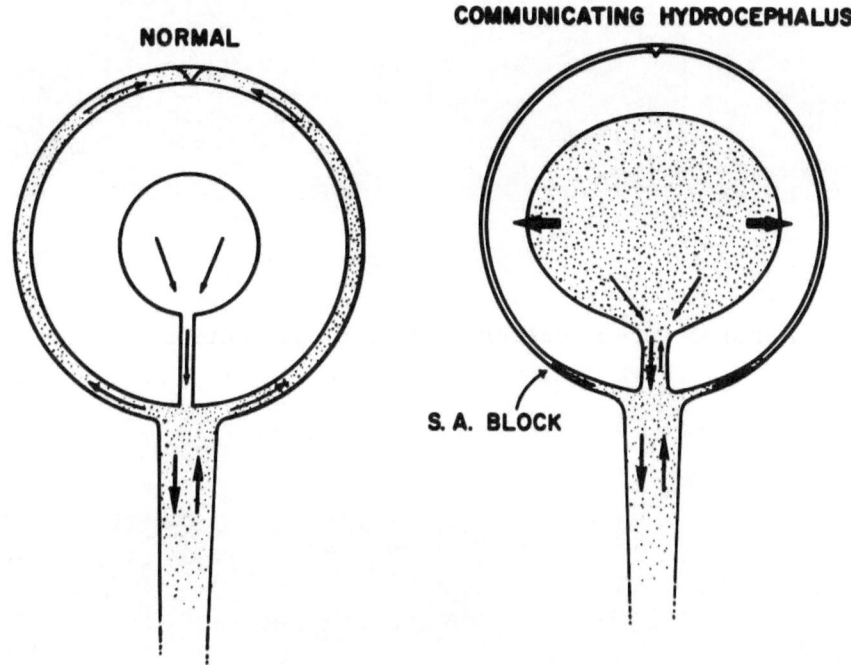

Fig. 1. Schematic representation of altered CSF pathways in communicating hydrocephalus (after E. R. HEINZ)

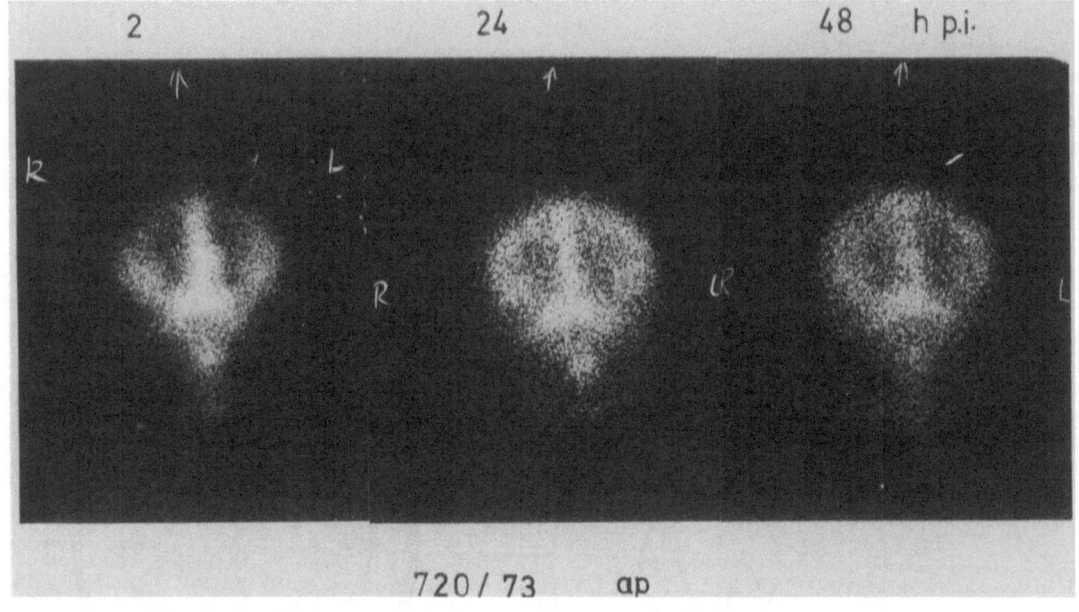

Fig. 2. Normal CSF-circulation in a. p.-projection

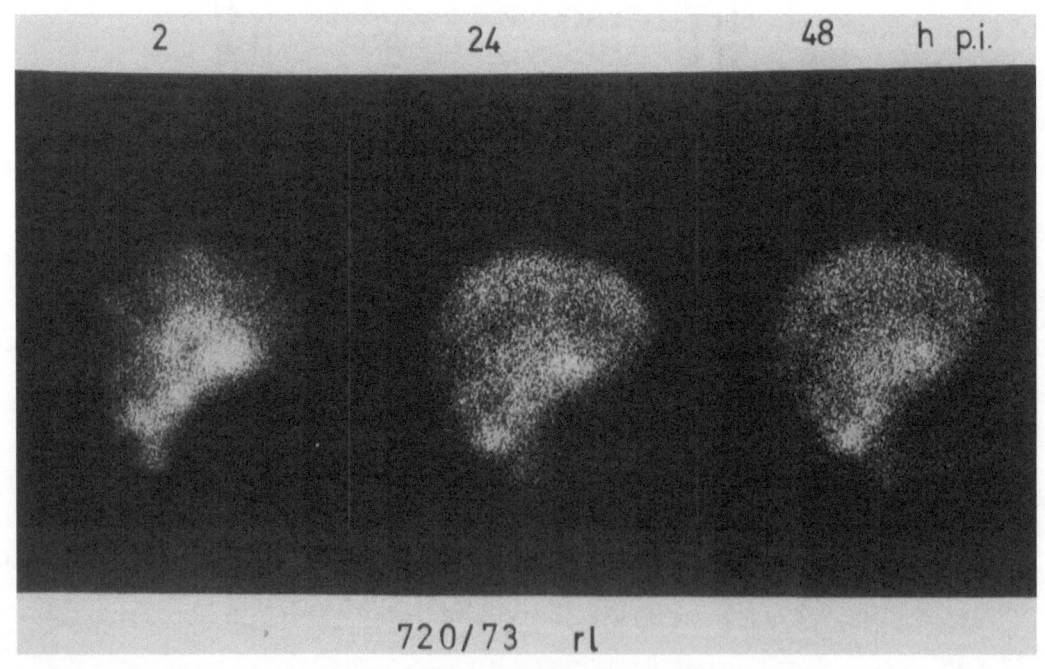

Fig. 3. Normal CSF-circulation in lateral projection

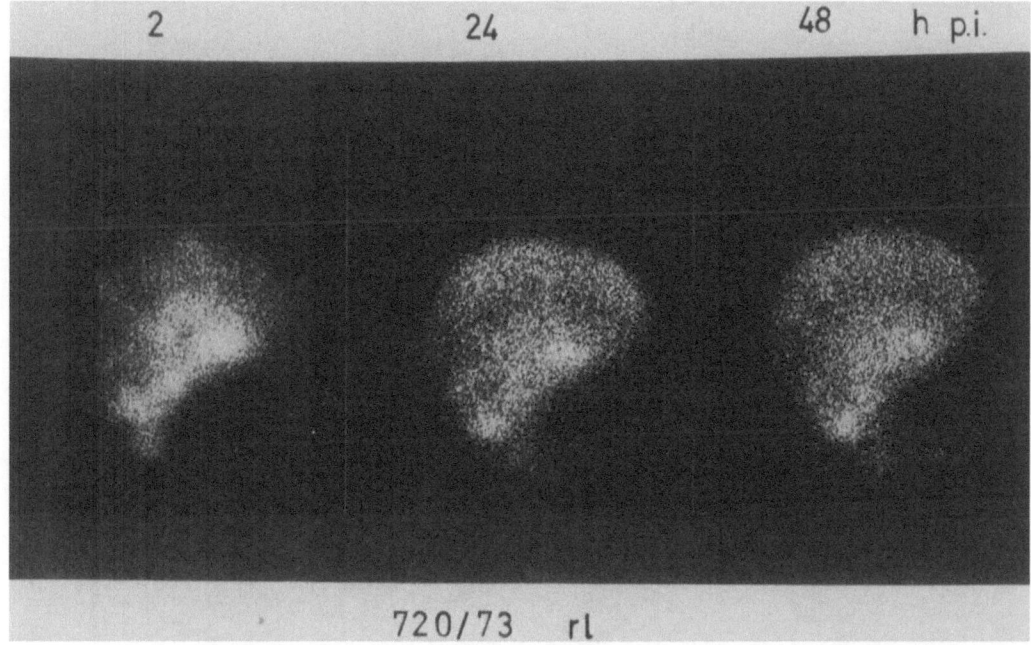

Fig. 4. Pathological CSF-circulation: ventricular reflux
                                    sufficient ventricular clearance
                                    activity over the surface

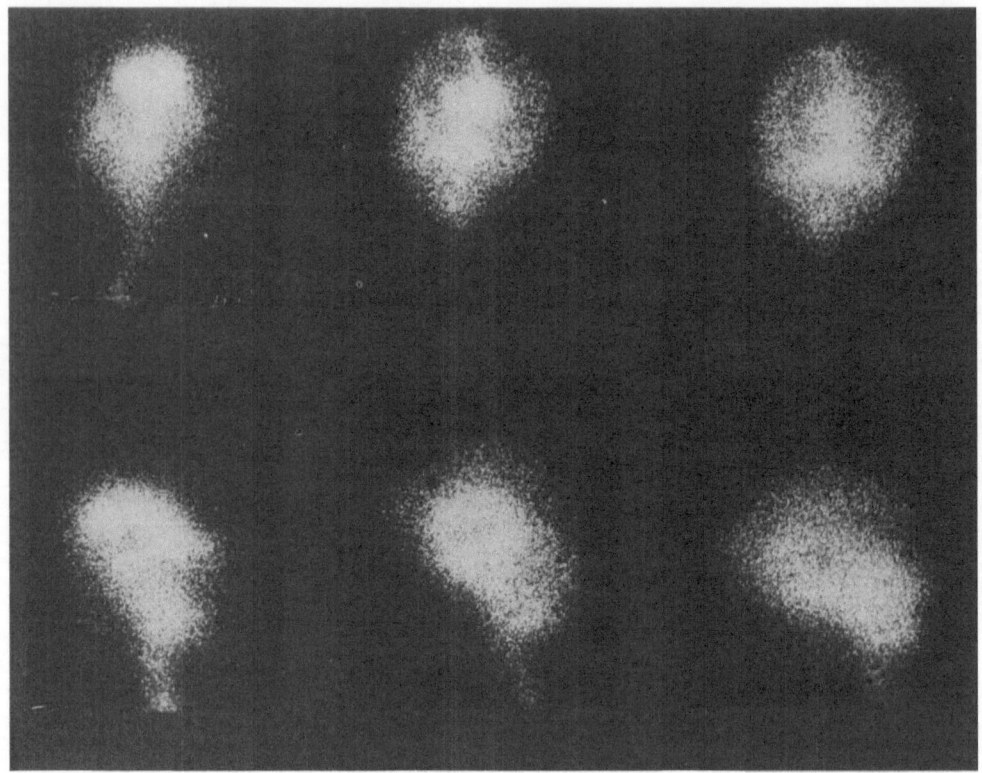

856 74   111 In HSA

Fig. 5. Pathological CSF-circulation:
ventricular reflux
insufficient ventricular clearance
no activity over the surface

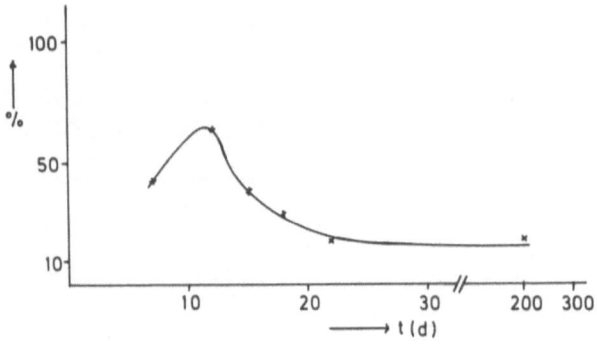

Fig. 6. Relationship between the incidence of disturbed CSF-dynamics
and time passed since spontaneous hemorrhage

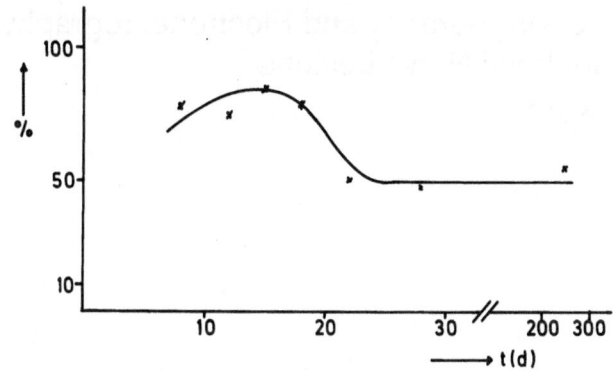

Fig. 7. Relationship between the incidence of disturbed CSF-dynamics and time since traumatic hemorrhage

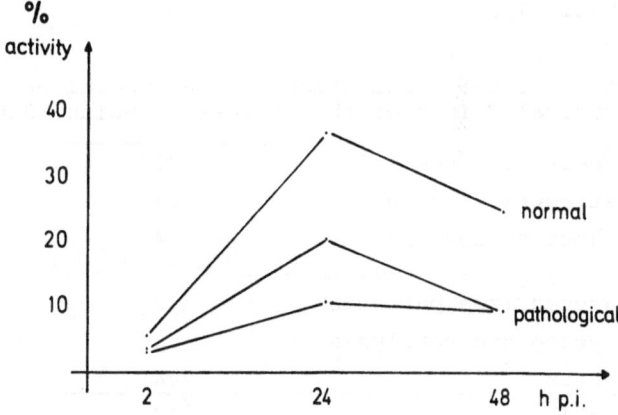

Fig. 8.: Quantitative cisternography: characteristic values in the case of a normal (upper curve) and a pathological (lower curve) qualitative cisternogram; the middle curve represents just adequate ventricular clearance

Electromyography and Electroneurography in the Appraisal of Peripheral Nerve Lesions

N. KLUG

In the expert appraisal of peripheral nerve lesions by specialists, electromyography (EMG) and electroneurography (ENG) play an important role.

During the last two years, 312 electromyographic examinations were carried out on patients with suspected peripheral nerve lesions in the Neurosurgical Department of the University Clinic of Mainz (Table 1).

Table 1. EMG examinations of peripheral nerve lesions at the Neurosurgical Clinic of the University Mainz (August 1972 - August 1974)

Expert evidence	38
Iatrogenic lesions	21
Injection lesions	4
Post-injection hematomas in marcumarized patients	3
Psychogenic paralysis	3
Others	244
Total	312

Repeated examinations and recordings from cranial nerves are not included in the table. In 38 cases (12 %) an expert opinion was provided.

A survey of the 38 cases supported by expert opinion is given in Table 2. In 14 cases, the nerve lesion or the suspected nerve damage was caused by industrial accidents and in 10 cases by road or household accidents. In 7 cases an expert opinion had to be given on disabled ex-servicemen. In 3 cases a nerve compression syndrome was verified, and in another 3 patients the nerve lesion was iatrogenic. In a single case a psychogenic paralysis was diagnosed. Of importance was the fact that in 5 cases an aggravation or malingering was demonstrated and that in 50 % of the cases the electromyographic examination decisively contributed to the establishment of the diagnosis and therapeutic course to be instituted.

With knowledge of the innervation scheme of the examined muscles as well as of the normal pattern of activity and the so-called "EMG pattern" of the neurogenic lesion, electromyography offers the possibility of objectively assessing the functional state of the peripheral nerves.

Table 2. Survey of 38 EMG expert opinions on peripheral nerve lesions at the Neurosurgical Clinic of the University Mainz (August 1972 - August 1974)

Causes	Number	Simulation	Decisive for Diagnosis	Treatment
Working accident	14	2	5	6
Trauma	10	-	3	6
Disabled exservicemen	7	3	5	2
Compression syndrome	3	-	3	3
Iatrogenic	3	-	-	1
Psychogenic	1	-	1	-
Total	38	5	17	18

Electromyography permits the diagnosis of lesions that are not identifiable by clinico-neurological means and, conversely, objectively disproves the claims of malingering patients. With the aid of electromyography it is also possible to differentiate inactivity-induced atrophy from that caused by nerve destruction and to differentiate a psychogenic paralysis from that of organic origin. With uncooperative patients, the simultaneous recording from agonists and antagonists and, in particular, stimulation neurography with the assessment of the duration of action potentials, the amplitude and morphology of the evoked action potential, as well as the determination of the motor and sensory nerve conduction velocity and the distal motor latency can prove to be of valuable assistance.

Specialists concerned with the establishment of expert opinions are, for the most part, faced with nerve injuries caused by direct trauma as a result of road or industrial accidents. Since such injuries usually result in a clearly defined neurological deficit, the electromyographic findings assist in objectivating the extent of the lesion and, by way of follow-up examination, in fixing the date for the operative therapy.

The so-called "occupational pareses" are more difficult to assess; they cover lesions of indirect traumatic origin in the case of chronic, occupation-dependent irritation of a nerve. During the last few years several authors have pointed out the possibility of clinically misdiagnosing a paresis of the motor branch of the median nerve with thenar atrophy or a typical motor paresis caused by the injury to the ramus profundus of the ulnar nerve with wasting of the small hand muscles caused by occupational chronic pressure. These conditions are not infrequently misdiagnosed as spinal muscular atrophy. An examination of neighbouring muscles and muscles of the contralateral extremity readily enables the physician to exclude a general neurological disease. By contrast, an accurate topical diagnosis can be established in a rapid and reliable manner in the case of isolated nerve lesions by electromyographic or electroneurographic studies. This also applies for the sulcus ulnaris syndrome, which can be reliably identified by the fractionated determination of the nerve conduction velocity and readily differentiated from a C 8 syndrome or a lesion of the lower brachial plexus.

The detection of a polyneuropathy which presents as exotoxic polyneuropathy with a specific local concentration in connection with

industrial toxins may prove difficult to diagnose clinically. Electromyography usually assists in establishing the diagnosis of polyneuropathy but the method frequently fails to give aetiological information.

In problematic cases, in which, for instance, expert opinion is required to decide whether the worsening alleged by the patient (disabled ex-servicemen) has developed independently of or as a consequence of the war injury, electromyography of peripheral nerve lesions
can be of great value.

Electromyography is a reliable method of verifying a psychogenic paralysis. Here, it is true, no pathological denervation activity is present. If the request to the patient to contract the muscles does not
result in a discharge of motor units, the next step is to perform
neurography, whereby normal motor latencies and normal nerve conduction velocities as well as physiological potentials are obtained.
Convinced of his paralysis, the patient is surprised to experience
strong muscle contractions in response to electrostimulation. The
examiner can make use of this effect by way of suggestion and this,
as a rule, induces the patient to carry out active movements at the
end of the examination with the action potentials failing to show
the typical signs of a neurogenic lesion. In the examination of a
psychogenic paralysis, we consider it important that the patient be
able to monitor the result of his efforts acoustically via a loud-
speaker and optically via an oscillograph.

Among our patients we frequently find cases in which it takes days
or weeks after application of a plaster cast to the lower leg or a
wire extension until the clinical diagnosis of a peronaeus paresis
is established. If, by means of electromyography, a neurogenic lesion
of the triceps surae group and the flexor of the lower extremity are
additionally identified, it appears justified to assume the presence
of a primary lesion of the sciatic nerve, for instance, an injury by
traction. In this case the assumption of an iatrogenic injury of the
peroneal nerve would be unlikely.

During the last 2 years we have seen 6 nerve lesions caused by injection. Two of them were of particular interest because the injections
were properly applied but performed on marcumarized patients. In both
cases extensive haematomas developed in the gluteal region followed
by uniform and partial denervation of the entire ischio-crural musculature. This denervation had been conclusively diagnosed electromyographically. In our view, this finding contrasts with the direct
injection injuries to the sciatic nerve which as a result of clinical
and electromyographic studies often predominantly affect the lateral
peroneal part of the nerve. The good spontaneous remission can be
regarded as a further characteristic of a sciatic nerve paresis
caused by an intragluteal haematoma. Prognostically this remission
is much easier to assess than the one associated with a direct injection injury. It would be interesting to learn whether similar
cases have been encountered by other colleagues, mainly because one
of the patients, a lawyer, intends to sue for damages caused by im-
proper injection.

In summarizing our observations, it can be said that electromyography
and electroneurography can be employed as an efficient and frequently
conclusive supplementary procedure in the appraisal of peripheral
nerve lesions.

Recovery of the Median Nerve in the Carpal Tunnel Syndrome – Electroneurographic Studies after Surgery and Local Corticosteroid Injections in 71 Cases

H. Assmus

The carpal tunnel syndrome (CTS), often misinterpreted as cervical brachialgia, is the most common entrapment neuropathy. Burning night pain and motor and sensory disturbances of the median nerve are the main symptoms. The diagnosis is verified by electromyographic investigations and nerve conduction studies. There is no doubt that the results of the surgical treatment are good (9, 14, 16, 17, 23). Preoperative neurophysiological evaluations had been more often published and with many more cases (1, 2, 6, 7, 8, 13, 22) than follow-up examinations (4, 5, 15, 18, 19).

In our series 71 hands of 48 female and 10 male patients with an average age of 53 years (31 - 77 years) were examined. Both hands were affected in 50 %. 58 hands had undergone surgery, 14 hands local beta- or dexamethasone injections into the carpal tunnel. The follow-up interval ranged from a few weeks to 17 years.

For stimulation of the mixed nerve at the wrist, surface electrodes and stimuli with a duration of 0,2 msec were used. The muscle action potential (MAP) was recorded with a concentric needle electrode from the thenar, the antidromic sensory nerve action potential (NAP) with ring electrodes (inter-electrode distance 30 mm) from the second finger. The technique was similar to that previously described (12).

Results

The clinical results have been briefly summarized in Table 1. After surgery all patients no longer had burning night pain. Only in a few cases did patients complain of tender scars, especially when a longitudinal incision was used. The sensory disturbances improved well, and in most cases only discrete numbness which could not be verified by routine clinical tests remained. Wasting and weakness did not improve as well. Patients treated by local beta- and dexamethasone injections which were tolerated without any complication often had only transient relief from pain. Sensory and motor disturbances remained essentially the same.

Postoperatively the distal motor latency (or motor conduction time) was improved by 2,8 msec during the first three months and by further 0,8 msec during the following 9 months. After a year and more, the average motor latency reached the upper level of normal range with 4,7 msec (Fig. 1). In regard to the average age of 62 years in the patients with latencies above 5,0 msec, it is justified to speak of approximately normalized motor values 12 months after surgery. The amplitude of the sensory NAP was also improved continuously during the first year postoperatively (Fig. 2). In a high percentage sensory NAPs could again be recorded after surgery. After corticosterioid in-

Table 1. The results of treatment in 71 hands with CTS

| | Surgical treatment (58 hands) | | Corticosteroid inject. (14 hands) | |
	preop.	postop.	pretr.	posttr.(<1 yr.)
Brachialgia	51 (87 %)	–	14	– a
Numbness / Dysesthesia	55 (94 %)	18 (31 %) b	8	unchanged
Weakness	35 (60 %)	14 (24 %)	3	unchanged
Thenar atrophy	40 (69 %)	16 (28 %)	5	unchanged

a = Only transient relief. b = Mild sensory disturbance

jections the motor latency improved slightly, and at the same time the amplitude of the MAP increased. This was also true for the latency and amplitude of the sensory NAP (Fig. 3).

In order to prove the differential diagnostic aid of the corticosteroid injections a group of patients with mild or moderate symptoms of a CTS was compared to that with brachialgia of other origin or borderline cases (Fig. 4). Those patients with motor latencies above 4,7 msec and amplitudes of sensory NAP less than 20 µV were relieved from pain by the injections whilst the others remained unaffected. The case history of a 56-year old house wife suffering from a traumatic CTS after COLLES' fracture and SUDECK's dystrophy should be given special mention. After giving three corticosteroid injections, the pain was relieved but the motor latency and amplitude of the MAP became worse. Only after surgery did the clinical symptoms and the neurophysiological findings improve (Fig. 5).

Discussion

The follow-up studies of other authors (4, 5, 18, 19) and our own series confirm that clinical improvement was approximately parallel to the neurophysiological findings. In motor disturbances the pathological latencies improved much better than the thenar atrophies. In severe cases with motor and sensory "block" improvement of the sensory disturbances can at least be expected. The number of good postoperative results may be increased by strict indication and exact neurophysiological examination. In mild cases and patients suffering only from numbness and dysesthesia the sensory NAP is a more sensitive indicator than the clinical examination (2, 6). Amplitude and latency of the antidromic sensory NAP (compared to that of the ulnar nerve) can easily be recorded and are in our opinion of some diagnostic value in clinical routine. Indeed BUCHTHAL et al.(1) found in 15 % and SEDAL et al. (20) in 39,3 % of their cases mild involvement of the ulnar nerve. A comparison of the NAP with that of the other hand will be of no use since both sides are affected in about 50 %. In borderline cases the local corticosteroid injection also has some diagnostic value (3, 6, 16, 17).

Prompt relief from burning night pain and improvement of the electrophysiological findings confirm the diagnosis "CTS". In most cases cutting-off the transverse ligament is essential for a good recovery of the median nerve.

Surgery is absolutely indicated in all cases with atrophies and moderate sensory disturbances (16, 17) and in most cases of traumatic CTS (24). When there is evidence of median nerve involvement in SUDECK's dystrophy, operation should be performed in order to eliminate the mechanical irritation of the vegetative fibres of the median nerve which probably favours the dystrophic process (11, 21). The technique of operation has no bearing on the result provided all fibres of the lig. carpi transversum are cut off and the muscular thenar branch is preserved. We now use a transverse incision in the distal flexion crease of the wrist and believe that under this technique less tender scars are observed than with longitudinal incisions.

Summary

The follow-up findings after surgery and conservative treatment for CTS in 71 cases are reported in order to show similarities of the clinical and neurophysiological findings during the recovery of the median nerve and to stress the diagnostic value of nerve conduction studies and corticosteroid injections in borderline cases. Finally the indication for surgery is discussed.

REFERENCES

1. BUCHTHAL, F., ROSENFALCK, A., TROJABORG, W.: Electrophysiological findings in entrapment of the median nerve at wrist and elbow. J. Neurol. Neurosurg. Psychiat. 37, 340 - 60 (1974).

2. DUENSING, F., LOWITZSCH, K., THORWIRTH, V., VOGEL, P.: Neurophysiologische Befunde beim Karpaltunnelsyndrom. Korrelationen zum klinischen Befund. Z. Neurol. 206, 267 - 84 (1974).

3. GOODMAN, H. V., FOSTER, J. B.: Effect of local corticosteroid injection on median nerve conduction in carpal tunnel syndrome. Ann. Phys. Med. 6, 287 - 294 (1962).

4. GOODMAN, H. V., GILLIATT, R. W.: The effect of treatment on median nerve conduction in patients with the carpal tunnel syndrome. Ann. Phys. Med. 6, 137 - 155 (1961).

5. HOGELL, A., MATTSON, H. S.: Neurographic studies before, after and during operation for median nerve compression in the carpal tunnel. Scand. J. Plast. Reconstr. Surg. 5, 103 - 109 (1971).

6. KAESER, H. E.: Diagnostische Probleme beim Karpaltunnelsyndrom. Dtsch. Z. Nervenheilk. 185, 453 - 470 (1963).

7. KEMBLE, F.: Electrodiagnosis of the carpal tunnel syndrome. J. Neurol. Neurosurg. Psychiat. 31, 23 - 27 (1968).

8. KEMBLE, F.: Clinical manifestations related to electrophysiological measurements in the carpal tunnel syndrome. Electromyography 8, 19 - 26.

9. LEVEN, B., HUFFMANN, G.: Das Karpaltunnelsyndrom. Klinische Erfahrungen. Münch. med. Wschr. 114, 1054 - 1059 (1972).

10. LOONG, S. C., SEAH, C. S.: Comparison of median and ulnar sensory nerve action potentials in the diagnosis of the carpal tunnel syndrome. J. Neurol. Neurosurg. Psychiat. 34, 750 - 754 (1971).

11. LYNCH, A. C., LIPSCOMB, P. R.: The carpal tunnel syndrome and COLLES' fractures. JAMA 185, 363 - 366.

12. MAVOR, H., SHIOZAWA, R.: Antidromic digital and palmar nerve action potentials. Electroenceph. clin. Neurophysiol. 30, 210 - 21 (1971).

13. MANZ, F.: Bestimmung der distalen Nervenleitzeit und Nadelelek-
    tromyographie beim Carpaltunnelsyndrom. Dtsch. med. Wschr. 95,
    1124 - 1127.

14. MAXION, H., WESSINGHAGE, D., LENG, E.: Untersuchungsbefunde nach
    konservativer und operativer Behandlung des Karpaltunnelsyndroms.
    Med. Welt 23, 913 - 915 (1972).

15. MELVIN, J. L., JOHNSON, E. W., DURAN, R.: Electrodiagnosis after
    surgery for the carpal tunnel syndrome. Arch. Phys. Med. Rehab.
    49, 502 - 507 (1968).

16. MUMENTHALER, M., SCHLIACK, H.: Läsionen peripherer Nerven. Diag-
    nostik und Therapie. 2. Aufl. Stuttgart: Georg Thieme 1973.

17. PHALEN, G. S.: Reflections on 21 years' experience with the car-
    pal-tunnel syndrome. JAMA 212, 1365 - 1367 (1970).

18. RICKENBACHER, M.: Karpaltunnelsyndrom. Spätergebnisse nach opera-
    tiver Behandlung des Karpaltunnelsyndrom. Klinische und elektro-
    myographische Nachkontrolle von 24 Fällen. Helv. chir. Acta 38,
    359 - 366 (1971).

19. SCHLAGENHAUFF, R. E., GLASAUER, F. E.: Pre- and postoperative
    electromyographic evaluations in the carpal tunnel syndrome. J.
    Neurosurg. 35, 314 - 319 (1971).

20. SEDAL, L., McLEOID, J. G., WALSH, J. C.: Ulnar nerve lesions
    associated with the carpal tunnel syndrome. J. Neurol. Neurosurg.
    Psychiat. 36, 118 - 123 (1973).

21. STEIN, A. H.: The relation of median nerve compression to SUDECK's
    syndrome. Surg. Gynecol. Obstetr. 713 - 720 (1962).

22. THOMAS, P. K.: Motor nerve conduction in the carpal tunnel syn-
    drome. Arch. Neurol. (Chic.) 10, 635 - 641 (1967).

23. WESSINGHAGE, D.: Klinik und Therapie des Karpaltunnelsyndroms.
    Dtsch. med. Wschr. 94, 2544 - 2547 (1969).

24. WILHELM, K.: Das Karpaltunnelsyndrom als Traumafolge. Arch.
    orthop. Unfall-Chir. 72, 87 - 93 (1972).

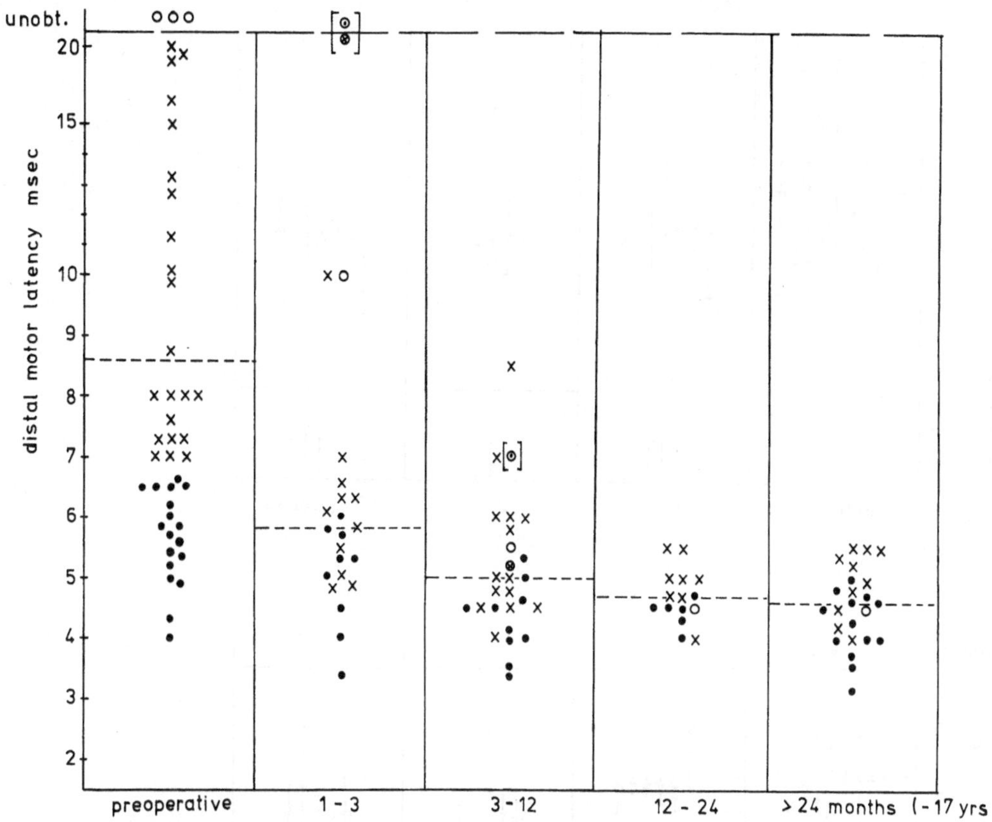

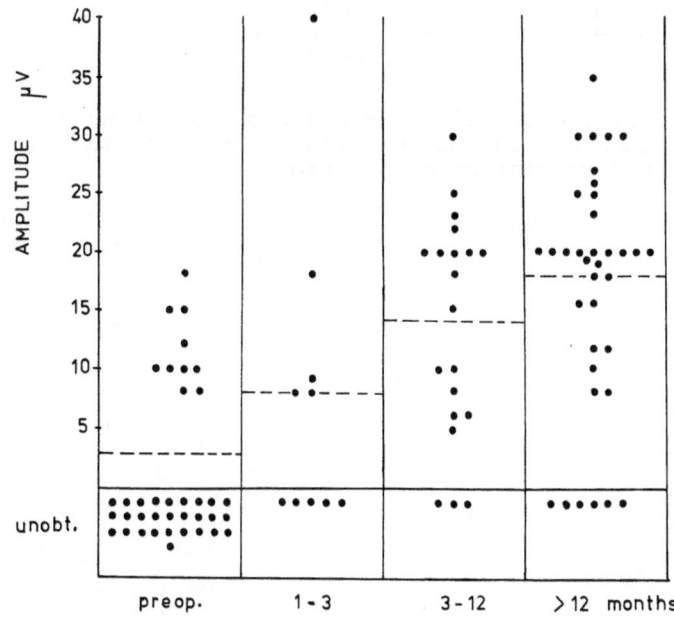

Fig. 1. Follow-up examination of the distal motor latency in patients with CTS: preoperative and postoperative findings divided into four intervals. · mild and moderate severe cases; x severe cases; o no MAP obtainable; (o) transient postoperative deterioration

Fig. 2.
Amplitudes of the antidromic sensory NAPs: pre- and post-operative values. Points under the line: no sensory NAP obtainable

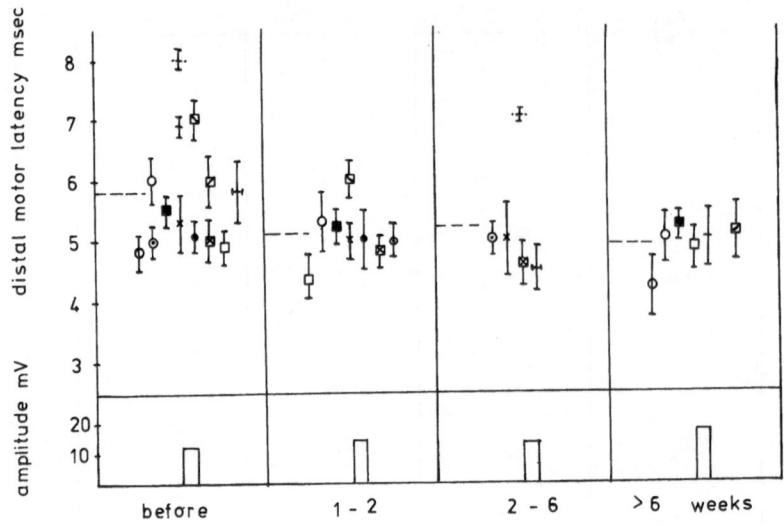

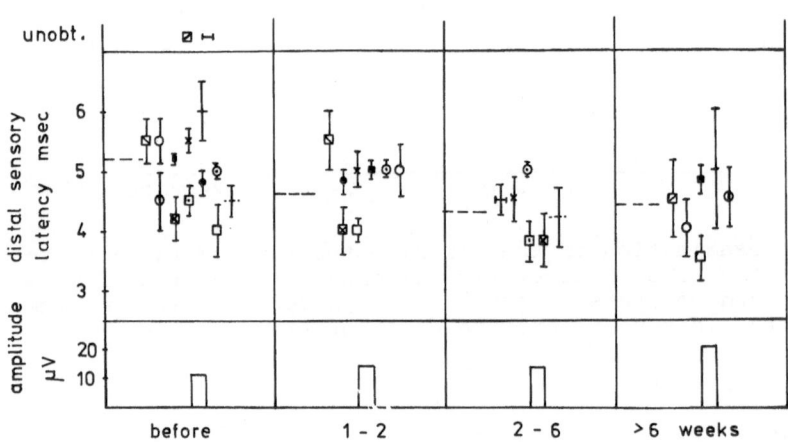

Fig. 3. Follow-up findings of the distal motor and sensory latencies
and amplitudes (vertical lines and columns beneath) of the evoked
potentials before and after corticosteroid injection

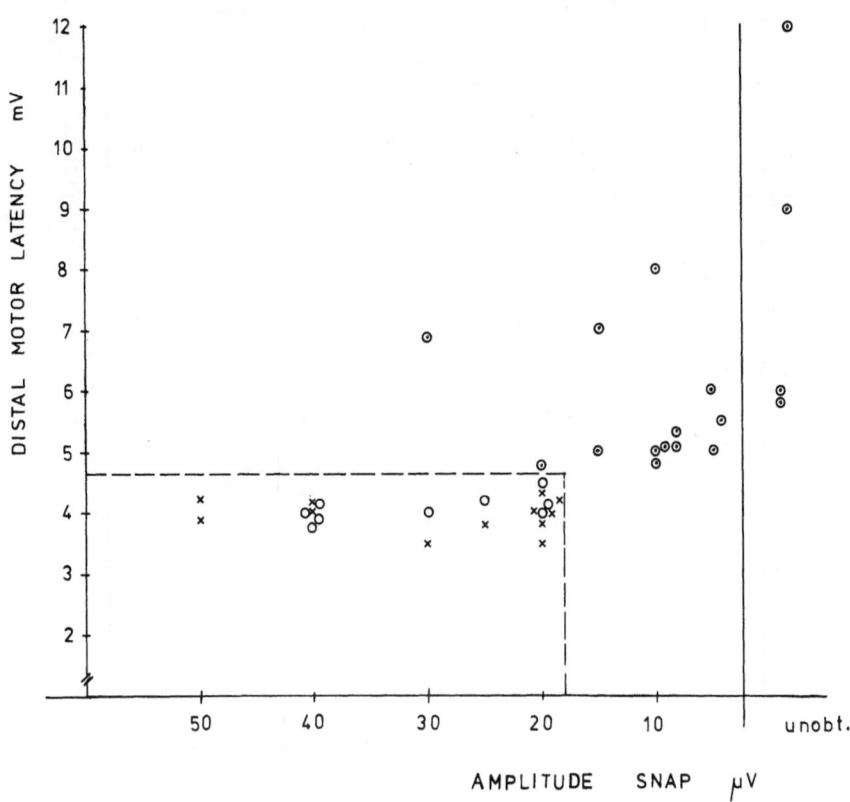

Fig. 4. Distal motor latencies plotted against the amplitudes of the sensory NAPs. ⊙ patients with CTS in which pain was relieved by corticosteroid injection; O borderline cases in which pain remained unaffected; · cases with brachialgia of other origin, no treatment

393

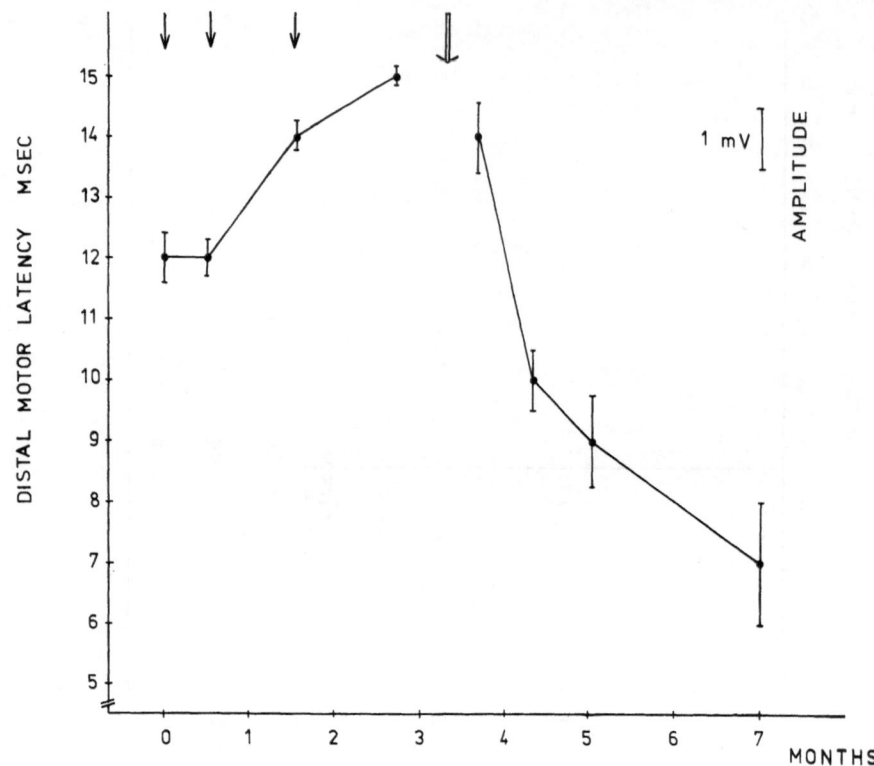

Fig. 5. Follow-up findings in a case of a 56-year old house wife with a traumatic CTS and SUDECK's dystrophy. Three corticosteroid injections are marked by small vertical arrows, the time of surgery by a large one

Arteriosclerotic Alterations of the Superficial Temporal Artery in Severe General Sclerosis

G. KLETTER, W. FEIGL, and H. SINZINGER

The increasing popularity of the anastomosis between the superficial temporal artery and the middle cerebral artery has motivated us to investigate to what extent the superficial temporal artery is actually suitable for this operation in the case of severe general arteriosclerosis. We were particularly interested in correlating these alterations with general arteriosclerosis, which affects the complete vascular system. Our investigations were concerned with the following four questions:

1. What are the degenerative changes that appear in the superficial artery?

2. Do these alterations correlate with those of general arteriosclerosis?

3. How does age influence these alterations?

4. Is the superficial temporal artery in view of the sclerotic alterations actually suitable for an extra-intracranial bypass operation?

Methods

In order to study the qualitative alterations, 40 cases of both sexes and of various ages were picked randomly from the routine material of the Institute of Pathological Anatomy of the University of Vienna and examined. In each case the temporal artery was taken from the left side immediately in front of its division into its two main branches. This point was considered to be histologically representative. Alongside these histological studies, comparative sections from the carotid bifurcation, the carotid siphon and from the middle cerebral artery of the same side were examined.

Concerning the correlation with general arteriosclerosis and the alterations according to age, we could refer to an extensive study on arteriosclerosis performed by the 1st Anatomical Institute of the University of Vienna, of which we used 136 cases in which the distribution of general arteriosclerosis had been examined.

H. E., van GIESON, ELASTICA, KOSSA, PAS and ALZIAN staining methods were used for the histological sections. Moreover Sudan III-sections were prepared from non-fixed autopsy material.

Results

Our histological findings were in accordance with those obtained by
LIE (1965) (1).

We observed that the ideal form of the artery is usually seen in the
small child, the endothelium being immediately adjacent to the internal elastic lamina. Already around the age of ten, the morphological
picture of the second stage according to LIE, of arteriosclerosis may
occur, i. e. ruptures of the internal elastic lamina (Fig. 1). With
advancing age, reduplications and proliferation of the elastic lamellae increase. Moreover a subendothelial layer, rich in cells and
poor in fibres, is formed (lamina musculo-elastica) (Fig. 2). During
the third stage, the intima grows nearly as thick as the media and
the alterations of the internal elastic lamina spread around the
whole interior vascular lumen. In the fourth stage calcareous infiltrations and foam cells are sparse, however their number is of no
importance. The most significant morphological finding obtained by us
was an increasing narrowing of the lumen by proliferation, however
simultaneously with senile ectasis (Fig. 3).

We saw that the sclerotic alterations of the superficial temporal
artery proceed at the same rate as in the other vessels of the organism, i. e. we could hardly find a difference in the extent of arteriosclerosis. A difference was only seen in the form of arteriosclerotic changes. While the superficial temporal artery was mainly
characterized by an increase of elastic lamellae and the formation of
a layer which is rich in cells and poor in fibres when simultaneous
senile ectasis occurred, considerable calcifications appeared in the
area of the internal carotid artery and of all other vessels examined,
causing sclerotic reductions of the vascular diameter, which in this
case were not compensated by ectases (Figs. 4 and 5). The middle
cerebral artery, which we investigated at its origin, was also affected by these alterations.

Arteriosclerosis increases continuously in all vessels, including the
superficial temporal artery. In cases with vascular risk, the superficial temporal artery - just as all the other vessels of the organism - is clearly more affected. It has already been mentioned that
senile arteriosclerotic vascular changes proceed in all vessels continuously and equally; it is, however, interesting that in the age
group of 70 to 80 the extent of the changes in the temporal artery
predominated. Thus we can conclude that the alterations in these vessels represent a continuous process which is directly proportional
to age.

Discussion

Using the routine material of the Insitute of Pathological Anatomy
and of the 1st Anatomical Institute we were in a position to examine
the alterations of the superficial temporal artery and to correlate
them very well with the changes in the rest of the vascular system.
From the surgical point of view we were particularly interested in
the changes of the lumen of the superficial temporal artery. Although
the use of histological sections calls for discrete judgement, since
only perfusion fixing of the arteries will permit precise judgement
of the size of the lumen, we may state rather safely that the lumen
of the superficial temporal artery hardly changes with increasing
age. Our preliminary results with arteries fixed by means of per-

fusion confirm this statement. Now we can answer the questions raised in the beginning as follows:

1. The degenerative alterations of the superficial temporal artery consist mainly in ruptures of the internal elastic lamina, in re-duplication and increase of the elastic lamellae and in the grad-ual formation of a thickened subendothelial layer which is rich in cells and poor in fibres. Simultaneously an ectasis of the ves-sel occurs, which compensates for the reduction of the lumen.

2. The alterations of the superficial temporal artery correlate with the changes of the other arteries of the organism with regard to the extent of alterations. However, the form of sclerosis is some-what different, since most of the other vessels experience a con-siderable reduction of the lumen by calcifications and deposition of lipoid substances.

3. The changes of the superficial temporal artery are directly pro-portional to the ageing process, risk factors, such as nicotine, diabetes, hypertension, causing a significant increase in the severity of sclerosis.

4. The superficial temporal artery, chosen by YASARGIL for the forma-tion of an artificial extra-intracranial shunt, is according to our studies excellently suitable for this operation. Although the alterations are of the same severity as those of the afferent ce-rebral vessels, no reduction of the lumen occurs in view of the simultaneously increasing senile ectasis of this vessel.

Summary

Using the autopsy material of large pathological and anatomical in-stitutes, form and severity of sclerotic changes of the superficial temporal artery were examined and correlated with the other vessels of the organism, particularly with the carotid artery, the aorta and the middle cerebral artery. No difference in the severity of arterio-sclerosis was observed, however, the different form of alterations results in a constant lumen of the superficial temporal artery, con-trary to the other vessels examined so that the superficial temporal artery appears to be very suitable for extra-intracranial artificial anastomoses.

REFERENCES

1. LIE, J. T., BROWN, A. L., CARTER, E. T.: Arch. Path. 90, 278 - 285 (1970).

2. YASARGIL, M. G.: Microsurgery applied to Neurosurgery. Stuttgart: Georg Thieme 1967.

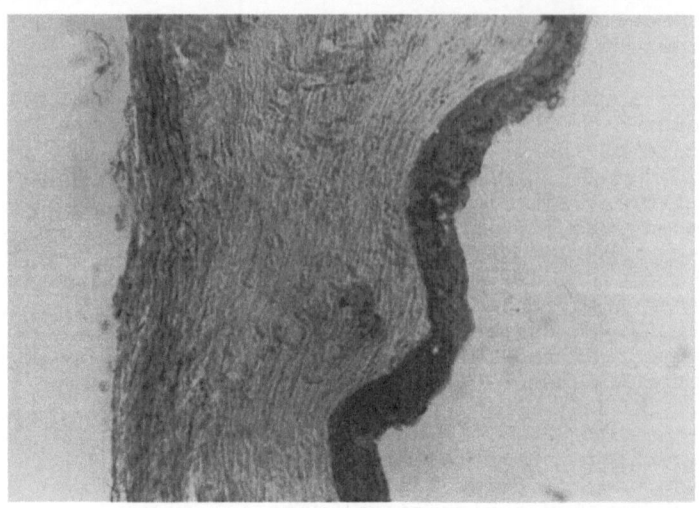

Fig. 1. Superficial temproal artery in second stage of arteriosclerosis. Reduplication and proliferation of the elastic lamella

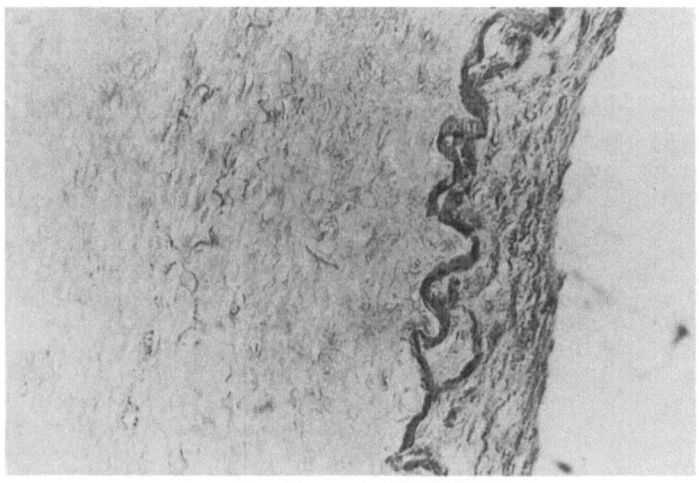

Fig. 2. Superficial temporal artery with formed "lamina musculoelastica"

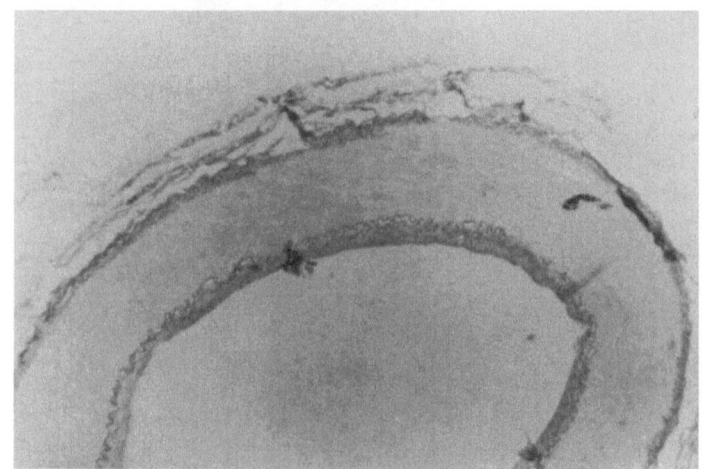

Fig. 3. Superficial temporal artery with thick wall but without calcareous infiltrations and without lipoids. The lumen is not reduced causing senile ectasis

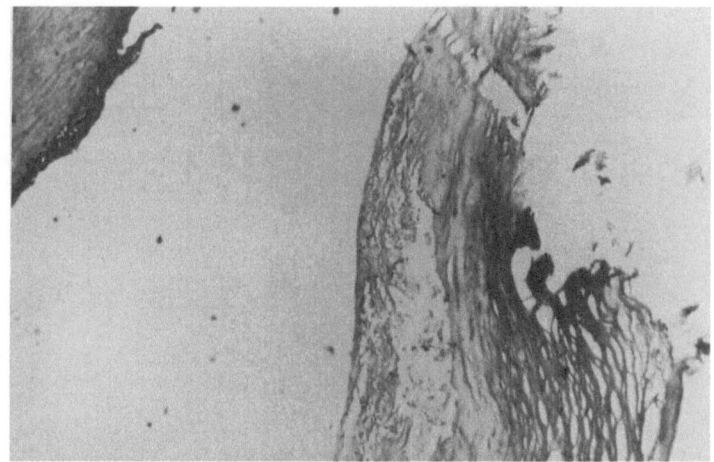

Fig. 4. Internal carotid artery with calcareous infiltrations and foam cells and reduction of the vascular diameter

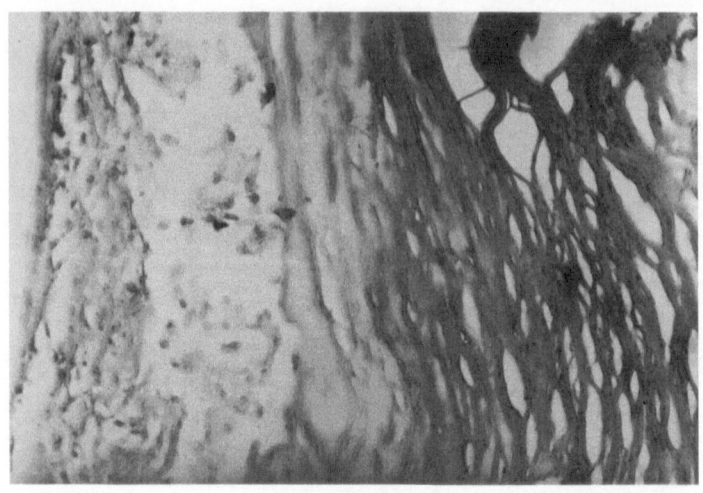

Fig. 5. Lipoids and foam cells in the wall of the internal carotid
artery

Tuberculous Abscess Formation in the Spinal Canal

M. Shaaban, H. Artmann, and E. W. Kienecker

It is difficult to diagnose tuberculosis of the spinal column because
of its slow onset, its limited clinical symptoms and the frequent absence of anamnestic indications. Furthermore, a survey of the litea-
ture indicates that a primary pulmonary tuberculosis can only be proved in about 52 % all cases of skeletal tuberculosis (5, 6, 11). Patients are admitted to hospital only when focal symptoms occur. In
case of gibbus formation and dropping abscesses diagnosis is not so
difficult, but if the symptomatology is limited exclusively to neurological symptoms, all spinal expansive processes must be considered
in the differential diagnosis (2, 11).

The majority of cases with spinal column tuberculosis have tuberculous spondylitis. It makes up to 52 % of skeletal tuberculosis and
tis greatest indicdence has been noted in patients aged between 25
and 40 years (5, 6, 11). Furthermore we find extremely few examples
of genuine tuberculogenous abscess formations in the literature.

On comparison, most adults do not exhibit any change in the general
good condition as do children who suffer from spinal column tuberculosis. Remarkable laboratory results are also often absent (11).

Although we did not have any patient showing spinal column tuberculosis since 1967, we have treated 2 cases with intraspinal tuberculous
abscesses in the last year. In the same period various cases of tuberculosis occurred in Bremen especially at schools. That is why we would
like to call your attention to the fact that spinal column tuberculosis must still be considered in the differential diagnosis.

In both cases we did not have any anamnestic indication of tuberculosis. The first one - a 34-years-old man - highly suspicious of
herniated lumbar disc, suffering already for one year from lumbago
and for one month from sciatic pain and pollacuria. Clinical examination revealed a compression syndrome of the cauda equina with acute
urinary retention and lack of signs of inflammation. The preliminary
roentgenological findings showed no particularity and especially the
lumbar roof plates seemed to be intact (Fig. 1). During the lumbar
puncture for myelographical examination, we were astonished to see
that the extradural space discharged pus. The subsequent laminectomy
of the L_4-arch exposed a medio-lateral abscess on the left side ,
covered by granular tissue which we were able to exstirpate bioptical-
ly. Only the postoperative tomogram revealed a beginning defect of
the roof plate of the 4th lumbar vertebral body (Fig. 2), similar to
the osseous defect of tuberculous spondylitis.

The 2nd case showed a 34-years-old Turkish patient with a node which
had developed in his neck 8 weeks before admission to hospital. A
general practioner who took it to be a furuncle, opened it by an in-

cision. 4 weeks later the patient was suffering from a chiefly left-sided tetraparesis. This had developed within 48 hours into a complete tetraplegia with paralysis of a great part of the respiratory muscles. He could only gasp by means of the auxiliary musculature. Clinical, roentgenological and myelographical examination revealed an expansive process with destruction at the spinal processes and at the arches of the cervical vertebrae 2 and 3 (Fig. 3) and complete stop of the contrast medium (Fig. 4). Considering the nature of the alteration and in reference to the first case, we included a tuberculous abscess among other possibilities in the differential diagnosis before the operation. It was afterwards confirmed by laminectomy of $C_1 - C_4$ and could be exstirpated.

In this case the tuberculous genesis in the first place had been taken into consideration whereas in the first case only the subsequent tomogram could provide us with decisive diagnostic hints.

The diagnosis was confirmed in both patients through histological and bacteriological examination. After the operation and the subsequent antituberculous therapy however we were surprised to notice, in a short period of three months, that the neurological symptoms vanished completely.

We can find similar cases in the literature where attention is especially focussed on the difficulty of differential diagnosis and the incidence of false diagnosis (2, 3, 12, 13). We could only find comparable notes of cases made by CHADDUCK, DECKER et al. and RAO et al. They too have demonstrated that the clinical findings, just as in our case, simulated a herniated lumbar disc (3, 12, 13).

For some years now according to KASTERT and other authors, early operation, combined with antituberculous medication, is recommended and it is pointed out that it results in a considerable shortening of postoperative treatment and an earlier recovery of working capability (1, 5, 6, 7, 8, 9).

Formerly the treatment was of about 700 days where as nowadays we only need 120 - 180 days. Almost in 100 % of all cases one can obtain a complete cure of the focus as far as children, adolescents and middle-aged adults are concerned. Only in the case of elderly patients and those of old age the percentage is about 80 - 90 % (1, 4, 5, 8).

Considering the favourable course of our patients as well as that of two other ones, personally known to us (10), we also believe that the indication for early operation is recommended. At least abscess formations of the described nature and of such dramatic courses as in our case, will probably exclude a comparable therapeutic success by antituberculous static medication alone.

REFERENCES

1. CARSTENSEN, E.: Grundsätzlicher Wandel in der Behandlung der Spondylitis tuberculosa. Chirurg. 40, 547 - 550 (1969).

2. CHADDUCK, W. M.: Intraspinal Tuberculous Abscess Simulating Lumbar Disc Disease. Virginia. med. mth. 99, 968 - 971 (1972).

3. DECKER, H. G., SHAPIRO, S. W., PORTER, H. R.: Epidural Tuberculous Abscess Simulating Herniated Intervertebral Disc. A Case Report. Ann. Surg. 149, 294 - 296 (1959).

4. JUDIN, Ja. B., GAIDUK, R. A.: Operatiwnoje letschenie tuberculesnowo spondilitita u poschilych. (Operative Behandlung der tuberkulösen Spondylitis bei älteren Menschen). Ortopedija 7, 49 (1969).

5. KASTERT, I.: Knochen- und Gelenktuberkulose (Skelett-Tbc). Chirurg.
40, 533 - 536 (1969).

6. KASTERT, I.: Die Behandlung der Spondylitis tuberculosa. Dtsch.
Med. Wschr. 97, 1356 - 1357 (1972).

7. KATERINITSCH, N. T.: O chirurgitscheskom letschenie tuberculesnowo
spondilitia. (Zur chirurgischen Behandlung der tuberkulösen Spondylitis). Ortopedija 12, 57 (1969).

8. MARTIN, N. S.: Tuberculosis of the Spine. J. Bone Jt. Surg. 52,
613 (1970).

9. MARTIN, N. S.: Pott's Paraplegia, a Report on 120 Cases. J. Bone
Jt. Surg. 53, 596 - 608 (1971).

10. PISCOL, K.: Seltener spinaler raumfordernder Prozeß: intramedul-
läres Tuberculom. Berl. ges. psych. neurol. Berlin (1959) u. per-
sönl. Mitteilung.

11. PITZEN, P., RÖSSLER, H.: Kurzgefaßtes Lehrbuch der Orthopädie, S.
34 - 54. München - Berlin - Wien: Urban und Schwarzenberg 1970.

12. RAO, S. B., DINKAR, J.: Extraosseous Extradural Tuberculous Granuloma Simulating a Herniated Lumbar Disc. Case Report. J. Neurosurg. 35, 488 - 490 (1971).

13. WALESZKOWSKI, J., RYDZEVSKY, W.: Zagadnienie Klinicznie odosobnio-
nych Gruzliczakow W Kanale Kregowym (The Problem of Clinically
Isolated Tuberculoma in the Vertebral Kanal). Neurol. Neurochir.
Psychiat. Pol. 21, 877 - 880 (1971).

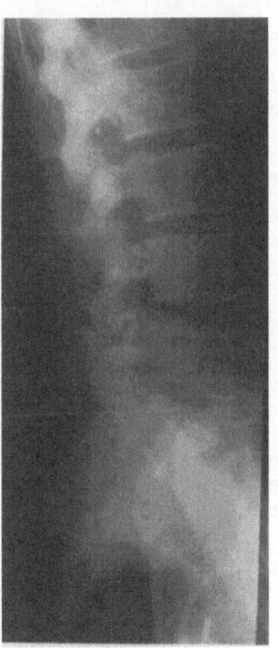 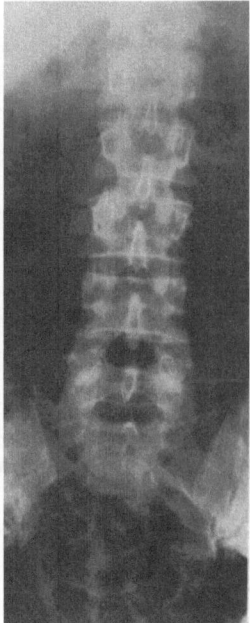

Fig. 1.
Case 1. Antero-posterior and
lateral view of the lumbar
portion of the spine showing
the roofplates of the vertebrae seemingly intact

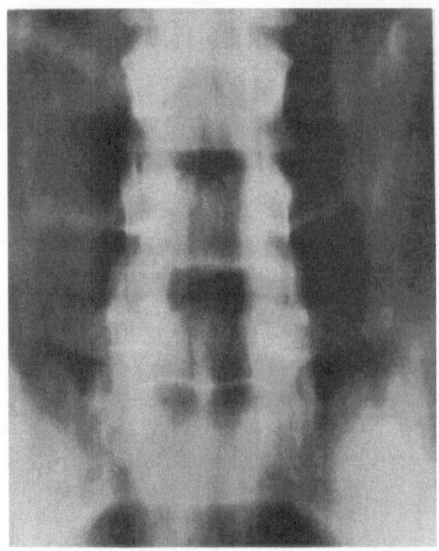

Fig. 2. Antero posterior tomogram of Fig. 1 after the operation. Notice the destruction of the roofplate of the 4th lumbar vertebral body

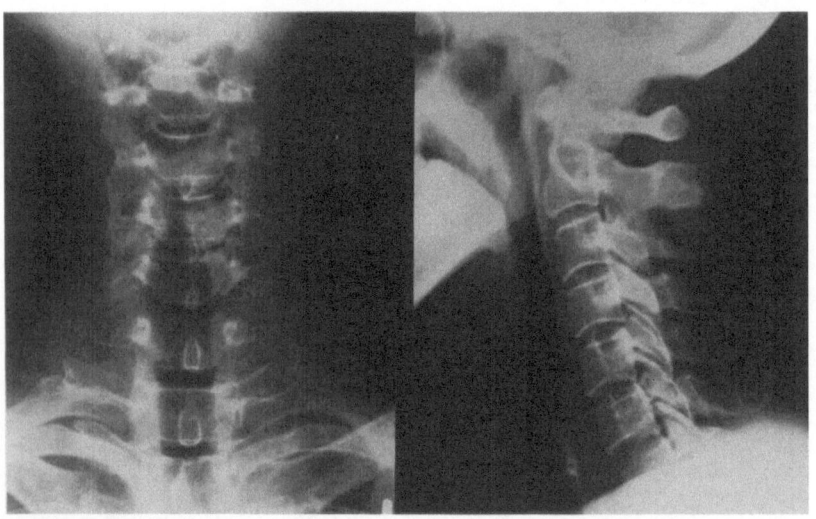

Fig. 3. Case 2. Antero posterior and lateral view of the cervical portion of the spine showing destruction of the spinal processes of the cervical vertebrae 2 and 3

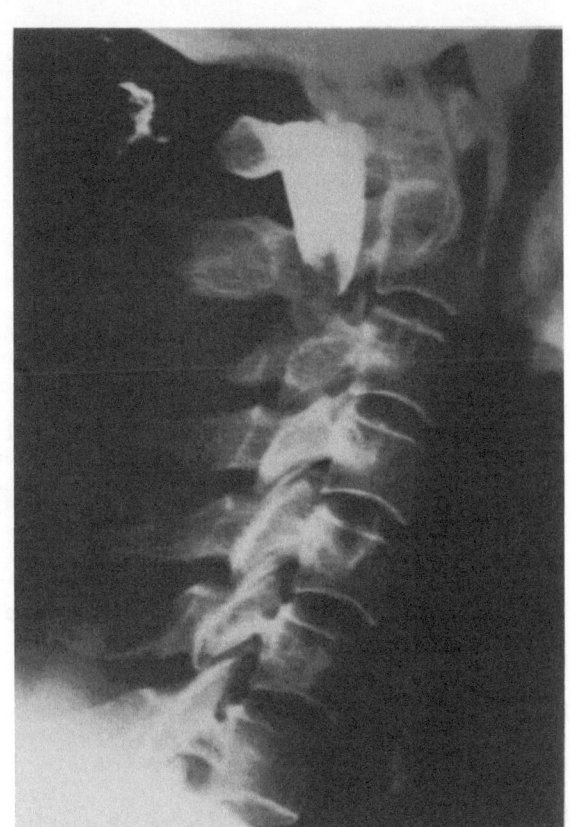

Fig. 4. Myelographic lateral view of case 2 showing complete stop of the contrast medium

Rudimentary Occipital Cephaloceles

J. KLEIN, K. V. PALM, and K. ABU BAKR

Between 10.9.1973 and 2.8.1974, that is just under a year, five babies
with cutaneous deformities over the small fontanelle were admitted to
the Neurosurgical Clinic in Bremen for surgery. We base our report on
this accumulation of similar cases, especially since praeoperatively
and macroscopically a reliable classification was not possible. The
diagnosis could only be made by means of a pathohistological examination.

The case in question involves three male and two female babies, four
of which were born on schedule and free of complications. The youngest
child was eighteen days old, the oldest eighty-five days old.

These alterations were observed at birth; they alone lead to admission
to the pediatric clinic and referral to us, with no other anomalies at
the time being under consideration.

The anomalies can be described as follows (Table 1):

Table 1.

Case No.	Age in days	Size and shape of cele	Surgical treatment	Histolog. diag.
1. M. S. ♂	18	Pfennig piece flat	Ovular skin excision	M C
2. M. Sch. ♂	25	Pfennig piece flat	Ovular skin excision	M C
3. F. Sch. ♂	40	Pfennig piece cupola shaped	Ovular skin excision, ligature	M E C
4. S. W. ♀	41	Zehnpfennig piece, flat	Ovular skin excision, coagulation	M E C
5. S. B. ♀	85	Mark piece, cupola shaped	Ovular skin excision, ligature, coagulation, CSF outflow	M E C

M C = meningocele, M E C = meningoencephalocele.

In all the case cutaneous anomalies were present in the area of the small fontanelle, ranging in size according to age from 1 cm to 3 cm in diameter; in three cases they were at skin level, in two cases they were cupola shaped. All were devoid of hair (Fig. 1), and showed a reddish colored area all around the anomaly, proportional in size to the anomaly (Fig. 2).

In all five cases the skin was thinned in the center, resembling silky paper, with a bluish transparency. All the children were operated under intubation anesthesia, in two cases we merely performed an ovular skin excision, as there was no evidence of a connection with the contents of the skull.

In two other cases, a solid cord of connective tissue which had an intracranial connection through a small fissure, was ligated and coagulated (Fig. 3).

In the fifth case a small lumen was present in the cord, through which CSF exuded to the exterior, whereupon the cele collapsed instantly (Fig. 4).

In three cases the histological examination yielded the typical picture of a meningocele; in two cases that of a meningoencephalocele, in which indeed only glial and no neural structures were found. In these two cases, there existed a connection with the skull contents as we observed during the operation.

As this time we wish to dwell upon two points which appeared especially important to us:

1. The differential diagnosis and

2. the question of the operative indications.

In the case of the first point it is interesting to note that exterior contrasting forms display themselves microscopically in a similar fashion: namely as a rudimentary dysrhaphic disturbance, in this case an occipital cephalocele. In the differential diagnosis the cephaloceles must be distinguished from sinus pericranii, hemangiomas, dermoids, dermal sinus as well as the congenital soft tissue defects of the cranium according to GERLACH (1, 2) et al. By a typical manifestation of cephaloceles, the diagnosis can often be determined by inspection or during the operation. In the case of sinus pericranii and hemangiomas, blood filling and connection to the intracranial vessels have to be tested by external appearance, through a compression test, or X-ray contrast examination, such as sinography.

Typical of a dermal sinus is a porus with an outflow of secretion, whereas dermoids and congenital soft tissue defects are to be differentiated by their appearance and the nature of their contents; as a rule they do not fulfil the criterion of the cephalocele, namely, resilent protuberance.

A bony defect was not observed by X-ray in any of our cases. In one case a sinus pericranii was excluded by sinography.

It was interesting to us and therefore worthy of mention, that the above mentioned soft tissue alterations which indeed had a common localization, despite such diverse external appearances, had a common origin: in all five cases a dysrhaphic disturbance must be assumed, whereby insignificant parts of the nervous system remained ectopic in an apparently very short interruption of the development process.

Nevertheless one cannot avoid viewing this group of deformities in relation with the larger cranial meningoceles and meningoencephaloceles.

The essential criterion of the group demonstrated by us is that an osseus occlusion has taken place, at least a defect could not be detected by X-ray although we found a fine cord in our cases No. 4 and 5 filled with CSF which communicated through a narrow bony apperture with the skull contents.

In order to denote the basic correlation between the large group of cephaloceles and characterize the specific properties of our cases, we have selected the germ rudimentary occipital cephaloceles in agreement with our neuropathologists.

The second point of view we wish to consider was the insecurity of the question of the therapeutic procedure. While in all of our cases parents pressured us to correct the skin alterations, the attending pediatrician took an insecure position toward the question of the operative indication and the time of the operation.

We decided to operate immediately because in all the cases the covering skin was so thin that the danger of injury with the possibility of infection by the slightest mechanical pressure was high. No larger osseus defect was to be seen. All the procedures were minor, of short duration, and were carried out without complications, by all means tolerable for the youngest infants. A progression of the alterations is possible, according to the literature; at least this course could not be excluded in case No. 5 with endocranial connection and CSF filling.

MEYER (3) reccomends operation of the small cephaloceles in the second half of the first year of life, provided that no special circumstances force earlier treatment. Based on our experience we would follow this procedure only in those cases where there is a significant osseus defect which is preoperatively provable, where an intracranial extension of the operation must be taken into account. We would advise immediate treatment of the group of rudimentary cephaloceles, for which the criterion is the lack of a radiological evidence of an osseus defect. This promotes normal conditions, removes the danger of infection - even meningitis - and frees the parents of understandable worry.

It is quite clear that we have not broached a momentous problem with the patients presented; this appears to apply to the statistical side as well. In Western Europe it is stated in the literature that in one to two births per thousand, dysrhaphic disturbances occur. According to GERLACH (1, 2) the occurrence of cephaloceles is only one-fifth to one-fiftieth of these. Contradictory to these statistics, we have observed five cases of rudimentary occipital cephaloceles within one year. Previously such cases were probably neglected, due to the insignificance of the anomalies.

REFERENCES

1. GERLACH, J.: Mißbildungen des Schädels und des Gehirns. In: Handbuch der Neurochirurgie, Bd. IV/1 (Hrsg. H. OLIVECRONA, W. TÜNNIS), S. 169 - 183. Berlin - Göttingen - Heidelberg: Springer 1960.

2. GERLACH, J., JENSEN, H.-P., KOOS, W., KRAUS, H.: Fehlbildungen des Schädels. Fehlbildungen des Gehirns. In: Pädiatrische Neurochirurgie (Hrsg. J. GERLACH, H.-P. JENSEN, W. KOOS, H. KRAUS), S. 215 - 265. Stuttgart: Geort Thieme 1967.

3. MEYER, E.: Mißbildungen und angeborene Störungen, Entwicklungs-
   störungen. In: Chirurgie des Gehirns und Rückenmarks im Kindes-
   und Jugendalter (Hrsg. K.-A. BUSHE, P. GLEES), S. 965 - 972.
   Stuttgart: Hippokrates 1968.

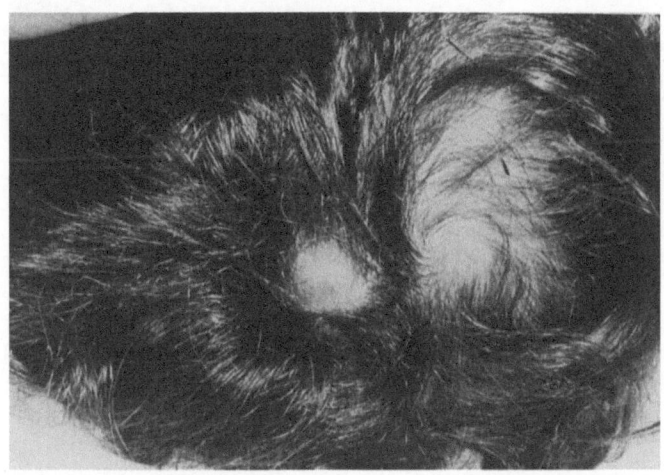

Fig. 1. Shows cupola shaped cutaneous anomaly without hair

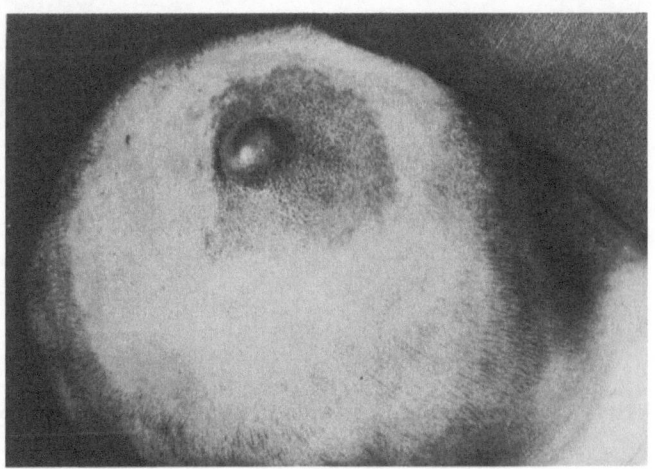

Fig. 2. Shows shaved head with reddish colored area around the cele

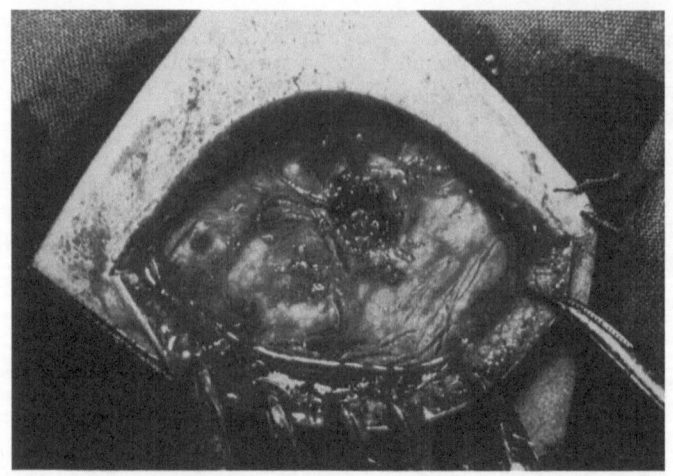

Fig. 3. Operative site shows ovular skin excision, ligated and coagulated cord of connective tissue

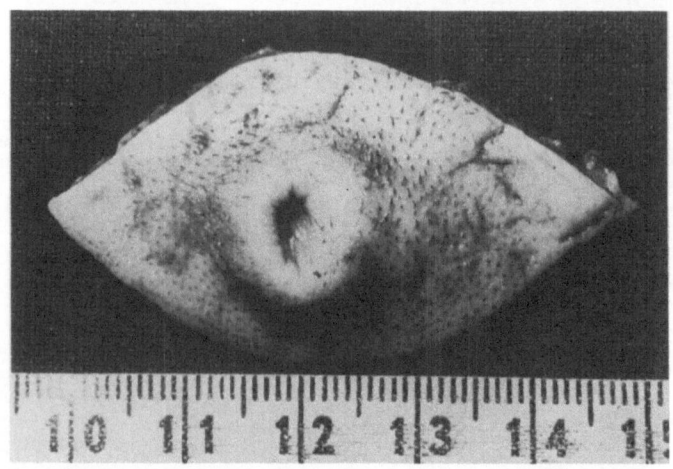

Fig. 4. Shows the collapsed cele after outflow of CSF

The Armoured Aneurysm Thread: A New Aid for the Surgical Treatment of Intracranial Aneurysms (With Technical and Clinical Notes)

K. PISCOL

The operation of an intracranial aneurysm has lost much of its original frightfulness but, still, must not be less exciting in some cases. The improved equipment and instrumentation in general, the possibility of optical magnification, bipolar coagulation etc. have most certainly contributed to this development. The sum of small technical modifications, even tricks and aids, which might seem simple enough, are of no less importance. To illustrate this point we would like to mention the intraoperative aspiration or compression of ruptured aneurysms, the finniking thread maneuvers to isolate the neck of the aneurysm, the artificial stenosis of the aneurysm neck by bipolar coagulation, the introduction of microinstruments, small metal plombs to avoid knotting and special clips for temporary exclusion of an aneurysm from the blood supply. These and other small achievements have essentially contributed to making the manipulation of the aneurysm proper safer, so that a direct complete exclusion has become the rule. Not only the operative results and patients' chances have improved, but at the same time the pre-, intra- and postoperative difficulties decreased. Among 45 patients operated on for an intracranial aneurysm at the Neurosurgical Clinic in Bremen between August 1st, 1972 and July 31st, 1974, only one case occurred, which was treated under hypothermia and compression of the interal carotid artery, due to inaccessible location and large size of the aneurysm. All other patients were operated on in the usual way under neuroleptanaesthesia. Special attention was given to blood pressure, which ranged around normal levels; values higher than normal were dealt with by means of drugs.

We would like to consider out "armoured aneurysm thread" among these small but helpful achievements. This instrument consists in a slightly hardened metal pin with a length of 10 mm and a diameter of 0,5 mm. The spherically shaped tip has a diameter of one millimeter. At the opposite end a 1 or 2 x 0 perma silk or coated polyesther (Ethiflex) thread is atraumatically fastened. Due to the lesser degree of hardness, the metal pin can be bent as required. On the other hand the pin is rigid enough to allow preparatory manipulations. The Ethicon Company has collaborated in the development and initiated the production of the armoured needle. As yet we have used two kinds of needle, which differ in the material of the globular tip: the first type consists of the same material as the needle itself, the second has a tiny plastic drop at its tip due to manufacture. reasons. The designation "armoured aneurysm thread" was chosen since the term "aneurysm needle", which was originally considered, is already used for a long ligature carrier and since the present name offers a more definite characterization (Fig. 1).

In certain situations there are definite reasons to prefer the thread to the clip when operating on an aneurysm, e. g. when there are important anatomical structures such as main vessels, cranial nerves or the optical nerve behind a sessile adherent aneurysm, and when there is the risk of injuring these structures by the clip due to insufficient visual control. The thread is also preferred, when the aneurysm has a sessile neck and artificial occlusion by bipolar coagulation is not possible or is too hazardous, or when a too large clip may lead to permanent alteration or irritation of the surrounding vessels or nerval tissue due to pulsation.

We also use the armoured aneurysm thread temporarily, e. g. when the neck of the aneurysm has its position behind an arterial vessel - mostly the internal carotid artery. Under such conditions the neck of the aneurysm is visualized by slightly pulling the thread and the clip can be placed more accurately. The same applies when the aneurysm neck has to be lifted or has to be encircled temporarily and final clipping is of greater advantage. Furthermore, temporary constriction of the aneurysm neck is basicaly favourable since it permits mastering the situation, when a clip injures the aneurysm wall or its position has to be adjusted. The "armoured aneurysm needle" also simplifies the removal of a huge aneurysmatical sack, whenever it compresses the adjoining structures such as the oculomotor or optic nerve.

Basically, we operate on all aneurysms with the aid of the operation microscope (microneurosurgical roof - unit from MÜLLER WEDEL). The optic system and the coaxial illumination make it possible to keep the way of access narrower than would be possible under a macroscopic operation or when using magnifying lenses. Therefore, there is less damage to the brain. When access is so narrow, the usual ligature carriers and aneurysm needles fail due to their stiffness and length. The very length is often hindering and can even be dangerous or make fine manipulation impossible. As compared to this, the armoured aneurysm thread has only advantages (Fig. 2). It can be bent according to the situation. The possibility of directing and seizing the armoured needle by means of a forceps or a needle gard offers great immobility in all directions and great variability even for encircling a vessel or other structures in a minimal space. In addition, not only does the globular tip of the armoured thread protect the aneurysm and its surroundings from injury, but it can also be used for preparation an dissection of adhesions and of the arachnoid. Recently we operated on a relatively sessile aneurysm of the internal carotid artery located beneath the posterior communicating artery, the exclusion of which would most certainly not have been possible without this new instrument. Only the slightly bent armoured thread allowed encircling the lower part of the internal carotid artery, so that the tip appeared in a small lacuna (Fig. 3) nearby the anterior clinoid process and could be seized there. In only one case an internal carotid aneurysm, partly located within the cavernous sinus, had to be encircled by a sling of temporal muscle fascia as suggested by KEMPE. This was only possible with the aid of the armoured thread, with which the fascial sling could be directed around the internal carotid artery underneath the deep posterior communicating artery.

The number of cases and the location of the aneurysms operated on with the aid of the armoured aneurysm thread are given in Table 1.

Among 42 aneurysms, four were located deeply infraclinoidal, and at the level of the base of the skull. In this group two patients were treated by ligature of the extracranial internal carotid artery, one by a circular sling of fascia, and one by reinforcement of the wall with histoacryl and encasement with muscle. The latter patient, who was operated on under hypothermia and extracranial ligature of the internal carotid artery, died two days later. It is the only case of operative death. All the remaining 38 aneurysms could be directly and completely excluded from the circulation. Two patients of this group died, one from myocardial infarct, and the other by superinfection after three weeks. The mortality in cases of direct exclusion of the aneurysm amounts to 5,3 %, the overall mortality to 7 %. No survivor had his clinical condition worsened by surgery. Two patients with pre-operative hemiplegia still present a regressing hemiparesis. One female patient operated on in stadium 4 is up to now little aconative.

Table 1. Aneurysma operations performed at the Neurosurgical Clinic in Bremen (August 1st, 1972 to July 31st, 1974)

Location	Right side		Left side		Total
A. carot. int., infraclinoid.	2	(1)	2	O	4
A. carot. int., supraclinoid. Ram. comm. posterior	7	6	3	2	10
A. cerebri anterior Ram. comm. anterior	9	4	4	2	13
A. cerebri media	7	3	6	2	13
A. vertebralis, A. basilaris	2	1	O	O	2
Total	27	14+(1)	15	6	42

The condition of all remaining patients can be classified as very good or good. 20 patients were treated with the aid of the armoured aneurysm thread and in one case a sling of fascia was directed around the internal carotid artery with the aid of an armoured thread. No case of death occurred in this group of patients as shown in Table 1. In our experience the armoured aneurysm thread prove to be excellent technical aid. It constitutes a good contribution towards more careful and controlled operations, so that it meets with the microneurosurgical principles.

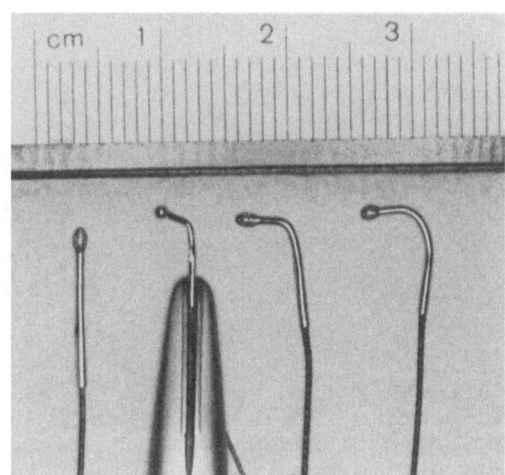

Fig. 1

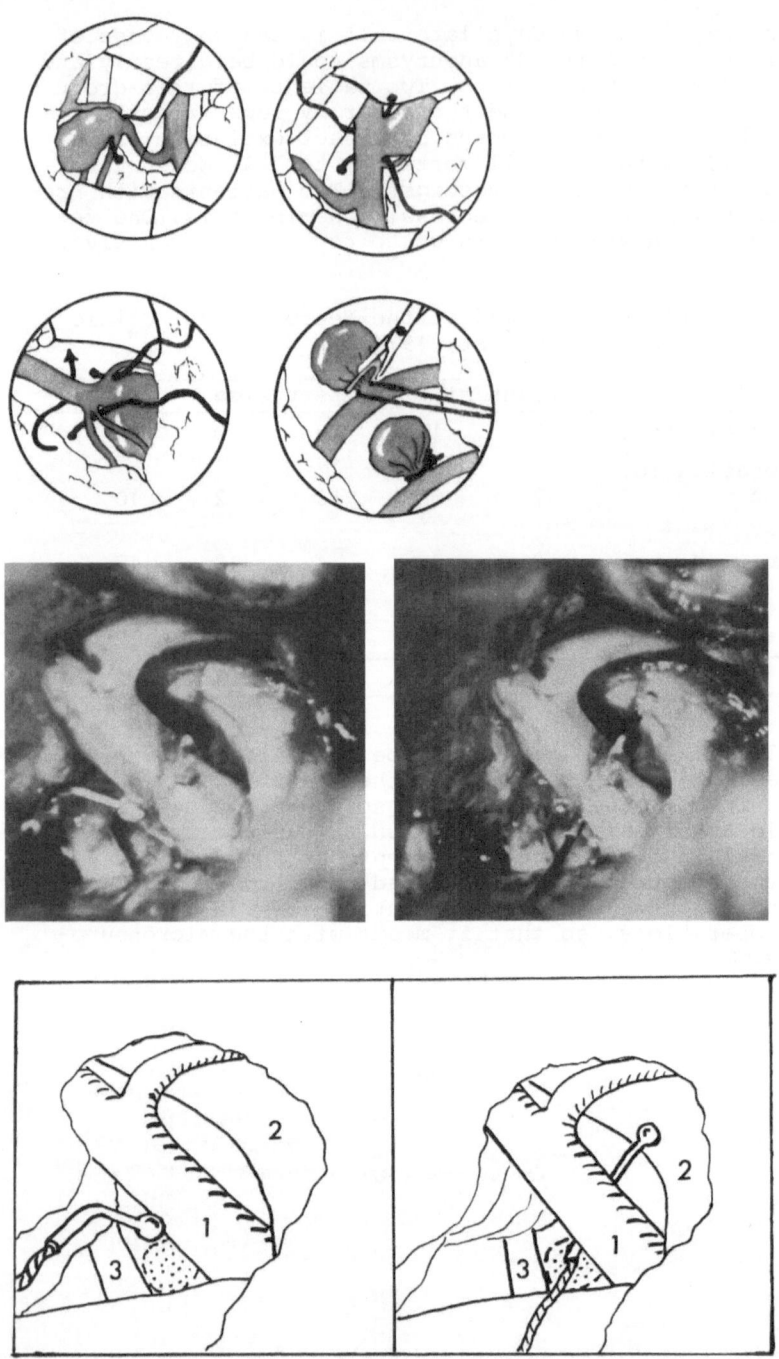

Fig. 3. The armoured aneurysm thread is passed around the internal carotid artery.
a) and c): The armoured thread lateral to the artery
b) and d): Armoured thread being passed around the vessel. The aneurysm can be recognized between the internal carotid artery and the occulomotor nerve.
1. internal carotid artery, 2. optic nerve, 3. occulomotor nerve

Longitudinal Myelotomy – Indications and Results

M. SCHIRMER, D. BARZ, and H. WENKER

Longitudinal section of the spinal cord in the frontal plane at the level of the lumbar intumescence was introduced by BISCHOF (1, 2) in 1951 for the treatment of high grade spastic paralysis of the lower extremities. The object of this operation is to interrupt the reflex arc in the spinal gray matter bilaterally, while preserving the sacral parasympathetic centre and the anterior and posterior horns of the spinal cord.

About 60 cases have been described in the literature so far, in which lateral longitudinal myelotomy was undertaken. In the majority of these patients the paraspasticity of the legs was caused by lesions of the spinal cord and to a lesser extent by diseases such as disseminated encephalitis, amyatrophic lateral sclerosis, myelitis, cerebral lesions of early childhood or even spinal tumors.

BISCHOF's lateral longitudinal myelotomy was undertaken in 7 female patients in the Neukölln Neurosurgical Department from 1970 to 1973.

Six of these patients suffered from multiple sclerosis: an intradural meningioma at Th$_5$ had been removed from a woman who was already 78 years old, after which the paraplegia arising from it regressed, but a spastic paraparesis of the lower extremities and painful spinal automatisms remained. All 7 patients were completely bedridden and consequently pure nursing cases.

We set the indication for lateral longitudinal myelotomy in order, on the one hand, to free the patients from their excruciating spasms and on the other hand - after elimination of contractures - to make them at least capable of using a wheel chair. The decision to advise this operation was facilitated by the fact that - with only one exception - the patients had already developed disturbances of the urinary bladder function as a result of the primary disease. The patients were instructed in detail about the problems of the myelotomy and the therapeutic effect to be expected.

We have performed the lumbar lateral longitudinal myelotomay strictly according to the information given by BISCHOF and mobilized the contracted joints immediately after the end of the operation, while the patient was still under anaesthesia and relaxation.

The previously marked spasticity of the legs could no longer be demonstrated, or only to a limited extent, in all 6 patients with multiple sclerosis immediately after the operation and mobilisation of the contracted joints; legs which had been fixed in extreme adduction and flexion preoperatively could be freely moved passively and fully extended. A moderate degree of spasticity recurred within the first year after the operation in only 2 patients. It gave no cause for re-operation in any case. In the six patients with multiple sclerosis there was neither restoration of voluntary motoricity nor a return of bladder function. Sensitivity disorders already present before the operation were demonstrated post-operatively, sometimes to an increased extent.

All 6 patients could already sit upright in bed or in an armchair for several hours within a few days after the myelotomy.

One patient died suddenly on the 23rd post-operative day and another ten months after the operation as a result of the far advanced primary disease. At the present time, four of the multiple-sclerosis-patients are still living and can move about in a wheel chair; the myelotomies were performed between one and three years ago.

Considering disseminated encephalitis as the primary disease, the therapeutic results obtained in the six patients previously mentioned were in accordance with our expectations, and were also assessed subjectively by the patients as good results.

The most gratifying operation result we obtained in the patient, now aged 82 years, who was operated on a spinal meningioma six months before the myelotomy. After the longitudinal myelotomy, both the paraspasticity and the painful spinal automatisms had disappeared. Post-operative incontinence of the urinary bladder and rectum disappeared again half a year after the myelotomy. Slight sensitivity disorders were dismissed by the patient as trifling. Since the second year after the myelotomy, the patient has been able to walk again with the help of a stick.

On the strength of our therapeutic results and the satisfaction of our patients with the therapeutic results achieved, we are of the opinion that BISCHOF's lateral longitudinal myelotomy should receive more attention for the treatment of high grade spastic paraparesenes of the legs.

REFERENCES

BISCHOF, W.: Die longitudinale Myelotomie. Zbl. Neurochir. 11, 79 - 88 (1951).

TÖNNIS, W., BISCHOF, W.: Ergebnisse der lumbalen Myelotomie nach BISCHOF. Zbl. Neurochir. 23, 29 - 36/120 - 132 (1962).

The Treatment of Spasticity by Foerster's Operation

F. Schepelmann

In 1908 FOERSTER introduced the section of the dorsal roots for the
treatment of a pathological increase of the contractile muscle tone
and involuntary movements after lesions of the central nervous system
(2). Failures of this operation were ascribed to several causes (6,
1). These failures suggest that the field of indication is limited.
Operative indication necessitates clarification of the pathophysiological mechanisms, which underlie the pathological phenomena of motor
activity in the individual case. The term spasticity in its clinical sense means increase of muscle tone which can be caused by different mechanisms. From the patho-physiological point of view gamma-
rigidity and alpha-rigidity can be differentiated. In this context
it is essential to state that gamma-rigidity comes into existence
through the gamma-loop, while the existence of alpha-rigidity is independent of the integrity of the peripheral reflex arc (9).

The motor activity in 2 cases of spinal spasticity was examined before and after the section of the dorsal roots. The first patient
had an operation for an extensive spinal angioma in the thoracolumbar
region. The second patient had spinal arachnopathy following meningitis. The clinical symptoms of the disturbed motor control in both
cases were severe paraparesis, increase of muscle tone, exaggerated
reflexes and frequent involuntary stereotype flexion of the legs. For
the treatment of these symptoms the section of the dorsal roots was
performed bilaterally in the first case from T 10 to S 1, and in the
second case from L 1 to S 2.

For the continuous quantitative recording of motor activity, the
electromyogram was recorded by surface electrodes simultaneously
from the M. tibialis anterior, M. gastrocnemius and M. semitendinosus
of both legs. With a time constant of 1 s the time-voltage-integral
of the 3 electromyograms, which were derived from either body side
was produced electronically. The average values of these integrals
were summed up numerically for a given time on the one hand and on
the other hand recorded continuously by a multi-pen-recorder. The
visible movements were registered.[1]

The comparison of the findings before and after the section of the
dorsal roots indicated that the quantity of the motor activity was
not at all reduced by this operation in the first case and only
partially reduced in the second case. The integral after 45 min. ran
up to 1561 in the first case and up to 6219 in the second case before
the operation; after the operation it came to 1597 in the first case
and to 1843 in the second case. The quantity of the involuntary movements corresponded to these numerical values. The approximate number

---

[1]A more detailed description of the method was given earlier (7).

of flexions of the legs over a period of 45 min. was 54 in the first case and 428 in the second case before the operation; after the operation it was 76 in the first case and 385 in the second case. The continuous recording of the course of motor activity revealed considerable fluctuations in both cases; in part these were rhythmic fluctuations of motor activity at a frequency of 2 - 4 per min. Such rhythmic fluctuations were found in both cases before as well as after the section of the dorsal roots. After the operation the frequency of the rhythm remained in the same range as before and only its amplitude was smaller and its shape smoothed (Figure).

In the first and probably also in the second case the lesion of the spinal cord was caused by circulatory disturbances. The results of animal experiments and clinical investigations suggest that asphyxia of the spinal cord can be followed by an increase of muscle tone, which is caused by the loss of spinal interneurones and is independent of the peripheral reflex arc (9). By compressing the aorta in rabbits KROGH (5) evoked an increase of muscle tone in the hind legs. GELFAN and TARLOV (3) obtained the same results in dogs by temporary occlusion of the thoracic aorta. Histologically it was found that up to 75 per cent of the spinal interneurones were destroyed by spinal asphyxia produced by this method, while nearly all motoneurones survived, however only 15 per cent of their axosomatic and 35 per cent of their axodendritic connections remained intact (4). This increase of muscle tone could not be eliminated by section of the dorsal roots as well in the dogs as in a corresponding clinical case in humans (8). In such cases spasticity has to be regarded as equivalent to alpha-rigidity. In accordance with this interpretation the integrals and the number of involuntary movements in 2 cases, which were examined here, demonstrate that interruption of the peripheral reflex arc by section of the dorsal roots did not eliminate the increase of motor activity and the inviluntary movements. Furthermore, the comparison of the course of motor activity before and after the section of the dorsal roots reveals that defined rhythmic fluctuations appear after as well as before the interruption of the peripheral reflex arc; this means that these phenomena are not primarily reflex processes. Peripheral afferences seem to cause an enlargement of the amplitude and a modulation of rhythmic increases of motor activity - probably through the gamma-loop in particular. However, the loss of peripheral afferences does not effect the disappearance of these increases of the motor activity.

In summary one can state that the spasticity, which is caused by circulatory disturbances of the spinal cord, is primarily not a reflex phenomenon and therefore FOERSTER's operation can not be expected to abolish this kind of spasticity.

REFERENCES

1. BISCHOF, W., SCHMIDT, H.: Behandlung der Verletzungen des Rückenmarks. In: Handbuch der Neurochirurgie, Bd. VII/1, (Hrsg. H. OLIVECRONA, W. TÖNNIS), S. 401 - 524. Berlin - Heidelberg - New York: Springer 1969.

2. FOERSTER, O.: Die Behandlung spastischer Lähmungen durch Resektion hinterer Rückenmarkswurzeln. Erg. Chir. 2, 174 - 209 (1911).

3. GELFAN, S., TARLOV, J. M.: Interneurones and rigidity of spinal origin. J. Physiol. 146, 594 - 617 (1959).

4. GELFAN, S.: Altered spinal motoneurons in dogs with experimental hind-limb rigidity. J. Neurophysiol., Springfield 29, 583-611 (1966).

5. KROGH, E.: The effect of the acute hypoxia on the motor cells of the spinal cord. Acta physiol. Scand. 20, 263 - 292 (1950).

6. PENZHOLZ, H.: Chirurgische Eingriffe am Nervensystem bei spastischen Lähmungen. Zbl. Neurochir. 16, 331 - 342 (1956).

7. SCHEPELMANN, F.: Dissociation of motoricity in cerebral lesions. In: Central-Rhythmic and Regulation (eds. W. UMBACH, H. P. KOEPCHEN), S. 295 - 301. Stuttgart: Hippokrates 1974.

8. TARLOV, J. M.: Rigidity in man due to spinal interneuron loss. Arch. Neurol. Psychiatr., Chicago 16, 536 - 543 (1967).

9. WIESENDANGER, M.: Pathophysiology of Muscle Tone. S. 1 - 46. Berlin - Heidelberg - New York: Springer 1972.

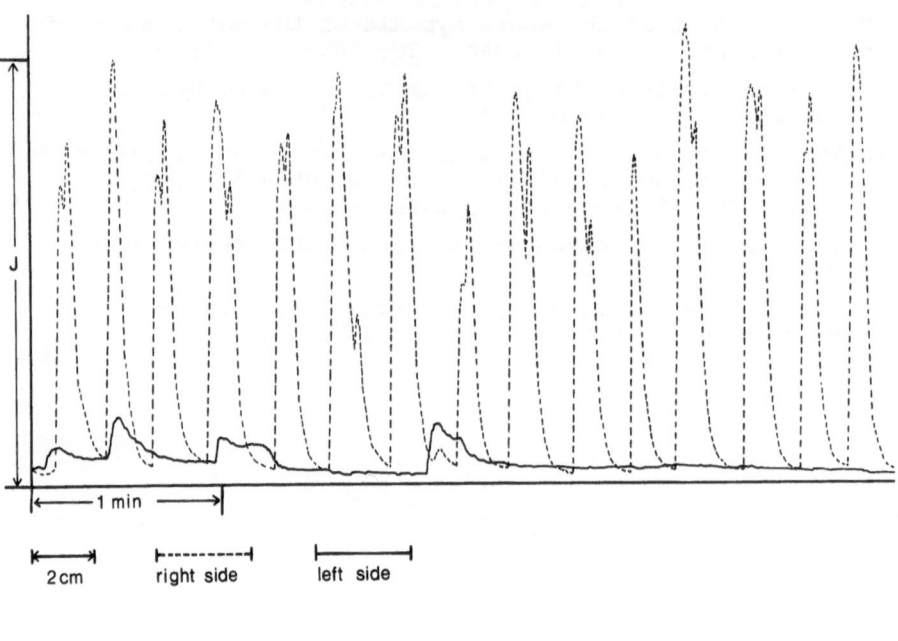

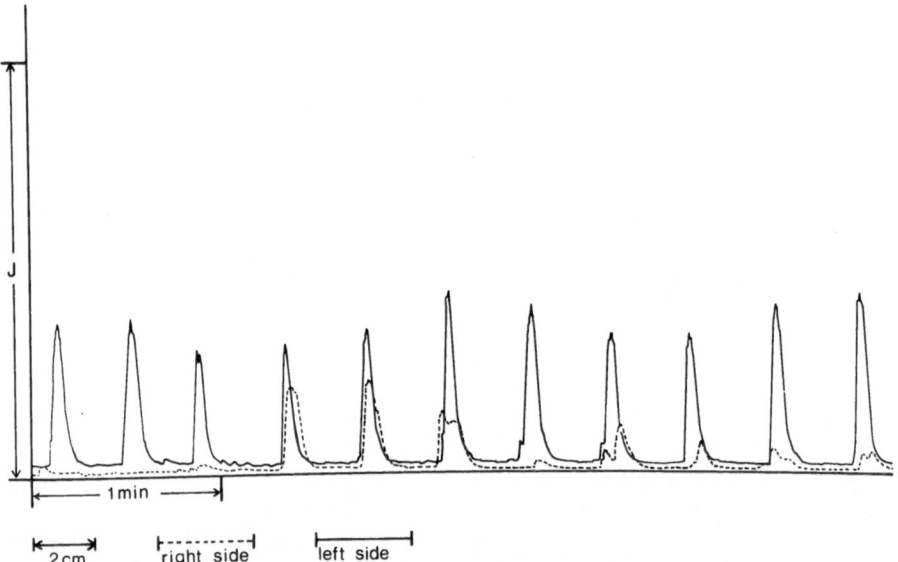

Fig. 1. Motor activity of the right and left leg. Integrated electromyograms derived from M. tibialis anterior, M. gastrocnemius, M. semitendinosus. Spinal arachnopathy due to meningitis before (upper
traces) and after (lower traces) bilateral section of the dorsal
roots L 1 - S 2. Rhythmic fluctuations of the motor activity at the
frequency of 2 - 4 per min. After posterior rhizotomy the rhythmic
increases of the motor activity do not disappear; only their amplitude is smaller and their shape is smoothed. For reason of recording-
technique the interrupted trace of the right side runs 1,5 mm behind
the continuous trace of the left side. The unit I corresponds to an
integral which is produced of a voltage of 100 µV and a frequency
of 100/s

420

Plastic Surgery in Bone Defects of the Posterior Orbital Cavity Using Palacos

Sch. Zamani

The reconstruction of the orbital cavity not only occupies eye, nose and throat specialists, surgeons specialising in facial traumata and oculists, but neurosurgeons also on occasions (1).

After the necessary evisceration of the orbita, it is tumors of the anterior cranial fossa in particular, with involvement of the orbital roof or the orbital wall that necessitate a reconstruction of the posterior orbita. In the field of traumatology, the increasing number of combined facial and cranial injuries also entail problems involving plastic reconstruction of the crushed posterior orbital wall and orbital roof (2, 3, 4, 5).

In quoting two cases, we shall here report upon the procedures we have selected.

Case 1: Pat. W., aged 49

On admission in June 1972, the patient stated that he had always somewhat protruding eyes. Towards the end of February 1972, it had been noticed by persons around him that there was a considerable protrusion of his right eye. In the course of examination, he complained about the occurrence of double vision in his right eye. The right eyeball was lower than the left one and restricted in its mobility, chiefly in an upward direction, and exhibited a distinct protrusion. There were no other neurological disturbances.

In radiography an extensive tumorous process was found in the orbital roof area. On 8th June, 1972, after right frontal osteoplastic trepanation, an entire 30 gram osteoma of the right superior and lateral orbital borders was macroscopically removed. The bone defect was equalized be a piece of suitably moulded Palacos (automyelizing polymethyl acrylate).

The postoperative healing process was without complication. In the ophthalmological check, a reduction in the exophthalmos of approximately 3 mm was measure. The right ocular levator muscle imbalance and double vision were no longer evident after operation.

Histology: Cavernous haemangioma of the osteoplastic type.

Case 2: Pat. St., aged 26

In a traffic accident, Mrs. St. sustained a severe facial and craniocerebral injury. On admission, the patient was found to be disorientated. She stated that seh was unable to see with the right eye.

External traumata included extensive haematomatous swellings of the right side of the face, "monocle" haematoma, total paralysis of the oculomotor nerve, suspicion of a traumatic optic nerve lesion on the right with simultaneous heavy bleeding into the anterior chamber. Retroposition of the facial cranium also existed.

The radiographs of the cranium revealed an extensive multiple fracture injury from crushing of the facial bones according to Le Fort II and III. The orbital roof and the posterior orbital wall had sustained multiple crushing.

The operation was conducted in cooperation with our facial surgery department. After right frontal osteoplastic trepanation, a multiple fracture of the orbital roof was ascertained. Some fragments of bone had penetrated the brain. After opening the dura, these were cautiously removed. The dura defects and the dura fissures were impermeably sealed by applying a suitably sized piece of lyophylized dura with a histoacrylic adhesive.

The defect in the orbital roof was filled by employing a very thin, multiply-perforated sheet of Palacos (polymerized methyl-acrylate). The surrounding bone borders were freshened prior to fitting in the implant, and the Palacos sheet itself was adhered with Histoacryl. Furthermore, an additional strip of lyophilized dura was adhered over the sheet of Palacos and secured by stitches. Following this, the facial surgeons took over and continued the operation. The evisceration of all pneumatized cavities in the facial part of the skull was carried out, the retro-positioned facial bones reset and fixed with wire sutures, in addition to which the nasal bones were reconstructed as far as possible.

Postoperative progress was without complications. With fully retained sight, there was a slight oculomotor paresis accompanied by a pronounced oedema of the right upper and lower eyelids. The radiographic check showed that the Palacos implant had adapted itself well to the roof of the orbita and to the contours of the anterior cranial base.

Discussion

The restoration of the orbital cavity after extensive tumor surgery and traumatic injury is being carried out by various clinics with the aid of autologous, homologous and heterologous transplants or implants (1, 2, 3, 4, 5, 6, 7, 8, 9, 10).

In view of the demands to be made on an implant, attention should be paid to tissue compatibility, material strength, good processing qualities and also sterilizability in cases of orbital roof reconstruction.

Autopolymerizing methyl acrylate (Palacos) meets a large number of these demands, even though the moulding qualities of the material leave much to be desired when solidifying too rapidly and being heated too strongly. Following the suggestions of various authors in the angloamerican literature, we have attempted, in both cases, to reconstruct the orbital roof with pre-moulded methyl acrylate sheets (8, 9, 10, 11, 12, 13, 14, 15). The difficulties arising when affixing the implants in the anterior cranial fossa we have tried to solve by sticking them over with Lyodura using Histoacryl as adhesive.

The tissue compatibility of the Palacos implant also proved to be
good when used in combination with several other plastics (Lyodura
and Histoacryl adhesive). Even with the concurrent use of Palacos,
Lyodura and Histoacryl adhesive we have met with no serious disturbances in the healing of wounds, so that in view of the facility
of handling these materials the use of these plastics provides genuine
advantages, particularly in the field of traumatology.

Three criteria must be fulfilled, however:

1. The Palacos sheet must be as thin as possible;

2. It must have multiple perforations;

3. It must be secured by soft tissue materials, adhesives or sutures.

REFERENCES

1. AICHMAIR, H., FRIES, R.: Kieferchirurgische und ophthalmologische
   Problematik gei Orbitabodenfrakturen. Fortsch. Kiefer-Gesichts-
   chir. 12, 145 - 152 (1967).

2. ABRAHAMS, I. W.: Repair of orbital floor defects with premolded
   plastic implant. Arch. Ophthal. (Chicago) 75, 510 - 512 (1966).

3. ANDERSON, M. F.: Blow-out fractures: report of a series. J. Oral
   Surg. 22, 405 - 407 (1964).

4. ANTHONY, D. H., FISHER, D. F.: Splint (stainless steel) orbital
   floor or rim fracture jackscrew. Trans-Amer. Acad. Ophthal.
   Otolaryng. 54, 379 - 380 (1950).

5. ABRAHAMS, I. W.: Repair of orbital defects with premolded plastic
   implant..Arch. Ophth. 75, 510 (1966).

6. BALLEN, P. H.: Rapidly polymerizing acrylic in reconstruction of
   the orbit. Amer. J. Ophth. 56, 378 - 386 (1961).

7. BALLEN, P. H.: Further experiences with rapidly polymerizing
   methylmethacrylate in orbital floor fractures. Plast. reconst.
   Surg. 34, 624 - 629 (1964).

8. BENNET, J. E., ARMSTRONG, J. R.: Repair of defects of bony orbit
   with methylmethacrylate. Americ. J. Ophthal. 53, 285 - 290
   (1962).

9. BROWNING, W. W., WALKER, R. V.: Reconstruction of post-traumatic
   orbital fractures with polyethylene. Amer. J. Ophthal. 52, 672 -
   677 (1961).

10. CONVERSE, J. M., SMITH, B., ØBEAR, M. F., WOOD-SMITH, D.: Orbital
    blowout fractures: A ten-year survey, Plast. Reconst. Surg. 39,
    20 (1967).

11. LIPSHUTZ, H., ARDIZONE, R.: The use of silicone rubber in the
    floor of the orbit. J. Trauma 3, 56 (1963).

12. NASTEFF, D.: Wiederherstellung des Orbitabodens. Zbl. Chir. 29,
    2207 - 2214 (1967).

13. SMITH, B., OBEAR, M., LEONE, C. R., Jr.: The correction of en-
    ophthalmos associated with anophthalmos by glass bead implantation.
    Am. J. Ophth. 64, 1088 (1967).

14. SHANNON, G. M.: Enophthalmos: foreign implants. Int. Symp.
    on Plastic and Reconstructive Surgery of the Eye and Adnexa,
    pp. 446 - 449. St. Louis: C. V. Mosby Comp. 1967.

15. WELDE, N. J., TUR, J. J.: Use of polyethylene plate in plastic surgery. Plast. Reconst. Surg. 33, 349 (1964).

Plastic Repair of Major Dura and Bone Defects by the Use of Lyophilized Dura and Autopolymerizing Acryl Derivatives (Palacos) in a Single Session

A. CASTRO

The closing of defects of the dura mater to prevent infections, the formation of liquor fistulae and cicatrizations, and to provide protection against external mechanical influences has always been one of the most important tasks to be carried out after neurosurgical operations (18).

The development of homoioplastic, lyophilized dura for the replacement of lost portions of the dura mater has, in the meantime, advanced to a stage where the employment of lyophilized dura has become a generally accepted practice in neurosurgery. The development in the field of filling bone defects, artificial or traumatic, has taken a similar course (3, 13, 14, 15, 16, 17).

The use of autopolymerizing acryl derivatives for this purpose (Palacos) has now become established, at least in Germany (2, 4, 5, 6, 7, 8, 9, 10, 12).

In view of the good experience gained with lyophilized dura and Palacos individually, we ventured to combine these two synthetic materials and report below on several patients in whom large cerebral dura defects and extensive bone defects were repaired with lyophilized dura and Palacos in a single session.

Case 1: Mrs. Franziska H., 79 years old

History: Progressive swelling of the right occiput, roughly 6 months to 1 year prior to hospitalization.

No subjective complaints.

Clinical History: Pulsating tumor having the size of a fist, behind the right ear. Radiographic appearance: area of bone destruction having the size of the palm of the hand, on the right, parieto-temporal. Surgical removal of a destructively growing tumor weighing 245 grams. Operative revision was necessary as a result of postoperative development of a liquor fistula. A large piece of Lyodura was inserted and sutured into place and the bone defect filled with moulded Palacos simultaneously. Wound healing free from complications.

Histological picture: infiltrative haemangio-pericytoma.

Case 2: Mrs. Waltraud B., aged 48

History: Hard tumor which slowly increased in size over a period of 7 years on the left frontally, located close to the median line. No subjective complaints. Absence of neurological disorders. Trepanation in the form of a bucket-handle section revealed an osteoma extending far beyond the midline to the right side, a developed meningioma underneath. The resulting dural and bone defects were closed in a single session with Lyodura and moulded Palacos material.

Histological picture: Meningotheliomatous meningioma and osteoma. Wound healing without complications and without seroma formation. A second puncture was not necessary.

Case 3: Mrs. Marianne S., aged 46

History: In 1970 removal of a 100 gram parasagittal meningioma on the left. Two years later removal of two recidivations originating from the sinus and the falx, weighing 60 and 70 grams, respectively. No complaints until August, 1973. Aggravation of hemiparesis. Psychopathological changes. Renewed operation in 1974: the recidivating growth had infiltrated the superior sagittal sinus over a length of 13.5 cm and had spread parasagittally more to the left than to the right. Resection of the superior sagittal sinus over the appropriate length. Removal of 135 grams of tumorous tissue. The osseous structure was infiltrated by the meningioma. Closing of the dural and bone defects with lyophilized dura and Palacos. Regression of the complete paresis of the right half of the body. Uneventful wound healing. Discharge from hospital with a slight right-sided hemiparesis.

Case 4: Mrs. Renate K., aged 40

History: Seven years prior to admission, removal of a 30 gram olfactory meningioma on the right, accompanied by meningiomatosis of the dura mater. Four years later, removal of a neurinoma of the left brachial plexus. A further two years later, the patient again began to suffer from headaches. Diagnosis: left occipital, process spreading supratentorially (meningioma recurrence).

Operation: Removal of a large number of minor thickenings of the dura mater (20 to 25 meningioma nodules) and of a tumor weighing roughly 76 grams originating in the tentorium. The dura and bone defects were covered with lyophilized dura and Palacos plastic in a single session.

Discussion

On the basis of the cases described, we have tried to demonstrate that the restraint exercised so far in using Lyodura and Palacos simultaneously need no longer be maintained

The customary prerequisites for the use of Lyodura or Palacos as a plastic filling material - such as the absence of a local infection, increased intracranial pressure or poor general health - will certainly apply also in the future, even though, in our opinion, they need no longer be regarded as absolute.

The development of a seroma reported after the use of Lyodura and Palacos was no longer often observed at our clinic. Punctures in the operated area were only occasionally necessary. Thus, an important source of infection was eliminated.

In performing the surgery we sued the technique described by WÜRINGER and THOMALSKE (19).

More recently, we have also started affixing the Lyodura with a histoacrylic glue (Blutyl II - cyanoacrylate glue) (1, 11, 17).

We have experienced no adverse effects resulting from the use of this third foreign body during surgery.

REFERENCES

1. ALBIN, M. S., D'AGOSTINO, A. N., WHITE, R. J., GRINDLAY, J. H.: Nonsuture sealing of a dural substitute utilizing a plastic adhesive methyl 2-cyanoacrylate. J. Neurosurg. 19, 545 (1962).

2. BALLEN, P. H.: Further experiences with rapidly polymerizing methylmethacrylate in orbital floor fractures. Plast. Reconstr. Surg. 34, 624 (1964).

3. BARANY: zit. nach H. JAKOBI. In: Ein Beitrag zur plastischen Duradeckung im Bereich der Lamina cribriformis. Z. Laryng. Rhinol. 34, 480 (1955).

4. BAUER, E., LANGEGGER, P. A.: Hinweise zur plastischen Deckung von Knochendefekten im Stirnbereich (Wien). Klin. Wschr. 50, 960 (1954).

5. CONTZEN, H., STRAUMANN, F., PASCHKE, E.: Grundlagen der Alloplastik mit Metallen und Kunststoff. Stuttgart: Georg Thieme 1967.

6. FLÖRKEN, H.: Großer traumatischer Defekt des Stirnschädels, Ersatz durch eine Plexiglasplatte. Chirurg. 27, 178 (1956).

7. GEIB, F. W.: Vitallium skull plates. J. Amer. Med. Ass. 117, 812 (1941).

8. GÜHRING, K.: Beitrag zur alloplastischen Deckung von Schädeldefekten mit einem autopolymerisierenden Kunststoff. Med. Klin. 23, 1020 (1960).

9. GÜNTHER, H.: Zur Indikation der Deckung von Stirndefekten mit autoplastischen Knochen, Knorpel und alloplastischem Material. Fortschr. der Kiefer- und Gesichtschir. Bd. XII, 247 (1967).

10. HERRMANN, K. O.: Die Ergebnisse der Behandlung von Knochendefekten mit Kunststoffplasten, 3 bis 5 Jahre nach der operativen Behandlung. Zentralblatt für Chirurgie, 86. Jahrg. 26, (1961).

11. HEISS, W. H., GUTHY, E., BECKER, H. M.: Experimentelle Untersuchungen zum Ersatz der chirurgischen Naht durch Klebstoff. Langenbecks Arch. klin. Chir., Bd. 308 (1964).

12. INGRAHAM, F. D., ALEXANDER, E., Jr., MATSON, D. D.: Polyethylene, a new synthetic plastic for use in surgery. Experimental applications in neurosurgery. J. Amer. Med. Ass. 135, 82 (1947).

13. JACOBY, W.: Statistische Übersicht über die Verwendung von lyophilisierter Dura in der Neurochirurgischen Universitätsklinik München. Med. Mitt. Bd. 43, Heft 112 (1969).

14. JACOBY, W., MARGUTH, F.: Erfahrungen mit lyophilisierter Dura. Beiträge zur Neurochirurgie, Heft 15.

15. JAKOBY, R. K.: The use of a methylmethacrylate seal in spinal fluid otorrhea and rhinorrhea. J. Neurosurg. 18, 614 (1961).

16. LOEW, F.: Experimentelle und klinische Erfahrungen mit lyophilisierter Dura und Histocoll T 100 B in der Neurochirurgie. Med. Mitt., Bd. 41, Heft 108 (1967).

17. PROBST, Ch.: Frontobasale Verletzungen. Pathogenetische, diagno-
    stische und therapeutische Probleme aus neurochirurgischer Sicht.
    Stuttgart: Hans Huber.

18. WORINGER, E., THOMALSKE, G.: Unsere Schädelplastik-Schnellmethode.
    Acta Neurochir. Suppl. $\underline{3}$, 11 (1955).

Experience with Meningiomas in the Posterior Fossa

G. LEDINSKI

Since the establishment of the Institute for Tumors and Allied Diseases in 1969, we have diagnosed and operated on four patients with meningiomas of the posterior fossa.

Two of the meningiomas were located in the lower part of the supratentorial space and in the infratentorial space, the larger part growing in the latter region. One of these went as far as the foramen magnum.

The third meningioma was located in the cerebello-pontine angle and the last tumor was found in the clivus.

All these tumors were successfully removed.

Meningiomas and Neighboring Structures

M. ZUMER

The author presented 4 interesting cases from a group of 12 meningiomas managed in his neurosurgical clinic during the year 1973.

Case 1. 64-year-old man with a very large olfactory meningioma subtotally removed. Six years later recurrence of the tumor which led to optic nerve compression. Total removal was achieved and recovery was good.

Case 2. 37-year-old man with bilateral parasagittal meningiomas. Carotid angiography showed partial narrowing of the superior sagittal sinus. The tumor was removed so that only small tumor remnants remained attached to the sinus - the adjacent falx was left in place. On the third day after operation, paraplegia occurred. Repeated carotid angiography now showed increased drainage from the intracranium through the posterior vertebral plexus in the late venous phase. Good recovery followed so that the patient was walking without a crutch six weeks later.

Case 3. 26-year-old lady with a hydrocephalus required an urgent Torkildsen operation. At surgery an obstruction of the aqueduct was ascertained 3 cm above the fourth ventricle. Her condition deteriorated 6 weeks after operation and vertebral angiography led us to suspect a pinealoma. At the second operation, a circumscribed tumor was found in the region of the lamina quadrigemina which could not be removed. Microscopic examination revealed the presence of a meningioma (fibroblastic type). Two months later the patient died. At autopsy the hydrocephalus was found to be due to a large midline meningioma extending to the posterior part of the third ventricle from the lamina quadrigemina and blocking the aqueduct.

Case 4. 43-year-old man with a large right temporal tumor, richly vascularized and therefore suspected of being a glioblastoma. At operation an excessively bleeding meningioma was removed which was partly thick and solid and partly flat "en plaque" extending from the frontal to the occipital region. Good recovery followed.

Scenes of Stone Cutting from the 16th and 17th Century

W. BRAUN

When confronted with the question as to who were the predicessors of
the present day neurosurgeons one is continually referred to the ad-
venturous pioneer work of a few 19th century surgeons and to the re-
lics of trepanation from ancient times in Peru or Egypt. True there
is some evidence of trepanations carried out in the centuries between,
e. g. the instruments as reviewed by GURDJIAN in his report on war
surgery. Whether or not trepanations were performed at that particular
time is not known today. Thus the question arises: Was there a period
of dormancy between then and present day surgery.

The observant visitor to the art galleries and print cabinets through-
out the world will certainly answer that he remembers seeing 16th and
17th paintings of head operations. Cannot these pictures be accpeted
as evidence of some form of development in the field of neurosurgery?
Are such pictures not as acceptable as written evidence? How can this
discrepancy between the numerous paintings and the almost complete
absence of historical-medical knowledge be explained?

The first example shows a painting by BARTHOLOMÄUS MATON (1640 - 1690)
from the Gallery in Karlsruhe (Fig. 1). We are shown into a quack's
practice and witness and operative intervention on a patient who has
come dressed in the style of the day. The fee for the medical attention would appear to be a duck and a basket of eggs which the patient
has brought with her. Whilst the patient's left hand is grasping the
arm of the chair in pain her right hand is balled to a fist. At the
same time the quack, with great concentration and feeling, is about
to incise the forehead. Are we here, concerned with a simple frontal
blood-letting or an incision e. g. that of a furuncle? It is not possible to pick out any details. From the whole situation, however, we
can with certainty assume that the cranium is respected as boundary.

An engraving by WEYDMANS (Fig. 2) from the first half of the 17th
century goes a little further: again it deals with a frontal intervention on a woman who is being held down by an assistant. On the
table we see a scalpel, a spatula and scissors, but no instrument
which would permit trepanation. Despite the small incision, for the
numerous tumors on the table, we may be sure that the physician's
effort are concerned with the removal of a tumor.

The procedure depicted in the painting by HEMESSEN (1504 - 1566)
(Fig. 3) from the Prado is quite clear. The foreign body which is
about the size of a plum is being scraped out with a large scalpel,
the handle of which is apparently made of some kind of horn. Whilst
the face of the surgeon reflects the success of the almost completed
intervention a relative prays desperately with arms out stretched to
heaven. The serious faced nurse holds the patient's head whilst a
second nurse prepares an ointment. In this very credible scene we

cannot find a surgical instrument which can give us any information
as to the extent of such operations. Are the round figures suspended
from string, swabs or are they trophies from earlier operations which
are supposed to indicate the ability and success of the wonder doctor.

An engraving by PIETER BREUGHEL (1528 - 1569) (Fig. 4) would appear
to give an insight into a real tumor clinic. Four patients are treated
simultaneously on four operating-chairs without being able to reduce
the throng of people seeking help. A fat monk with a small tumor in
the glabella is being carried in and he can expect the same treatment
as those already in the operating-chairs. The tumors or foreign bodies,
always localized in the frontal area, are removed with a scalpel or
forceps.

The frequency with which they are removed is somewhat unusual as some
are already spread out on a cloth on the floor. A hammer, chisel and
pliers are recognizable on the instrument table. There are none, however, that would serve for a trepanation.

At that particular time there was not only an out-patient department
but also private patients. One such patient is undergoing a very painful operation in a painting by JAN DE BRAY (Fig. 5) from the Boymans-
van Beuningen Museum in Rotterdam. It is a very impressive scene, the
care with which the famous surgeon, according to the diplomas decorat-
ing the wall and even his hat, is about to remove, apparently without
any loss of blood the tumor from the shouting and struggling patient
with the aid of a scalpel and forceps. The concentration required for
such an intervention is depicted by the protruding lower lip of the
surgeon. As a precaution the patient's valuable robe has been covered
with a towel. Practically nothing can be said about the extent and
depth of the incision. As a result, it is quite clear that the artist
was not concerned with a subtile reproduction of a surgical intervention, but rather with the confrontation of the physiognomies between physician and patient. A young moor watches the procedure with
awestruck eyes. He is holding a bowl ready to receive the tumor. And
since this plate is already filled with tumors, all round and potato-
like, we slowly begin to doubt that this scene is concerned with a
real operation.

This question is answered by looking at this painting by JAN STEEN
(1626 - 1679) also from Rotterdam Museum (Fig. 6). A peasant is tied
down in a chair and is being operated on by a charlatan who is assis-
ted by a smugly smiling old hag. The surgeon feigns to produce a vast
number of stone-like foreign bodies from a wound behind the ear of
the shouting patient and throws them into a vessel. Where those stones
originate from is quite clear: a boy is passing them to him to the
undisbuised and malicious joy of the onlookers and those looking in
through the window. The only person who does not see through this
swindle is the patient himself. Thus it is quite clear that we are
dealing with a sham intervention which according to the number of
historical painting must have been general practice in elementary
medicine in 16th and 17th century Holland. Here, in this masterpiece,
the humorous JAN STEEN was able to perpetuate this on canvas for all
prosperity.

It is concerned with socalled "stone cutting" i. e. the pretentious
removal of foreign bodies from the body cavities particularly from
the skull. In quackery of that time this intervention was a panacea
for innumerous complaints particularly melancholia and insanity. Ul-
timately stone cutting apparently developed to a symbolism and even
to a proverb as in Germany one speaks today of "Stechen eines Stars"
which means to open a person's eye to something.

The last figure, an engraving by BREUGHEL (Fig. 7) which considers the moral consequences rather than the specific events, can be considered a pictorial quintessence of this eronious belief. Today we are no longer in a position to interpret, with any accuracy, the scenes depicted in the paintings of that period. Therefore, without prejudice, let us look at some of the details. A large crowd is gathered round a witch in the market square. In her left hand she is holding up a stone whilst her right arm is round the neck of a fool. An assistant illuminates a stone on the forehead of the fool. Another person is tied down in a chair. A man is pouring a liquid over this patient's head to reveal the "tumors" covered by the hair. A knife is already inserted under the headband. In the pouch attached to the belt around the witch's waist only scissors are visible. A fool with a very large stone is being dragged forward by two assistants. His defensive movements inadvertently empty an assistant's money bag scattering his wages to the ground. Birds of fantasy of the type created by HIERONYMUS BOSCH populate this uncanny scene. The owl is no longer the symbol of wisdom but rather that of shortsightedness and stupidity.

In an egg, both surgeon and fool are equally obsessed with the crazy deed: There is not enough space in their small world for all the fool's stones. Everywhere in this picture one can see the same depressing view of life as if the artist, with the add of this "neurosurgical" painting, wished to demonstrate the uncanny ubiquity of human stupidity and shortsightedness. Finally, all that is left for us is the hope that the painting would have been less sarcastic if BREUGHEL had been able to attend this congress.

REFERENCES

1. GURDJIAN, E. St.: The treatment of penetrating wounds of the brain sustained in warfare. A historial review. J. Neurosurg. 39, 157 - 166 (1974).

2. HOLLÄNDER, E.: Die Medizin in der klassichen Malerei. S. 398 - 418. Stuttgart: Enke 1913.

3. HOLLÄNDER, E.: Die Karikatur und Satire in der Medizin. S. 198 - 204. Stuttgart: Enke 1921.

4. VAN GILS, I. B. F.: Het snijden van den kei. Nederl. Tijdschr. Geneesk. 14, 57 - 64 (1940).

5. MEIGE, H.: L'opération des pierres de tête. Aesculape 22, 50 - 62 (1932).

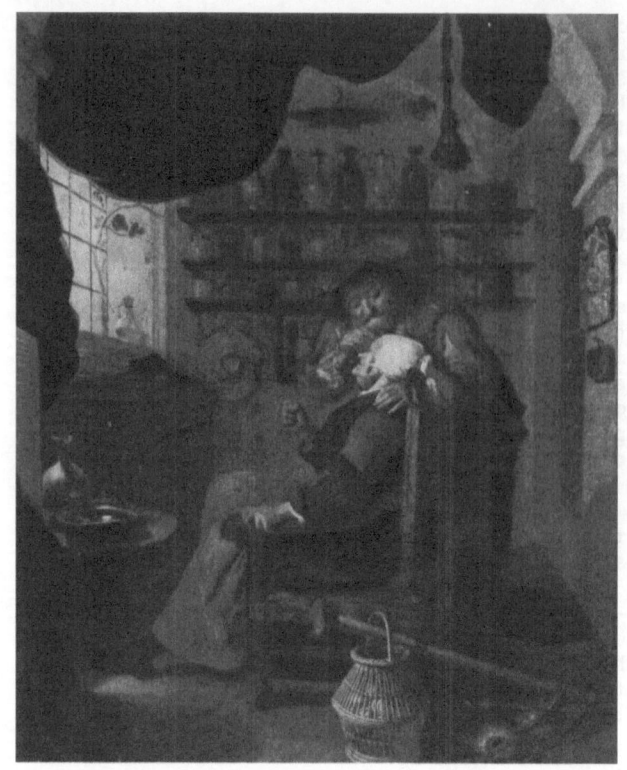

Fig. 1.
Bartholomäus Maton,
1640 - 1690
(Gallery of Karlsruhe)

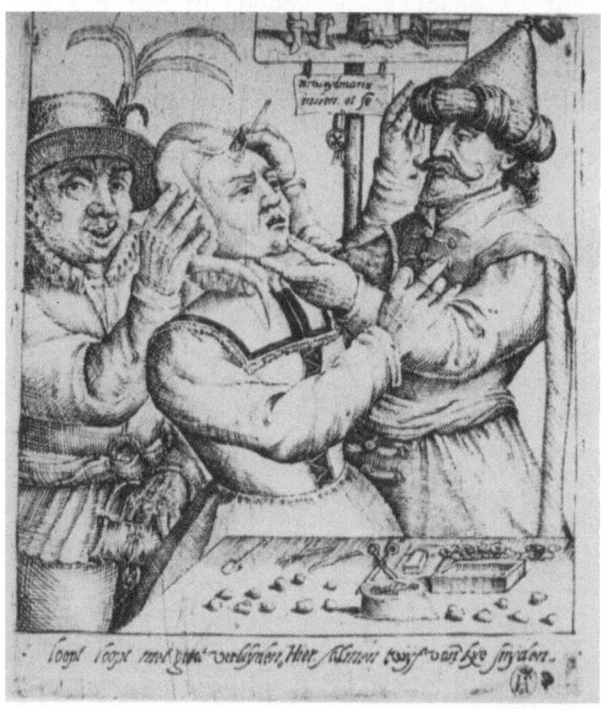

Fig. 2.
Weydmans (Boymans-van
Beuningen Museum in
Rotterdam -
'Kupferstichkabinett')

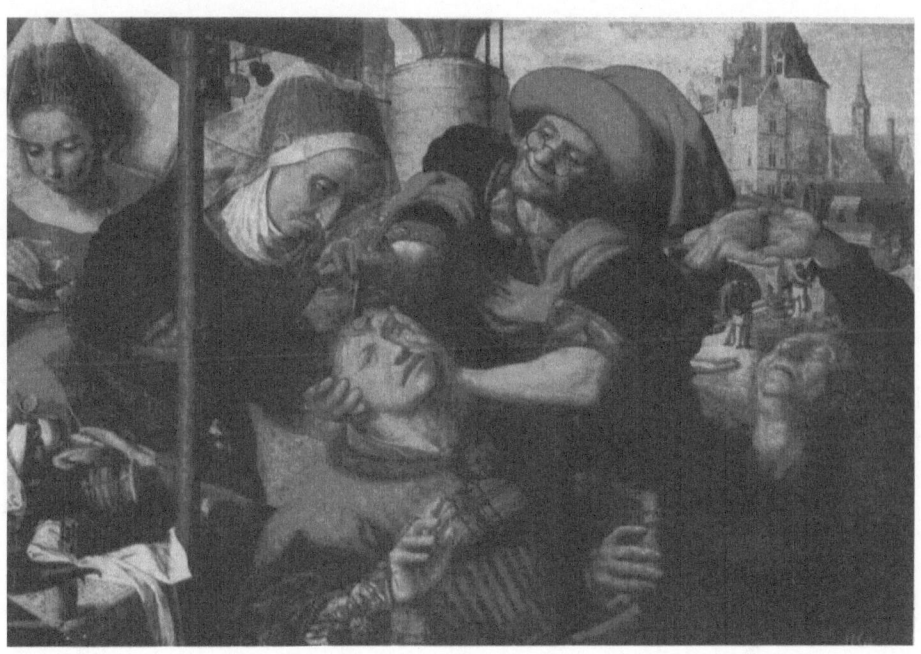

Fig. 3. Hemessen, 1504 - 1566 (Prado, Madrid)

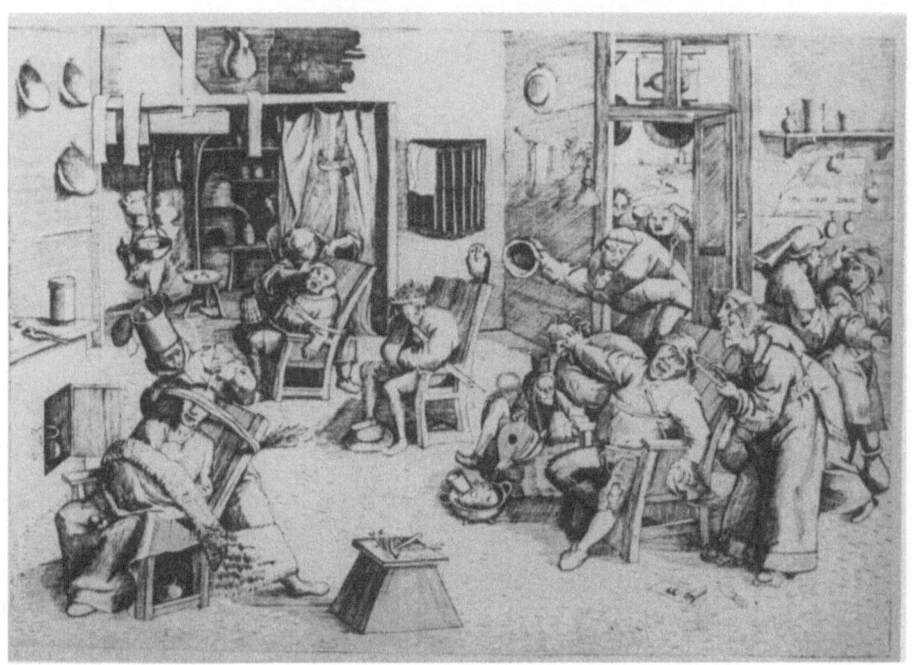

Fig. 4. Pieter Breughel, 1528 - 1569 (Boymans-van Beuningen Museum in Rotterdam - 'Kupferstichkabinett')

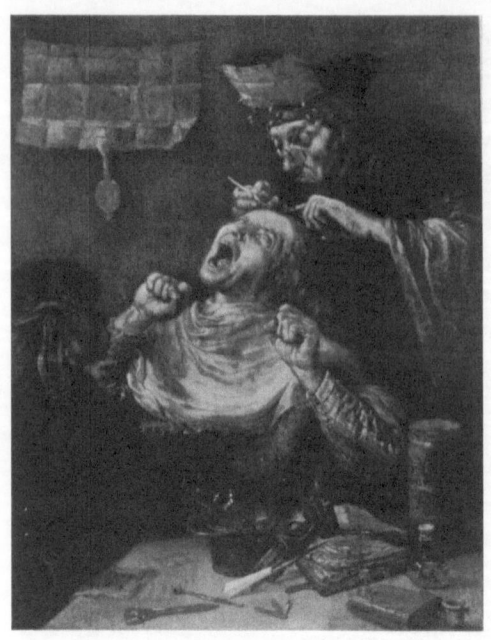

Fig. 5. Jan de Bray
(Boymans-van Beuningen Museum
in Rotterdam)

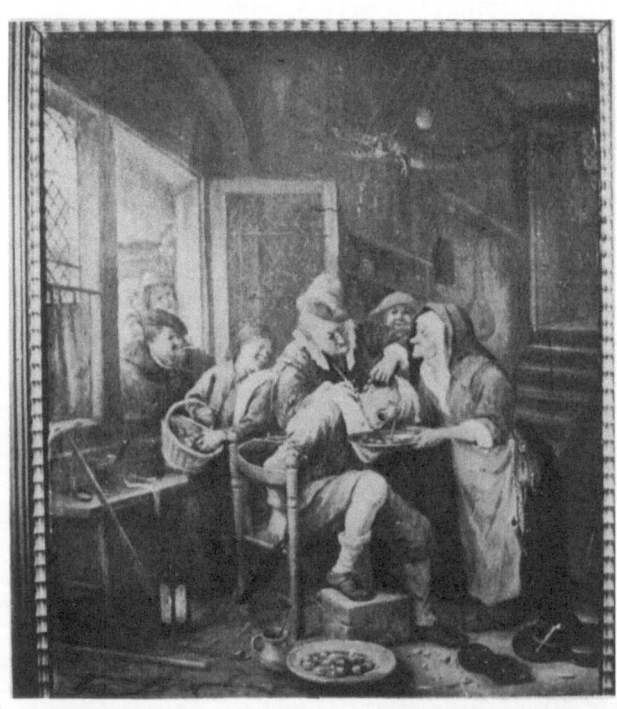

Fig. 6. Jan Steen, 1626 - 1679 (Boymans-van Beuningen Museum in
Rotterdam)

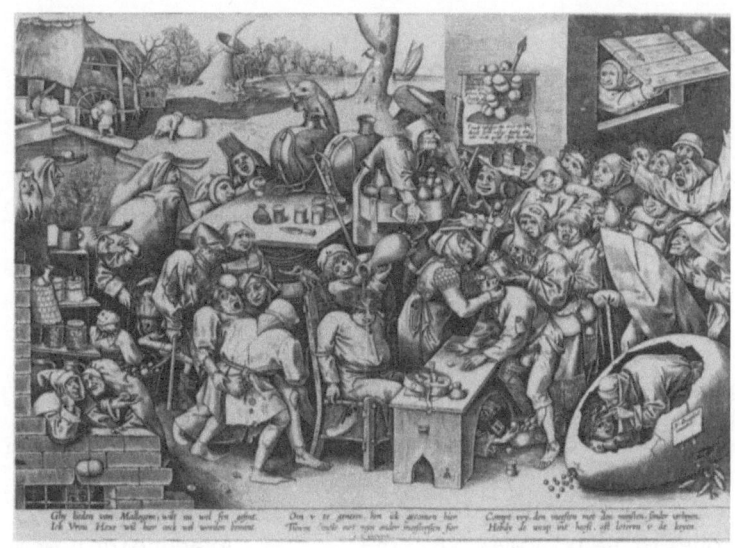

Fig. 7. Pieter Breughel, 1528 - 1569 (Reichsmuseum in Amsterdam -
'Kupferstichkabinett')

Subject Index

Electrophoreses 154
Electrostimulation 386
Encephalitis, parainfectious 129
Encephalitogenic protein 131
Encephalomyelitis, allergic 130
- disseminata 55
   s. Multiple sclerosis
Epidermoid 85
Epilepsy 112, 150
   s. Jacksonian fits 169
   s. seizures
   s. spasmodic fits 207
Exophthalmos 32, 33, 35, 69
-, progressive 51
   s. protrusion of eyeball 207
Experiments, animal 318
-, cats 314
-, chemotherapeutic 319
-, study 322
-, rats 318 - 319, 322
Extramedullary tumors 202

Facial paresis 51
Falx meningiomas 34, 51, 45, 122,
   239, 245, 246
Fatty acids, unsaturated 129
Fibroblastic tumors 3
Fibrosarcoma 6, 8
Foerster's operation 417 - 418
Follicle stimulating hormone
   (FSH) 327
Fontanelle 406
-, small 406
Forensic problems, neuro-
   surgery 273
Four-vessel angiography 251
Funicular myelosis 184

Gamma camera 219
Gasserian ganglion 80
German Civil Code 282, 296
Gibbus formation 401
Glioblastoma 5, 6, 30, 171, 231,
   318 , 319, 367
Glioma, chemically induced 318
-, transplanted 318
Gliomas of childhood 29
-, subependymal 129
Gliosis 128, 129
Grading of meningiomas 1
Gram-negative germs 343
Growth hormone 327

Headaches 34, 175, 206
-, hydrocephalic 35
Hemangioblastoma 1, 172
Hemangioma, cavernous 421
Hemangiopericytic meningioma 6
Hemangiopericytoma 1, 425
Hematoma echoes 368
-, monocle 422

Hemianopia 55, 60, 108
Hemiparesis 34, 94, 176
Hemisphere, dominant 93
Hemorrhage, subarachnoid 374
Hg-compounds 230
Histiocytosis-X 121, 122
Histoacryl 412
Histochemical studies 29
Histogram 361
-, pressure 310
Histological studies 395
Hormone, concentration 327
-, replacement therapy 327, 330
Hospitalism 343
Hydrocephalus, communicating 374
Hydrocortisone 305
Hyperbaric oxygenation treatment
   (HOT) 262, 268
----, function 268
Hyperosmolar solutions 310
Hyperostosis 32, 33, 215, 219
Hypothermia 411

Immunodiffusion 154
Immunoglobulin 154
Immunological reactions 152
Infection 425
-, rate 343
Infundibulum 62, 63
Infusion, angiotensin 315
-, noradrenalin 315
Injections, intramuscular 295
-, intravenous 295, 296
Injection, lesions 384
Instruction to patient 278 - 281,
   287
Intensive care, neurosurgical
   343
--, unit, organisation 343
--, units 295
Internal carotid artery 206
Intervertebral disc polapse 201
Intracranial meningioma 23
-, pressure 310
--, increased 374
Intramedullary tumors 185, 187,
   202
Intraoperative, management 257
Isotope, cisternography 374 - 378
-, diagnosis 108
-, diagnostic 318

Jacksonian fits 169
Judgement
-, physician's 285

Klebsiella 343
- meningitis 343
- pneumonia 343

Laminectomies 183, 401

Advances in Neurosurgery

Vol. 1:
Brain Edema. Pathophysiology and Therapy
Cerebello Pontine Angle Tumors. Diagnosis and Surgery

Editors: K. Schürmann, M. Brock, H.-J. Reulen, D. Voth
187 figures. XVII, 385 pages. 1973
ISBN 3-540-06486-6 DM 69,–
ISBN 0-387-06486-6 (North America) $23.10
Distribution rights for Japan: Nankodo Co. Ltd., Tokyo

Cerebral Angiomas
Advances in Diagnosis and Therapy

Editors: H.W. Pia, J.R.W. Gleave, E. Grote, J. Zierski
161 figures. VIII, 285 pages. 1975
ISBN 3-540-07073-7 DM 58,–
ISBN 0-387-07073-7 (North America) $23.80
Distribution rights for Japan: Maruzen Co. Ltd., Tokyo

L.G. Kempe: Operative Neurosurgery

Vol. 1:
Cranial, Cerebral, and Intracranial Vascular Disease

335 figures, some in color. XIII, 269 pages. 1968
ISBN 3-540-04208-3 Cloth DM 190,–
ISBN 0-387-04208-3 (North America) Cloth $55.60
Distribution rights for Japan: Nankodo Co. Ltd., Tokyo

Vol. 2:
Posterior Fossa, Spinal Cord, and Peripheral Nerve Disease

290 figures, some in color. VIII, 281 figures. 1970
ISBN 3-540-04890-1 Cloth DM 190,–
ISBN 0-387-04890-1 (North America) Cloth $77.60
Distribution rights for Japan: Nankodo Co. Ltd., Tokyo

Radiological Exploration of the Ventricles
and Subarachnoid Space

By G. Ruggiero, J. Bories, A. Calabrò, G. Cristi, G. Scialfa,
F. Smaltino, A. Thibaut. With the cooperation of G. Gianasi,
G. Maranghi, C. Philippart, E. Signorini
90 partly colored figures (279 separate illustrations)
XIV, 152 pages. 1974
ISBN 3-540-06572-5 Cloth DM 148,–
ISBN 0-387-06572-5 (North America) Cloth $60.70
Distribution rights for Japan: Igaku Shoin Ltd., Tokyo

Springer-Verlag
Berlin
Heidelberg
New York

Prices are subject to change without notice

Cerebral Circulation and Stroke II
Newer Contributions of the Salzburg Conference
In preparation

Intracranial Pressure
Experimental and Clinical Aspects
Editors: M. Brock, H. Dietz
142 figures. XVI, 383 pages. 1972
ISBN 3-540-06039-1 Cloth DM 86,—
ISBN 0-387-06039-1 (North America) Cloth $29.30
Distribution rights for Japan: Igaku Shoin Ltd., Tokyo

A. Wackenheim, J.P. Braun
Angiography of the Mesencephalon
Normal and Pathological Findings
128 figures. XI, 154 pages. 1970
ISBN 3-540-05266-6 Cloth DM 120,—
ISBN 0-387-05266-6 (North America) Cloth $33.10

K.J. Zülch
Atlas of Gross Neurosurgical Pathology
379 figures. V, 228 pages. 1975
ISBN 3-540-06480-X Cloth DM 120,—
ISBN 0-387-06480-X (North America) Cloth $49.00
Distribution rights for Japan: Nankodo Co. Ltd., Tokyo o

Journal

Acta Neurochirurgica
Official Organ of the European Association
of Neurosurgical Societies
Editorial Board: A.A. Jefferson, G. Lazorthes,
L. Leksell, F. Loew, P.E. Maspes, S. Obrador,
H. Verbiest, G. Weber
Editor for E.A.N.S.-Affairs: J. Brihaye
Springer-Verlag Wien-New York

Sample copies as well as subscription and back-volume
information available upon request.

Please address: or   Springer-Verlag
Springer-Verlag   New York Inc.
Werbeabteilung 4021   Promotion Department
D 1000 Berlin 33   175 Fifth Avenue
Heidelberger Platz 3   New York, N.Y. 10010

Springer-Verlag
Berlin
Heidelberg
New York

Prices are subject to change without notice